Visit our website

to find out about other books from Mos[...] and our sister companies in Harcourt He[...]

Register free at
www.harcourt-international.com

and you will get

- **the latest information on new books, journals and electronic products in your chosen subject areas**

- **the choice of e-mail or post alerts or both, when there are any new books in your chosen areas**

- **news of special offers and promotions**

- **information about products from all Harcourt Health Sciences' companies including Baillière Tindall, Churchill Livingstone, Mosby and W. B. Saunders**

You will also find an easily searchable catalogue, online ordering, information on our extensive list of journals...and much more!

Visit the Harcourt Health Sciences' website today!

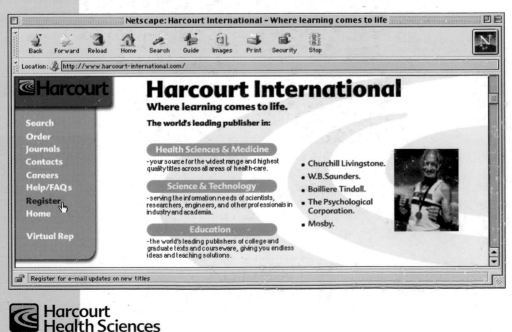

Harcourt Health Sciences

Mosby's Color Atlas and Text of

Obstetrics and Gynecology

(i) Revise placentation. ✓

Commissioning Editor: Ellen Green
Project Development: Gina Almond, Maria Stewart, Fiona Conn
Project Management: Fiona Conn, Frances Affleck
Design Direction: Judith Wright

Mosby's Color Atlas and Text of

Obstetrics and Gynecology

Ian A Greer MD FRCP (Glas) FRCP (Edin) FRCOG MFFP
Muirhead Professor and Head of Department of
Obstetrics and Gynaecology, University of Glasgow
and
Honorary Consultant Obstetrics and Gynaecology,
Glasgow Royal Infirmary, Glasgow, UK

Iain T Cameron BSc MA MD FRCOG MRANZCOG
Professor and Head of Department, Obstetrics
and Gynaecology, University of Southampton,
Southampton, UK

Henry C Kitchener MD FRCS (Glas) FRCOG
Professor of Gynaecological Oncology, University of
Manchester, St Mary's Hospital, Manchester, UK

Andrew Prentice BSc MD MRCOG
University Lecturer in Obstetrics and Gynaecology,
University of Cambridge Clinical School
and
Honorary Consultant Obstetrician and Gynaecologist,
Addenbrooke's Hospital, Cambridge, UK

Mosby

EDINBURGH LONDON NEW YORK PHILADELPHIA ST LOUIS SYDNEY TORONTO 2001

MOSBY
An imprint of Harcourt Publishers Limited

© Mosby International Limited 2001

M is a registered trademark of Harcourt Publishers Limited

The right of Ian A Greer, Iain T Cameron, Henry C Kitchener and Andrew
Prentice to be identified as authors of this work has been asserted by them
in accordance with the Copyright, Designs and Patents Act 1988

First published 2001

ISBN 0723424357

British Library Cataloguing in Publication Data
A catalogue record for this book is available from the British Library

Library of Congress Cataloging in Publication Data
A catalog record for this book is available from the Library of Congress

Note
Medical knowledge is constantly changing. As new information becomes
available, changes in treatment, procedures, equipment and the use of
drugs become necessary. The authors and the publishers have taken care to
ensure that the information given in this text is accurate and up-to-date.
However, readers are strongly advised to confirm that the information,
especially with regard to drug usage, complies with the latest legislation
and standards of practice.

The
publisher's
policy is to use
**paper manufactured
from sustainable forests**

Printed in China

Contents

Preface

Although there are a number of established textbooks of obstetrics and gynaecology and several colour atlases, there are few books which have combined the information contained within a traditional textbook with the visual imagery of colour atlases. This text aims to provide such a combination. Furthermore, rather than dealing with matters by a subject-based approach, this book adopts, where possible, a problem-orientated approach to diagnosis and management. This is in keeping with the philosophy in the undergraduate medical curriculum which has moved away from a traditional subject-based teaching method to problem-based or problem-orientated learning techniques and examinations. Similar changes have occurred in postgraduate education.

The intended readership of this book will include clinical medical students studying obstetrics and gynaecology, but will also be suitable for those in the early years of training in obstetrics and gynaecology. While the authors acknowledge that the management described reflects their own UK practice, the principles of the presenting problems and management are common worldwide and we anticipate that this text will be of value further afield than the U.K.

Thus, we hope this book will provide valuable learning support to the clinical teaching of obstetrics and gynaecology and, perhaps most of all, that those who read it enjoy it.

I.A.G., I.T.C., H.C.K., A.P. 2000

Acknowledgements

Professor Greer would like to thank Dr N. Macklon for provision of ultrasound images; Dr A. MacCuish for slides illustrating the section on diabetes; Dr P. Clark and Dr I.Walker for illustrations of blood films; Dr H. Gray, for ventilation-perfusion lung scan images; Dr A. Reid, for slide of X-ray venography; Dr G. Kohnen, for pathological slides relating to early pregnancy complications; Professor J. Neilson, for a slide illustrating fetal abnormality; Dr M. Rogers (for Fig. 4.1); Dr J. Gibson (for Fig. 4.7); and Dr A. Thomson (for Fig. 7.6). The figure on the arrangement of the fetal vessels in the terminal villi of the placenta is used with the permission of Professor P. Kaufmann and the publisher, Springer Verlag GMBH & Co. KG. This figure was originally published in Pathology of the Human Placenta (3rd edition, p. 136, Fig. 77) by K. Benirschke and P. Kaufmann. A figure from Contributions to Gynaecology and Obstetrics, 1985:13:5–17 is used with permission from Professor P. Kaufmann and Karger, AG, Basel

Professor Cameron would like to acknowledge the help of Dr H. Lyall, Dr T. Johnston and Dr F. Mackenzie, for contributions to the text on labour, reproductive endocrinology and infertility; Professor S. Franks and the Department of Audiovisual Services, Imperial College School of Medicine at St Mary's Hospital., London (for Fig. 2.12); U. Acharya (for Figs 2.14, 3.12 and 3.16); Dr M. A. Lumsden (for Figs 2.19 and 2.26); Leiras Oy, Turku (Fig. 2.21); Dr C. Stewart (Figs 2.23, 2.27, 3.1 and 3.3); Dr C. Barratt (Fig. 3.6); Dr S. Campbell (Fig. 3.9); and Dr P. Matson (Fig. 3.17).

Dr Prentice would like to acknowledge Dr S. Goodburn, Dr J. Compston and Mr C. J. Sutton, for slides; and Mr. L. Mascarenhas, for help with the text on contraception. He would also like to acknowledge the use of illustrations produced by Bayer PLC, Unipath Ltd, Ciba Pharmaceuticals (now Novartis), and the Sanofi Winthrop slide tutorial service on the menopause and HRT prepared by Miss J. Rymer. The figure illustrating the laparoscopic distribution of endometriosis is used with permission from the American College of Obstetricians and Gynecologists (Obstetrics & Gynecology 1986:67:335–338). The revised Fertility Society classification of endometriosis is used with permission from the American Society for Reproductive Medicine (Fertility and Sterility, 1985:43:351).

Professor Kitchener would like to thank Dr M. Cruikshank, for preparation of the sections on general gynaecology; Dr Hilary Buckley, Reader in Pathology, University of Manchester, for the gynaecological cancer pathology illustrations; and Dr Louise Smart for Fig. 11.17.

The authors are particularly indebted to Mr. Farook Al Azzawi; Professor V. Tindall; Professor C. D. Forbes and Dr William F. Jackson; and Dr M. Macpherson and Professor M. Symonds, for permission to use illustrations from their excellent illustrated atlases published by Mosby.

chapter 1

History and Examination in Obstetrics and Gynaecology

The principles of history-taking in obstetrics and gynaecology are no different from those of medicine and surgery. History-taking in obstetrics and, more particularly, in gynaecology, however, may require the type of questioning that many patients find difficult or embarrassing, and therefore must be approached with sensitivity. When taking a history, the clinician must be aware that different ethnic groups have a variety of taboos relating to sexual function and practice, and these should be respected at all times. The other major difference is that, with the exception of the oncological or very old patient, the majority of patients are relatively young, and therefore, fit and healthy. Thus, history-taking must be modified to meet the demands of the individual patient's condition.

Although obstetrics and gynaecology are discrete subject areas, there are a number of core questions that must be asked when taking either a gynaecological or obstetric history. It is a routine part of the obstetric and gynaecological history to enquire about the menstrual cycle. The key questions to be asked are listed in **Figure 1.1**. In gynaecology, the

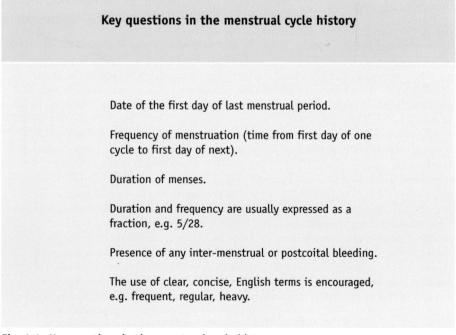

Key questions in the menstrual cycle history

Date of the first day of last menstrual period.

Frequency of menstruation (time from first day of one cycle to first day of next).

Duration of menses.

Duration and frequency are usually expressed as a fraction, e.g. 5/28.

Presence of any inter-menstrual or postcoital bleeding.

The use of clear, concise, English terms is encouraged, e.g. frequent, regular, heavy.

Fig. 1.1 *Key questions in the menstrual cycle history.*

Examples of expressing parity

A woman has had three pregnancies and books in her fourth pregnancy. The first pregnancy was ectopic, the second pregnancy was twins, with both born alive, and the fourth was stillborn at 36 weeks.

She is gravida 4 para 2+1.

A woman books in her first pregnancy.

She is gravida 1 para 0. She may be described as nulliparous.

Fig. 1.2 *Examples of expressing parity.*

importance of the menstrual history may be to investigate a menstrual disorder, to arrange the appropriate timing of investigations or to establish the possibility of pregnancy. In obstetrics, the timing of the last menstrual period and the regularity of the cycle are important in dating a pregnancy and arranging investigations at specific gestations.

Usually, a detailed past obstetric history is also taken. This history should include the number of pregnancies and their outcome. The number of pregnancies is described in terms of gravidity and parity. Gravidity is usually used only when a patient is pregnant. A patient in her first pregnancy is thus a primigravida or gravida 1 and in her second pregnancy gravida 2 and so on. Parity is a term that causes more confusion but is actually simple. A patient's parity is the number of pregnancies that have reached a registrable outcome. It is important to note that it is the number of pregnancies, not the number of offspring. A woman who has had a single twin or triplet pregnancy is para 1, just the same as a woman who has given birth to a singleton. Registrable outcomes are livebirths and stillbirths, whereas pregnancies that miscarry, ectopic gestations or are terminated are not registrable. It is however usual to record these other outcomes: a woman whose only pregnancy was terminated would be described as para 0+1 (**Fig. 1.2**). The past obstetric history is not just about the number of pregnancies, it is usual to enquire about the dates of pregnancies, the place of confinement, duration of the pregnancy, duration of labour, the mode of delivery, the fetal size and any complications (**Fig. 1.3**).

The third common element to the obstetric and gynaecological history is the use of contraception and a history of sexual activity. Although many forms of contraception involve the use of hormones, most patients do not consider these to be drugs and will not mention them on routine questioning about drug usage. Equally, it is important to ask about sexual activity (with tact and discretion) as this may help in the differential diagnosis, e.g. the diagnosis of pelvic infection is untenable when a patient is not sexually active. When seeing a patient who has never been sexually active, it may not be possible or desirable to perform a vaginal examination.

Record of past pregnancies

Pregnancy		Labour and Birth							Infant							
Weeks	Problems	Onset	Hours	Preparation	Delivery	Perineum	3rd Stage	Puerperium	Birthweight	Outcome	Condition	Present state	Cong Anomaly	Feeding		

Date 6/1/93	39	(N)	Sp		Vx	N	N	N	N	3700 g	(Live)	(Live)	(Well)	N	Br
Place St Thomas's		P	Ind		0th	Ass	P	P	P		0th	Died	0th	P	(Bot)
Case notes seen Yes/No						(CS)					Girl Boy		Name		
						Elective CS - Breech							Alex		

Date 7/95	9	N	Sp		Vx	N	N	N	N	g	Live	Live	Well	N	Br
Place Rosie		P	Ind		0th	Ass	P	P	P		0th	Died	0th	P	Bot
Case notes seen Yes/No						CS					Girl Boy		Name		
		9 week miscarriage													

Date 20/12/96		(N)	(Sp)		(Vx)	(N)	N	(N)	(N)	3900 g	(Live)	(Live)	(Well)	N	(Br)
Place Rosie		P	Ind		0th	Ass	(P)	P	P		0th	Died	0th	P	(Bot)
Case notes seen Yes/No						CS					(Girl) Boy		Name		
						Episiotomy							Alice		

Date		N	Sp		Vx	N	N	N	N	g	Live	Live	Well	N	Br
Place		P	Ind		0th	Ass	P	P	P		0th	Died	0th	P	Bot
Case notes seen Yes/No						CS					Girl Boy		Name		

Date		N	Sp		Vx	N	N	N	N	g	Live	Live	Well	N	Br
Place		P	Ind		0th	Ass	P	P	P		0th	Died	0th	P	Bot
Case notes seen Yes/No						CS					Girl Boy		Name		

Date		N	Sp		Vx	N	N	N	N	g	Live	Live	Well	N	Br
Place		P	Ind		0th	Ass	P	P	P		0th	Died	0th	P	Bot
Case notes seen Yes/No						CS					Girl Boy		Name		

Ethnic origin

White ☑ Black Afri ☐ Black Carrib ☐ Ind ☐ Pak ☐ B'dash ☐ Chin ☐ Medit ☐ Other (Specify) ☐

Country of Birth United Kingdom

Hepatitis Screening...................... Yes (No)
Result:
Electrophoresis .... Yes (No)
Result:

ALLERGIES: None

Fig. 1.3 *Recording a past obstetric history.*

GYNAECOLOGICAL HISTORY-TAKING

In many respects the gynaecological history is very similar to a history taken from a medical or surgical patient. The major differences are the questions that elucidate the patient's menstrual bleeding pattern, highlight abnormalities in the functional anatomy of the genitourinary tract and point towards endocrine disorders affecting the hypothalamo–pituitary–ovarian axis.

The majority of consultations for gynaecological problems relate to menstrual disorders. An accurate history of menstrual function is also important in the management of problems of early pregnancy. Traditionally, menstrual disorders have been described using Latin terms. Other than the most obvious of these (menorrhagia – heavy periods), many of the terms are misused and are only confusing. It is suggested that clear, concise, English is used to describe menstrual problems. The basic menstrual history should elucidate the frequency and regularity with which menstruation occurs. This menstrual history is often recorded as the last menstrual period (LMP), which is the day on which menstruation last commenced, and the cycle is expressed as a fraction (**Fig. 1.1**). When this convention is used, the menstrual cycle is annotated as K, the numerator is the number of days that menstruation lasts and the denominator is the time from the first day of one menstrual period to the start of the next. The normal menstrual cycle may vary from 21 to 35 days and individuals may vary from one cycle to the next. The numerator and denominator may therefore be expressed as ranges (e.g. K=3–5/25–30). As well as recording the exact numerical details of the menstrual cycle, descriptive terms to define the frequency and regularity of the cycle may be employed. The perceived heaviness of the flow should also be assessed. This can be done by asking the patient about the number of tampons and towels she uses each day, whether double towels or a towel and tampon have to be used to contain the flow and how this has changed with the development of her symptoms. It is acknowledged that this does not correlate well to the actual volume of blood loss but it does give a measure of how it affects the woman's life. The patient may have kept a record of her menstrual cycle which may be of value in assessing the situation. A complete menstrual history should also record the age at first menstruation (menarche) and age at last menstruation (menopause) when appropriate.

The menstrual cycle is not the only history of genital tract bleeding that should be sought. Bleeding after intercourse (postcoital bleeding) should always be enquired about. Generally, a history of postcoital bleeding suggests a cervical problem. This may be a significant cervical pathology or nothing more sinister than a cervical ectopy, often described as an erosion (**Fig. 1.4**). Another feature also enquired about is bleeding between menstrual periods. Intermenstrual bleeding may suggest an endometrial pathology.

Fig. 1.4 *A cervical erosion or ectropion.*

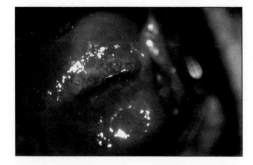

Menstruation may be associated with pain and discomfort. Pain associated with menstruation is termed dysmenorrhoea. The pain does not need to be confined to the days on which the patient menstruates but may precede the onset of menstruation for a few days. Cyclical pain unrelated to menstruation may also be of significance and a careful history should consider that lower abdominal pain may be of gastrointestinal or urinary origin. One other specific symptom that should also be enquired about is pain during or after intercourse – dyspareunia. This topic should always be approached with sensitivity and respect. Some patients will state that intercourse is not painful when, in fact, they are no longer sexually active because intercourse has become too painful to tolerate. Dyspareunia is subdivided into superficial and deep. Superficial dyspareunia relates to symptoms experienced around the introitus and lower vagina, whereas deep dyspareunia suggests pathology within the pelvis. When pain is the presenting symptom, infection is a potential underlying cause. Vaginal discharge is another symptom that may be associated with infection. Patients should be asked specifically about the colour of vaginal discharge and whether the discharge smells or causes irritation.

Some patients will present with irregular or absent menstrual periods (**Fig. 1.5**). When the gap between successive menstrual periods is greater than 6 weeks this is termed oligomenorrhoea. When the gap between periods extends to beyond 6 months or periods are completely absent, then the patient has amenorrhoea. It should always be remembered that the most common causes of amenorrhoea are pregnancy and the menopause. However, stress due to major life events, such as examinations or bereavement, can also be associated with amenorrhoea. Generally, a regular menstrual cycle implies regular ovulation and a normally functioning hypothalamo–pituitary–ovarian axis and, conversely, an irregular or absent menstrual cycle implies an ovulatory disorder. For these patients, further questions related to specific symptoms are required in the attempt to elucidate potential underlying causes.

Another endocrine-based disorder that may present to the gynaecologist is hirsutism: excessive hair growth. The important features of hair growth are age at onset, family history, ethnic group, rapidity of onset, menstrual pattern and other features that suggest excessive androgen production, such as seborrhoea or acne. A complete examination of the hirsute patient will include an objective assessment of the degree of hirsutism using a Ferriman–Gallwey score (**Fig. 1.6**).

Urinary incontinence and prolapse are also important in history-taking, particularly for older women. Prolapse may present with a sensation of 'something coming down'. An enquiry should always be made about urinary symptoms. If the patient complains of incontinence, it is important to determine whether this is stress incontinence or urge incontinence. Stress incontinence occurs after coughing, sneezing, laughter or exercise when the abdominal pressure is raised. Usually only small volumes of urine are lost. A history of genuine stress incontinence without other urinary symptoms is suggestive of weakness of the pelvic floor and may occur with prolapse. It should be noted that an increased frequency of micturition may occur as the woman tries to keep her bladder empty to avoid incontinence.

Urge incontinence is when urine is lost because of an inability to delay micturition. Urgency is the sensation to void immediately the bladder feels full. If the woman does not reach the toilet in time, she will be incontinent. Although the bladder feels full, the volume will be small and thus frequency and nocturia will occur. She may be unable to interrupt the urinary stream. These symptoms should be sought specifically in patients with a history of incontinence. These symptoms suggests an unstable bladder with involuntary contractions of the detrusor muscle. Other symptoms of importance in the incontinent patient are the presence or absence of dysuria and haematuria, and whether there is any difficulty voiding which may be in keeping with outflow obstruction due to prolapse. Stress and urge incontinence may coexist.

Disturbances in menstruation

Symptom	Possible abnormality	Confirmatory test
Galactorrhoea	Hyperprolactinaemia	Serum prolactin, pituitary imaging
Visual disturbance	Distortion of optic chiasma by pituitary tumour	Visual field testing, pituitary imaging
Medication (e.g. phenothiazines)	Hyperprolactinaemia	Serum prolactin
Temperature preference	Thyroid dysfunction	Thyroid function test
Hirsutism	Polycystic ovarian syndrome, hyperandrogenism	Ultrasound, serum androgens
Acne and seborrhoea	Polycystic ovarian syndrome, hyperandrogenism	Ultrasound, serum androgens
Hot flushes, decreased libido, headache	Low oestrogens, menopause	Serum follicle-stimulating hormone
Weight gain or loss	Hypothalamic dysfunction or polycystic ovarian syndrome-type picture	Body mass index

Fig. 1.5 *Disturbances in menstruation.*

EXAMINING THE GYNAECOLOGICAL PATIENT

A general examination of the gynaecological patient will include an assessment of their wellbeing, the presence of stigmata of endocrine conditions such as hirsutism and a breast examination, including an assessment of galactorrhoea if appropriate. It may be useful to

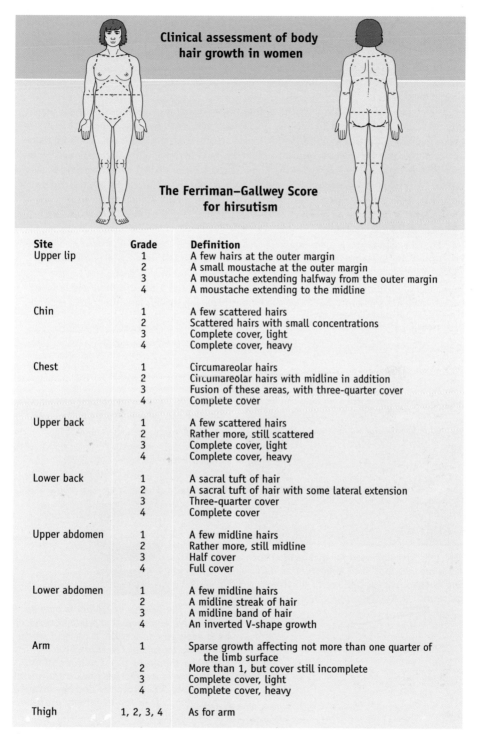

Clinical assessment of body hair growth in women

The Ferriman–Gallwey Score for hirsutism

Site	Grade	Definition
Upper lip	1	A few hairs at the outer margin
	2	A small moustache at the outer margin
	3	A moustache extending halfway from the outer margin
	4	A moustache extending to the midline
Chin	1	A few scattered hairs
	2	Scattered hairs with small concentrations
	3	Complete cover, light
	4	Complete cover, heavy
Chest	1	Circumareolar hairs
	2	Circumareolar hairs with midline in addition
	3	Fusion of these areas, with three-quarter cover
	4	Complete cover
Upper back	1	A few scattered hairs
	2	Rather more, still scattered
	3	Complete cover, light
	4	Complete cover, heavy
Lower back	1	A sacral tuft of hair
	2	A sacral tuft of hair with some lateral extension
	3	Three-quarter cover
	4	Complete cover
Upper abdomen	1	A few midline hairs
	2	Rather more, still midline
	3	Half cover
	4	Full cover
Lower abdomen	1	A few midline hairs
	2	A midline streak of hair
	3	A midline band of hair
	4	An inverted V-shape growth
Arm	1	Sparse growth affecting not more than one quarter of the limb surface
	2	More than 1, but cover still incomplete
	3	Complete cover, light
	4	Complete cover, heavy
Thigh	1, 2, 3, 4	As for arm

Fig. 1.6 *The Ferriman–Gallwey Score for hirsutism.*

examine the thyroid gland. Gynaecological patients will in addition to an abdominal examination usually require a vaginal or bimanual examination to be performed. Vaginal examination is an intimate procedure and should always be carried out in the presence of a chaperone. At all times the patient must be treated with courtesy and respect and, when possible, if a patient requests that a female doctor undertakes the examination, this request should be met.

The abdominal examination of the gynaecological patient is performed with particular interest in the lower abdomen, but uses inspection, palpation and percussion just as in any abdominal examination. A definition of masses arising from the pelvis may be more easily achieved by using the left as opposed to the right hand with the more sensitive edge of the index finger being used to delineate the upper edge. A mass arising from the pelvic organs is dull to percussion unless a loop of bowel is in front of it. In women with masses, ascites should be looked for as this can be a feature of ovarian tumours. Palpation of the inguinal nodes must be remembered when appropriate. It is best if the bladder is empty for the purposes of the examination.

Vaginal examination is a two-stage procedure. The first stage of the procedure involves visualizing and inspecting the vulva, including the clitoris, followed by inspection of the cervix and vaginal walls with the aid of a speculum. Normally this procedure is carried out in the dorsal position using a bivalve speculum (**Figs 1.7** and **1.8**) lubricated with a water-based lubricant. The procedure may also be performed in the left lateral or Sim's position.

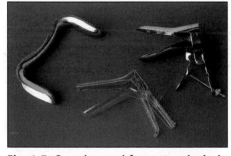

Fig. 1.7 *Speculae used for gynaecological examination. Top: Sim's speculum; middle and bottom: plastic and metal bivalve speculae.*

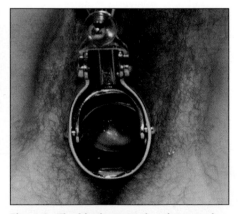

Fig. 1.8 *The bivalve speculum is opened and locked. The normal cervix and cervical os is exposed and visible. A cervical smear can easily be taken. The lubricated speculum should be inserted directly into the vagina in a direction toward the sacral promontory, i.e. backward and downwards, if the woman is in the lithotomy position. (From Tindall, V. R. 'A Colour Atlas of Clinical Gynaecology' (Wolfe Medical Publications Ltd 1988), with permission.)*

This position is more often used to assess vaginal prolapse when direct visualization of the anterior vaginal wall and descent of the cervix can be directly assessed with the aid of a Sim's speculum (**Fig. 1.9**). The patient can be asked to cough or bear down to assess the degree of prolapse and presence of stress incontinence. A cervical smear may be performed in the course of speculum examination (**Fig. 1.10**), as can swabs for bacteriology if infection is suspected, including high vaginal and cervical swabs. When taking a smear, the spatula is applied firmly to the cervix and firmly rotated around 360° in order to collect adequate exfoliated cells. Sometimes this causes a little bleeding. Too much bleeding (e.g. the presence of menstrual blood) or an inadequate collection of cells (e.g. in an atrophic cervix) can render the smear unsatisfactory for examination. Sometimes the position of the cervix can be awkward for a good application of the spatula onto the cervix.

After the first stage, bimanual examination of the pelvic organs is performed. The procedure should be considered to be a bimanual procedure as much more information is obtained from the abdominal hand than from the vaginal hand. For this procedure the labia are gently separated to allow two fingers of the right hand to be gently inserted into the vagina. Occasionally, only one finger may be used if the patient is tender or tense, often after insertion of one finger the patient may gain confidence and relax allowing a second finger to be inserted. Initially, these fingers are used to palpate the lower end of the vagina and to assess the presence of any swelling in the glands surrounding the vaginal introitus and the laxity of the superficial pelvic muscles. The two fingers are then inserted further into the vagina and turned palmar surface up. The cervix can normally be felt. The pelvic organs can be steadied and pushed up with these fingers so making it easier for the abdominal hand to feel the organs. At this point, the left hand is placed on the abdomen

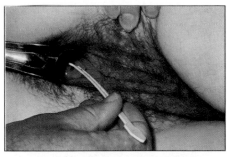

Fig. 1.9 *Left lateral position. A Sim's speculum has been inserted. With the buttocks held up there is a good exposure of the anterior vaginal wall and cervix. In this case a cervical smear is being taken. (From Tindall, V. R. 'A Colour Atlas of Clinical Gynaecology' (Wolfe Medical Publications Ltd 1988), with permission.)*

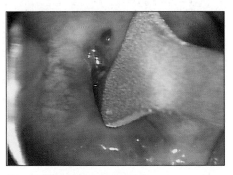

Fig. 1.10 *Taking a cervical smear.*

initially at the umbilical region then moved down to the suprapubic region to identify the uterus and bimanual palpation of the pelvic organs is undertaken (**Fig. 1.11**). The position of the cervix often gives an indication of how the uterus is lying, i.e. anteverted (cervix 'points' to sacrum) or retroverted (cervix 'points' to pubic symphysis: a retroverted uterus occurs as a normal finding in approximately 15% of women). In turn, the vaginal hand should be moved into each fornix of the vagina and the abdominal hand should also be moved towards each iliac fossa to obtain the maximum information. The information that is sought includes the size, position and mobility of the uterus, the presence or absence of masses in the adnexae (the tubes and ovaries) and the presence of tenderness in the pelvis. It should be noted that normal ovaries may not always be felt on examination. The detection of extreme tenderness when the cervix is gently moved from side to side, cervical excitation, is an indicator of pelvic peritonism. At all times the patient should be treated with respect and any discomfort should be minimized. For some patients it is not possible or desirable to undertake vaginal examination, e.g. children or virgins. With such patients, information may be obtained from bimanual examination with a single finger inserted in the rectum or on rectal examination alone.

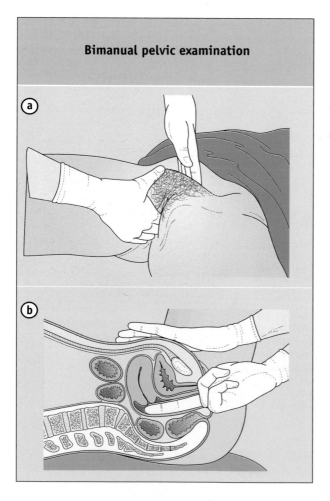

Bimanual pelvic examination

(a)

(b)

Fig. 1.11 *Bimanual examination in the dorsal position. The fingers in the vagina steady the pelvic organs and the structures palpable in the midline are felt between the abdominal hand and the vaginal fingers.*

OBSTETRIC HISTORY-TAKING AND EXAMINATION

History-taking of the obstetric patient is an important component of the screening process of the booking appointment during antenatal care. This aspect of history-taking is addressed in the section on antenatal care. During later pregnancy and labour, an important part of assessment is determining fetal growth, fetal lie, position and presentation.

BOOKING EXAMINATION

At booking it is traditional to conduct a general, cardiovascular, respiratory, breast and abdominal examination. Booking weight and height are also recorded. The most important component of the cardiovascular examination is recording a baseline blood pressure measurement. Abdominal examination should include inspection for the presence of scars and palpation for the fundal height, although the uterus is not usually palpable in the abdomen until 12 weeks' gestation when it is felt just above the pubic bone. Traditionally, obstetricians performed a bimanual examination to estimate uterine size, gestation and to attempt to detect adnexal swellings. However, with the advent of routine ultrasound in early pregnancy there is no point in subjecting patients to a vaginal examination which many women find distressing, unless a particular problem is identified that requires such an examination. Nevertheless, the opportunity to perform a cervical smear if it is indicated or due should not be missed.

EXAMINATION IN THE SECOND AND EARLY THIRD TRIMESTER

A major part of antenatal care is directed towards screening for hypertension and fetal growth. Examination in the clinic during the second trimester or early third trimester usually involves a measurement of blood pressure (**Fig. 1.12**), urinalysis by dipstick (**Fig. 1.13**) and examination of the abdomen to assess fetal growth (**Fig. 1.14**).

Preparation for examination

Tell the patient what you plan to do, indicate that you will not cause her pain and reassure her if required. Ask her to lie down, removing excess pillows, but have some lateral tilt or prop up the head of the examination couch in order to avoid her lying flat because supine hypotension may ensue. This occurs later in pregnancy and is caused by compression of the inferior vena cava by the gravid uterus, resulting in reduced venous return, tachycardia and hypotension. If such hypotension occurs, the patient will feel faint: roll her on to her side and allow the patient to recover. Fold the draw sheet down to the level of the symphysis pubis, exposing the abdomen from the xiphisternum to the pubic region. Ask her to place her hands by her sides and breathe quietly.

Examination of the abdomen: inspection

Abdominal examination will include inspection for scars (e.g. previous caesarean section), fetal movements, the shape of the uterus, which may give a clue as to whether the lie is transverse or longitudinal, the presence of stretch marks, eversion of the umbilicus and the linea nigra may be noted. This is a pigmented line running from the umbilicus to the pubic symphysis over the linea alba. It is normal in pregnancy because of increased pigmentation.

Examination of the abdomen: palpation

Palpation at this gestation concentrates on the fundal height. Of less importance at this gestation is the fetal position and presentation (unless preterm labour is a possibility). The

Measurement of blood pressure in pregnancy

Use a bell stethoscope to give optimal amplification of Korotkoff (K) sounds.

Use appropriate cuff size (too small and blood pressure will be overestimated; too large and blood pressure will be underestimated).

Take measurements with the patient sitting after a period of rest with the arm supported at heart level, or in a lying position with a lateral tilt with the arm at heart level.

During the first inflation of the cuff, obtain an approximate systolic pressure by palpation of the radial pulse.

Inflate the cuff to approximately 20 mmHg above the systolic pressure determined by palpation. The systolic pressure is then recorded as the level at which repetitive sounds are first heard (K1), rounded up to nearest 2 mmHg.

Traditionally, the diastolic pressure is recorded at the point of muffling of these sounds (K4), however K5, when sounds disappear, provides a more accurate measurement. Thus, practice changes to record diastolic pressure at K5.

Fig. 1.12 *Measurement of blood pressure in pregnancy.*

fundal height is often measured in centimetres from the symphysis pubis to the uterine fundus, the highest point of the uterus. It is usual to use the ulnar border of the left hand, working down from the xiphisternum, to identify the fundus. It is not always in the midline and is often found on the right side because of dextro-rotation of the uterus caused by the sigmoid colon in the pelvis. Some clinicians prefer to measure 'blind' using the measuring tape in such a way that they cannot see the figures in order to avoid potential bias. Between 14 and 34 weeks, the measurement in centimetres will approximate the number of weeks gestation but there is substantial variability. With complications such as transverse lie, the accuracy of the measurement is poor. Clearly, in situations such as twin pregnancy or polyhydramnios, such measurements are not useful in estimating fetal growth. When serial measurements are made by the same observer, there is greater accuracy in assessing growth. Liquor volume should also be assessed in the course of the palpation. It is difficult to feel fetal parts with polyhydramnios and, conversely, it is usually easy with oligohydramnios. A fluid thrill may be felt in polyhydramnios. To elicit this, the ulnar border of an assistant's hand is placed longitudinally in the midline and gentle pressure applied. This will damp vibrations through subcutaneous fat. A fluid thrill is then elicited.

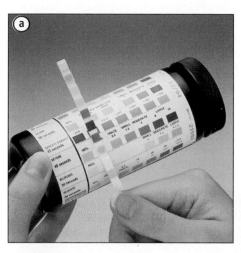

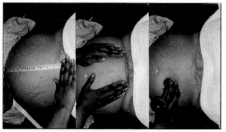

Fig. 1.13 *(a) Dipstick examination of the urine. (b) In obstetrics the presence of protein and glucose are particularly important.*

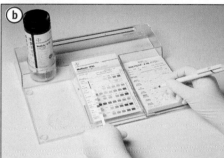

Fig. 1.14 *Examination of the abdomen in late pregnancy. Note on inspection the striae gravidarum ('stretch marks'). The symphysis-fundal height is measured, the presenting part and engagement determined and the fetal heart auscultated with a Pinard stethoscope.*

Examination of the abdomen: auscultation

The Pinard stethoscope should be used to detect the fetal heart. It is placed on the abdomen and at right angles to it. The ear is placed firmly against it and the hand removed from the stethoscope. It is usual to place the stethoscope initially in the subumbilical area in the midline and then move it until the fetal heart (120–160 beats/min) is heard. At later gestations, when the fetal lie and position are known, the stethoscope should be placed over the anterior shoulder. Ultrasound devices have largely replaced the Pinard. They have the additional benefit of allowing the mother to participate in hearing the fetal heart. Other sounds that may be heard are the funic (cord) souffle and uterine souffle.

Assessment of oedema

Oedema should be assessed on the lower limbs and hands where rings may be tight and may have been removed. Abdominal wall oedema may also be seen after removal of the Pinard stethoscope for auscultating the fetal heart.

EXAMINATION IN THE LATE THIRD TRIMESTER

In addition to the features assessed on examination in the second and early third trimester (particularly fundal height), in the late third trimester, and indeed in early labour, other features of abdominal palpation become prominent.

The lie

The relationship of the longitudinal axis of the fetus to the longitudinal axis of the uterus is described as the lie. The lie can be longitudinal (normal), transverse or oblique. When the whole uterus is lying obliquely, tilted to one side (usually the right) and the fetus lies longitudinally within the uterus, this is still a longitudinal lie and must not be confused with an oblique lie.

The presenting part

For a longitudinal lie, two types of presentation are described: breech or cephalic.

The fetal head may present as a vertex (the area bounded by the anterior and posterior fontanelles and the parietal eminences), deflexed head, brow or face. The 'attitude' describes the degree of flexion of the head. A well-flexed head will present as a vertex, the smallest diameter to present to the pelvis, so facilitating labour. Whereas a fully extended head will present as a face and partially extended as a brow. The diameters of the fetal head are shown in **Figures 1.15** and **1.16**.

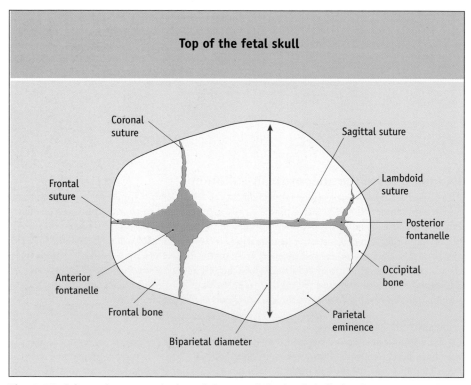

Top of the fetal skull

Coronal suture

Sagittal suture

Frontal suture

Lambdoid suture

Posterior fontanelle

Anterior fontanelle

Occipital bone

Frontal bone

Parietal eminence

Biparietal diameter

Fig. 1.15 *Schematic representation of the top of the fetal skull showing sutures and fontanelles.*

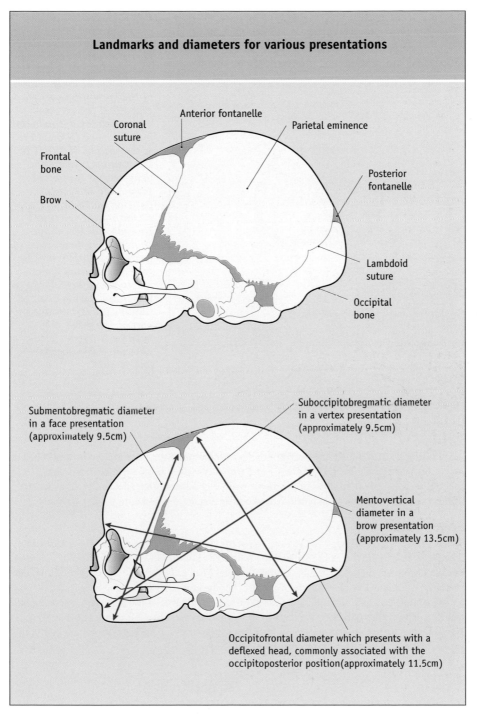

Landmarks and diameters for various presentations

Fig. 1.16 *Schematic representation of the fetal skull showing landmarks and diameters for various presentations in a term fetus.*

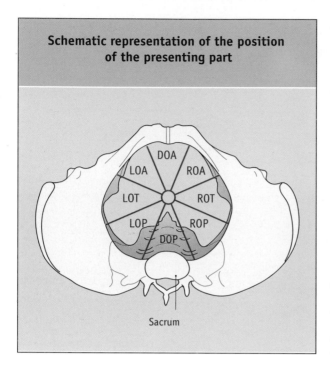

Schematic representation of the position of the presenting part

Sacrum

Fig. 1.17 *Schematic representation of the position of the presenting part. The pelvis is divided into eight segments for the description of the position of the presenting part. For example if the vertex is presenting the denominator is the occiput (if breech it is the sacrum, if face it is the mentum), where the denominator is directed toward the sacrum the position would be direct occipito-posterior (DOP) position (for breech the equivalent is direct sacro-posterior position, and for face presentation direct mento-posterior). If the presenting part is directed towards the left anterior part of the pelvis the position is left-occipito-anterior (LOA) position and so on.*

Position

The position is the relationship between the denominator of the presenting part and the pelvis as shown in **Figure 1.17**. Anterior and transverse positions are more common, accounting for more than 80% of positions, probably because this allows a greater degree of flexion. The most common is left–occipito–transverse (approximately 40%).

Engagement

When a head is presenting, it is usual to assess the degree of engagement of the fetal head by describing how many fifths of the head are palpable abdominally. The fetal head is engaged when its broadest diameter (the biparietal diameter) has passed the pelvic inlet. For a breech presentation it is the bi-trochanteric diameter. The head is usually divided into fifths, corresponding to an adult hand. When two fifths are palpable in the abdomen, the head is engaged. The vertex will be at the level of the ischial spines when engagement occurs (**Fig. 1.18**). Engagement tends to occur in a primigravida in the last 2 weeks of pregnancy but in parous patients it may not occur until labour.

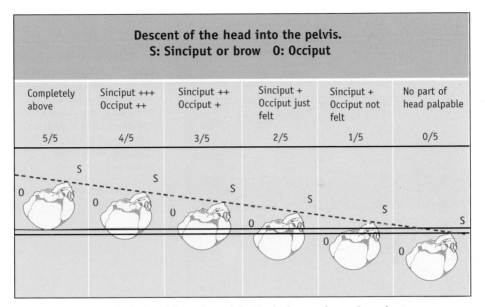

Completely above	Sinciput +++ Occiput ++	Sinciput ++ Occiput +	Sinciput + Occiput just felt	Sinciput + Occiput not felt	No part of head palpable
5/5	4/5	3/5	2/5	1/5	0/5

**Descent of the head into the pelvis.
S: Sinciput or brow   O: Occiput**

Fig. 1.18 *Descent of the head into the pelvis. S: sinciput or brow; O: occiput.*

Abdominal examination

Preparation, inspection, measurement of fundal height and assessment of liquor volume have been described. At 36 weeks, the fundus should be close to the xiphisternum, but at term may be slightly lower than this as the head enters the pelvis. After measuring the fundal height, the fundal contents are determined by palpation (**Fig. 1.19**). Both the examiner's hands are laid flat on the abdomen on either side of the fundus. Lateral palpation of the body of the uterus is performed to determine where most resistance is, indicating the location of the fetal back. The back can also be felt using Fairbairn's walk. In this manoeuvre one hand then the other hand 'step' in turn as they 'walk' with gentle fingertip pressure over the abdomen from one side to the other (**Fig. 1.20**); the soft concavity over the fetal front and limbs is felt in contrast to the resistance and convexity of the fetal back. This is useful to determine where to auscultate the fetal heart. The fetal pole at the lower end of the uterus is then palpated using the thumb and fingers of the right hand (**Fig. 1.21**), while steadying the fundus with the other hand. A decision should not be made about the presentation until both fetal poles have been palpated for their shape and consistency to determine which is the head. The head, it should be noted, is also ballotable if not in the pelvis. To determine the degree of engagement the examiner turns to face the patient's feet and presses deeply on either side of the lower pole of the uterus containing the fetal head with three fingers of each hand (**Fig. 1.22**). An estimate can be made of the degree of flexion of the head and also the number of fifths of head (finger breadths) in the abdomen. During this manoeuvre it is best to watch the patient's face to determine whether you are causing her discomfort.

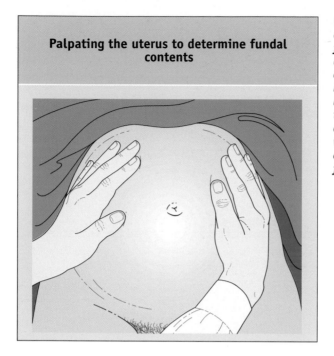

Palpating the uterus to determine fundal contents

Fig. 1.19 *Both of the examiner's hands are laid flat and relaxed on the abdomen to assess the contour of the uterus, the lie of the fetus, and the level of the fundus. With the tips of the fingers, the examiner then assesses which part of the fetus occupies the uterine fundus.*

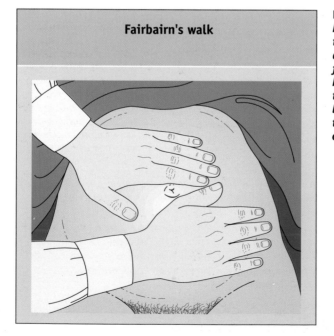

Fairbairn's walk

Fig. 1.20 *By moving the hands backwards (towards the examiner) one hand at a time, pressing with the fingertips of the other hand, it is easy to locate the convexity of the fetal back and the concavity of the fetal front which contains the small parts.*

Palpating the fetal pole

Fig. 1.21 *The fetal pole above the symphysis pubis is grasped gently but firmly with the thumb and fingers of the right hand. The contour and consistency of the fetal pole which occupies the lower part of the uterus can then be examined and compared with the other pole in the fundus.*

Assessing engagement of the fetal head

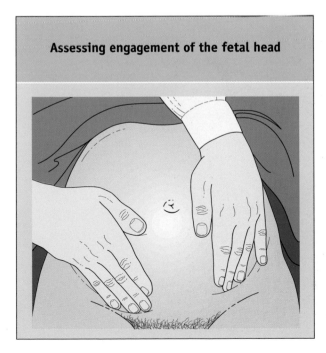

Fig. 1.22 *If the presentation is cephalic, the examiner faces the mother's feet and presses with the first three fingers of each hand on the sides of the fetal head, in the direction of the pelvic inlet. The fingers of one hand usually manage to slip in the direction of the pelvic inlet, whilst those of the other hand, being alongside the cephalic prominence, are obstructed. The manoeuvre helps to assess the degree of flexion of the fetal head.*

chapter 2

Menstrual Disorders and the Menopause

CONTROL OF MENSTRUATION AND PUBERTY

HYPOTHALAMO–PITUITARY–OVARIAN AXIS

Regular menstrual bleeding is the outward manifestation of cyclical ovarian activity and is regulated by a complex feedback system involving the hypothalamus, pituitary and ovary (**Fig. 2.1**). In the reproductive years, hypothalamic gonadotrophin-releasing hormone (GnRH) is delivered to the pituitary gland by portal capillaries. The releasing hormone is secreted in pulses at intervals of about 90 minutes. In turn, this pulse generation is controlled by opioid, catecholamine and other neuronal influences from higher centres of the brain. The binding of GnRH to pituitary receptors stimulates the synthesis and release of the gonadotrophins, follicle-stimulating hormone (FSH) and luteinizing hormone (LH). These hormones enter the systemic circulation to reach the ovary to initiate folliculogenesis, to trigger ovulation and to maintain the corpus luteum. The pulsatile release of GnRH is

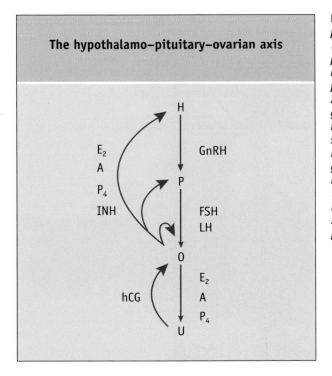

The hypothalamo–pituitary–ovarian axis

Fig. 2.1 *The hypothalamo–pituitary–ovarian axis. (hypothalamus: H; pituitary: P; ovary: O; uterus: U; oestradiol: E_2; progesterone: P_4; androgen: A; inhibin: INH; gonadotrophin-releasing hormone: GnRH; follicle-stimulating hormone: FSH; human chorionic gonadotrophin: hCG; luteinizing hormone: LH). (After Yen, S. 'Reproductive Endocrinology' (W. B. Saunders 1986), with permission.)*

crucial for normal pituitary function. Continuous administration of synthetic GnRH analogues results in a paradoxical inhibition of gonadotrophin release by impeding the availability of pituitary GnRH receptors. The consequent hypo-oestrogenic state has been exploited therapeutically for the treatment of a variety of ovarian steroid-dependent diseases.

THE MENSTRUAL CYCLE

Before the widespread availability of effective contraception, most women experienced a limited number of ovulatory cycles interspersed with episodes of pregnancy followed by lactational amenorrhoea. The monthly '28-day' menstrual cycle is now regarded as the norm and a woman can expect to have about 400 ovulatory cycles between puberty and the menopause. If the oocyte is not fertilized after ovulation, the corpus luteum is programmed to regress (luteolysis). The consequent fall in the circulating concentrations of oestradiol and progesterone initiates menstruation and stimulates increased secretion of pituitary FSH. FSH triggers the growth of a cohort of pre-antral follicles which in turn begin to produce oestradiol. At first, the increasing oestradiol concentrations exert negative feedback to the pituitary and hypothalamus to reduce the secretion of FSH. However, by mid-cycle the continued output of increasing amounts of oestradiol from the dominant follicle activates the LH surge by positive feedback. Ovulation follows and the dominant follicle, now the corpus luteum, begins to produce progesterone in increasing amounts (**Fig. 2.2**).

PUBERTY

Neuroendocrine events

There has been a gradual fall in the mean age of the menarche, which now occurs between the ages of 10 years and 16 years in developed countries. Progressively earlier activation of the ovarian and menstrual cycles is thought to be due to improved socioeconomic conditions and, more particularly, to improved nutritional status. The increased activity of

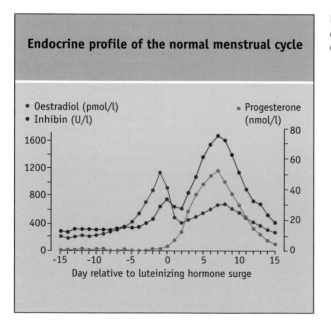

Endocrine profile of the normal menstrual cycle

- Oestradiol (pmol/l)
- Inhibin (U/l)
- Progesterone (nmol/l)

Day relative to luteinizing hormone surge

Fig. 2.2 *Endocrine profile of the normal menstrual cycle.*

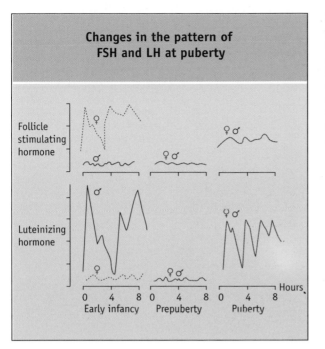

Changes in the pattern of FSH and LH at puberty

Follicle stimulating hormone

Luteinizing hormone

0   4   8   0   4   8   0   4   8   Hours
Early infancy   Prepuberty   Puberty

Fig. 2.3 *Changes in the pattern of FSH and LH secretion at puberty. After Klein, K. Oerter and Cutler, G. B. In Hillier, S. G., Kitchener, H. C. and Neilson J. P. (eds.) 'Scientific Essentials of Reproductive Medicine' (W. B. Saunders, 1996), with permission.*

GnRH-secreting neurons and the release of pulses of GnRH occur some years before the physical changes of puberty are seen. Maturation of the hypothalamo–pituitary–ovarian axis follows and increasing gonadotrophin concentrations stimulate ovarian activity (**Fig. 2.3**) which, in turn, initiates endometrial growth. As the final maturation of the oestradiol–pituitary/hypothalamus positive feedback mechanism is a late event, early menstrual bleeds result from withdrawal of oestradiol alone and are often erratic and unpredictable.

Physical changes

Although the timing of the appearance of the phenotypic changes associated with puberty is very variable, the acquisition of normal secondary sexual characteristics can be characterized by the development of four main physical features: breast growth, pubic hair growth, axillary hair growth and increase in height. In general, breast growth is oestrogen-dependent, whereas the appearance of hair is caused by increased androgen secretion from the gonads and the adrenal glands. The staging system developed by Tanner is invaluable not only for the assessment of normal children (**Fig. 2.4**), but for the management of women presenting with amenorrhoea, for which the stage of development provides a reflection of ovarian (testicular) and adrenal function.

MENSTRUAL INTERVAL

The maturation of the hypothalamo–pituitary–ovarian axis at puberty leads to the initiation of regular ovulatory cycles. If the oocyte is not fertilized, the corpus luteum regresses. The resultant fall in the circulating concentration of progesterone causes sloughing of the functional endometrium and menstrual bleeding. In women ovulating on a regular basis, the normal interval between menstrual periods is 28 days, with a range of 21–35 days (**Fig. 2.5**). The larger interval between periods at the extremes of reproductive life is due to the

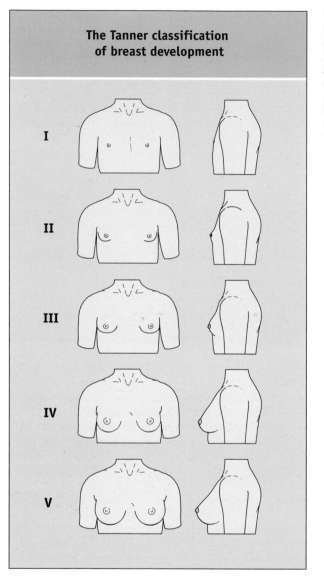

**The Tanner classification
of breast development**

I

II

III

IV

V

Fig. 2.4 *The Tanner classification of breast development. After Klein, K. Oerter and Cutler, G. B. In Hillier, S. G., Kitchener, H. C. and Neilson J. P. (eds.) 'Scientific Essentials of Reproductive Medicine' (W. B. Saunders, 1996), with permission.*

increased number of anovulatory cycles. Inherent programming of the corpus luteum means that the luteal phase of the cycle is relatively constant (about 14 days in length). Thus, variation in the menstrual interval is determined primarily by changes in the length of the follicular phase. When assessing ovulation by measuring the circulating concentration of progesterone, blood must be taken in the midluteal phase of the cycle, defined as 7 days before the next period and not necessarily 21 days after the last period, unless the woman has a 28-day cycle.

NORMAL MENSTRUAL BLOOD LOSS

The menstrual period usually lasts for 5–7 days. Whether the degree of blood loss is normal or heavy, 90% of the menstrual loss takes place within the first 3 days of bleeding. The

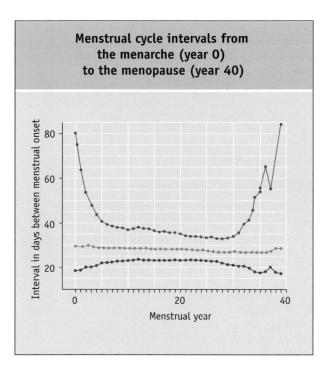

Fig. 2.5 *Menstrual cycle intervals from the menarche (year 0) to the menopause (year 40). The lines show the median interval with the 5th and 95th centiles. (After Treloar et al. 'Variation of the human menstrual cycle through reproductive life' (International Journal of Fertility, 1967, 12: 77–126), with permission).*

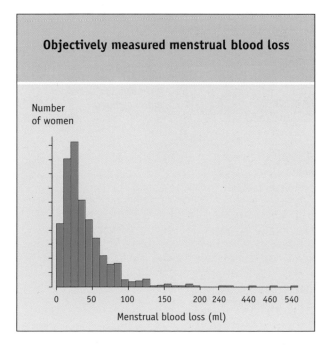

Fig. 2.6 *Objectively measured menstrual blood loss: a population study. (After Hallberg et al. Acta Obst. Et Gynec. Scandin. 1967, 45: 333 (Munksgaard International Publications Ltd), with permission).*

degree of menstrual blood loss can be measured by extracting blood from soiled sanitary wear. In the most widely used method, towels and tampons are soaked in sodium hydroxide and the resultant alkaline haematin derivative is quantified against a known volume of peripheral blood. Average (mean and median) monthly menstrual blood loss is between 30 ml and 40 ml. The distribution of menstrual blood loss is skewed to the right, with some women losing in excess of 500 ml each month (**Fig. 2.6**). Excessive menstrual bleeding (menorrhagia) is diagnosed objectively when the monthly menstrual loss exceeds 80 ml. These women are at increased risk of iron deficiency anaemia. Although objective measurement of blood loss is not used routinely in clinical practice, it should be noted that 50% of women complaining of heavy periods have a blood loss of less than 80 ml/month.

AMENORRHOEA AND OLIGOMENORRHOEA
Definition and aetiology
Amenorrhoea is the absence of menstrual bleeding for 6 months (**Fig. 2.7**). For oligomenorrhoea, the interval between periods ranges from 35 days to 6 months. Although the onset of menstruation can be delayed constitutionally beyond the age of 16 years in some normal individuals, it is particularly important to investigate girls presenting in their middle teens with primary amenorrhoea and absent secondary sexual characteristics. A crucial difference between patients with primary and secondary amenorrhoea is that the latter have already shown that they have a uterus with a patent outflow tract and that the endometrium has previously responded to cyclical ovarian steroids. Polycystic ovary syndrome (PCOS) is the most common diagnosis of normogonadotrophic women presenting with secondary amenorrhoea. Hypogonadotrophic hypogonadism is usually the result of abnormal GnRH pulses and is very rarely caused by isolated defects in the synthesis or release of FSH or LH. In Asherman's syndrome, damage to the basal endometriums prevents endometrial regeneration. The problem is usually caused by vigorous curettage (after delivery or early pregnancy loss) or endometritis (sometimes tuberculous). Pregnancy and lactation are common causes of amenorrhoea and should always be borne in mind.

Fig. 2.7 *Classification of primary and secondary amenorrhoea.*

Classification of primary and secondary amenorrhoea	
Primary amenorrhoea	Ovarian failure
	Hypothalamo-pituitary failure
	Other (outflow obstruction)
Secondary amenorrhoea	Physiological (pregnancy, lactation)
	Hyperprolactinaemia
	Normal gonadotrophins
	Low gonadotrophins
	Extraovarian disease (thyroid, adrenal)
	Other (Asherman's syndrome)

**Initial endocrine assessment of women
presenting with amenorrhoea or oligomenorrhoea**

Pituitary	Follicle-stimulating hormone
	Luteinizing hormone
	Prolactin
	Thyroid-stimulating hormone
Ovary	Oestradiol
Ovary and adrenal	Testosterone

Fig. 2.8 *Initial endocrine assessment of women presenting with amenorrhoea or oligomenorrhoea.*

Endocrine assessment

The initial endocrine assessment (**Fig.** 2.8) of women with amenorrhoea or oligomenorrhoea is the same. For patients with oligomenorrhoea, blood should be taken in the follicular phase of the cycle (day 3 to 7) to avoid misinterpretation of results due to the 'midcycle' LH surge. An elevated concentration of FSH suggests ovarian failure, whereas low or normal gonadotrophins usually signify inappropriate release of GnRH. An increased LH concentration may be found in women with PCOS. This is often associated with an elevated concentration of testosterone. Measurement of circulating thyroid-stimulating hormone (TSH) provides a good screen for thyroid disease; women with hypothyroidism or hyperthyroidism usually present with amenorrhoea as opposed to oligomenorrhoea. Hyperprolactinaemia is seen in 15–20% of women with secondary amenorrhoea. The upper limit of normal for prolactin concentrations is about 350 mU/L, but the concentration is increased by stress (including that of venepuncture) and is rarely associated with significant pituitary pathology unless the value exceeds 1000 mU/L.

Primary amenorrhoea: Turner syndrome

A syndrome of short stature, primary amenorrhoea and sexual infantilism in females was described by Henry Turner in 1938. Subsequent cytogenetic studies showed that many of these individuals have a 45XO karyotype whereas others are mosaic (such as 45X/46XX or 45X/46XX/47XXX). The 45XO karyotype is thought to be the most common chromosome abnormality in humans, seen in 0.8% of all zygotes, however, less than 3% of these pregnancies survive to term. Besides the classical triad of features, other abnormalities include webbed neck, high arched palate, prominent low-set ears, epicanthal folds, increased carrying angle (cubitus valgus), wide-set nipples, shortening of the fourth and fifth digits and hypoplastic nail beds (**Fig.** 2.9). There is a predisposition to renal and cardiovascular abnormalities (particularly coarctation of the aorta), pigmented naevi and lymphoedema. The long-term management requires the prescription of ovarian steroid

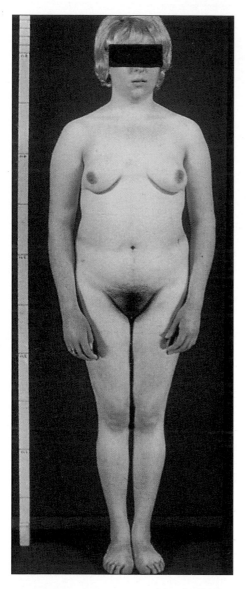

Fig. 2.9 *Features of Turner's syndrome. This patient was 162.6 cm (5' 4") in height. One of the commonest forms of mosaicism in Turner's syndrome is sex chromatin positive gonadal dysgenesis (XO/XX mosaic). This was the reason for this patient's gonadal dysgenesis. The secondary sexual characteristics were reasonably well developed despite her prime symptoms of amenorrhoea and infertility. (From Tindall, V. R. 'A Colour Atlas of Clinical Gynaecology' (Wolfe Medical Publications Ltd 1988), with permission.)*

replacement therapy to protect against osteoporosis and cardiovascular disease. Oocyte donation offers the best treatment option for fertility.

Secondary amenorrhoea: hypogonadotrophic hypogonadism

Endocrine assessment results show (**Fig. 2.10**) low concentrations of FSH, LH and oestradiol, a normal concentration of TSH (biochemically euthyroid) and a marginally elevated prolactin concentration (within the 'stress' range and not indicative of a pituitary tumour). The most likely problem is defective GnRH pulsatility caused by inappropriate input to the hypothalamus from higher brain centres. There may be associated weight loss or anorexia. If the woman has been amenorrhoeic for more than 12 months and no specific cause has been found, imaging should be considered to exclude organic pathology in the

The endocrine profile of a 26-year-old woman with hypogonadotrophic hypogonadism

Fig. 2.10 *The endocrine profile of a 26-year-old woman with hypogonadotrophic hypogonadism.*

Follicle-stimulating hormone	1.5 mU/L
Luteinizing hormone	<1.0 mU/L
Prolactin	450 mU/L
Thyroid-stimulating hormone	3.5 U/L
Oestradiol	110 pmol/L

pituitary and hypothalamus. The treatment of hypogonadotrophic hypogonadism is determined by the woman's wishes with regards to fertility. If pregnancy is sought, ovulation should be induced using pulsatile GnRH or gonadotrophins. Otherwise, ovarian steroid replacement is advisable to protect against the problems of hypo-oestrogenism (hot flushes, vaginal dryness, osteoporosis and cardiovascular disease). The combined contraceptive pill or standard hormone replacement therapy (which is not reliably contraceptive) are convenient therapeutic options.

Secondary amenorrhoea: hyperprolactinaemia

The synthesis and secretion of prolactin from the pituitary is under the inhibitory influence of dopamine released by the hypothalamus into the portal vessels. Hyperprolactinaemia is seen in 15–20% of women presenting with secondary amenorrhoea. One third of these will have a radiologically detectable pituitary tumour. Other causes of hyperprolactinaemia are pregnancy and medications (phenothiazines, metoclopramide, reserpine, methyldopa). There may be a prolactinoma (macro- or microadenoma) (**Fig. 2.11**) or a nonfunctioning pituitary tumour causing hyperprolactinaemia by preventing access of dopamine to the prolactin-secreting cells ('stalk effect'). Such nonfunctional tumours usually exhibit circulating prolactin concentrations between 1000 mU/L and 3000 mU/L, and surgery is the best therapeutic option. The consequences of hyperprolactinaemia are infertility (ovulation is suppressed by disrupting pulsatile GnRH release), hypo-oestrogenism (hot flushes, vaginal dryness and decreased libido in the short term; osteoporosis and probable cardiovascular morbidity later) and pressure effects (to the optic chiasma and cavernous sinuses). Medical treatment comprises the prescription of dopaminergic agonists, such as bromocriptine or the longer-acting cabergoline, to shrink the tumour and induce ovulation, or the correction of the hypo-oestrogenic state with exogenous steroids.

HIRSUTISM

Definition and aetiology

Hirsutism describes the presence of excess facial (**Fig. 2.12**) or body hair in women. This should not be confused with virilism, in which hirsutism is accompanied by other androgenic features (including clitoromegaly, deepening of the voice, increased muscle mass and loss of normal body contours) and which is usually caused by adrenal hyperplasia or androgen-secreting tumours of the adrenal or ovary. Hirsutism can result from an increase in sexual or nonsexual hair. By definition, sexual hair is hair that responds to sex steroids. The growth of sexual hair is stimulated by androgens and inhibited by oestrogens. Besides the hair found in the axillary and pubic regions, sexual hair is located primarily on the face, chest and abdomen. Under the influence of androgens, hair in these areas becomes longer, thicker and increasingly pigmented. This androgen-stimulated effect is maintained even after the androgen source has been withdrawn, a point which has important practical implications for clinical management.

Diagnosis

Excess body hair is a subjective complaint. Objective documentation is useful for both initial assessment and to monitor the effects of treatment. Measurement of actual hair growth by determining the length or weight of shaved hair, while used as a research tool, is not practical for everyday management. If available, clinical photography can be employed. Alternatively, the degree of hirsutism can be charted semiquantitatively using the Ferriman–Gallwey scoring system (**Fig. 1.6**). Different parts of the body are allocated a score from 0 (no hair) to 4 (heavy, dark hair). The total score is usually less than 10 in normal women. It should be noted that there is a wide range of 'normal' body hair pattern. This is under genetic control and varies markedly between different races. For example, women from the Mediterranean or India tend to be more hirsute than women from Scandinavia or the Far East.

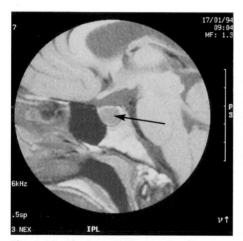

Fig. 2.11 *Pituitary MRI scan showing a prolactin-secreting pituitary macroadenoma.*

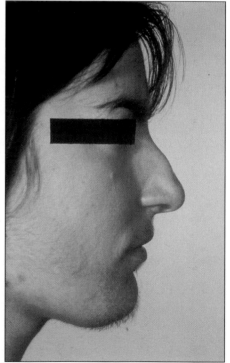

Fig. 2.12 *Idiopathic hirsutism with excess facial hair.*

Investigation

The investigation (**Fig. 2.13**) of women with hirsutism aims to exclude underlying organic disease, particularly adrenal hyperplasia or androgen-secreting tumours of the adrenal or ovary. History-taking should ascertain whether the woman has any relevant drug history (e.g. danazol or androgen-based synthetic progestogens). Rapidly advancing hirsutism and signs of virilism (clitoromegaly is a particularly sensitive marker) would suggest the presence of an androgen-secreting tumour. This is often associated with a circulating testosterone concentration greater than 6 nmol/L. Many women with hirsutism also present with oligomenorrhoea. Besides assessment of gonadotrophins, prolactin and TSH, the measurement of testosterone provides a useful screen (in the normal adult female the ovary and adrenal gland contribute equally to circulating testosterone concentrations). If the testosterone concentration is elevated, determination of dehydroepiandrosterone sulphate and 17-hydroxyprogesterone concentrations will help to reveal whether the adrenal gland is the source of excess androgen. The endocrine profile in the box (**Fig. 2.13**) shows elevated concentrations of testosterone and LH, compatible with a biochemical diagnosis of PCOS.

Polycystic ovary syndrome

A syndrome of oligomenorrhoea (or amenorrhoea), hirsutism and infertility, sometimes associated with obesity, was first described by Stein and Leventhal. Recent studies have shown that many women with PCOS are insulin resistant. Indeed, women with PCOS are at increased risk of developing noninsulin-dependent diabetes mellitus and long-term cardiovascular disease. The precise cause of PCOS is not known but the syndrome may be caused by an underlying metabolic disorder, of which, abnormal ovarian function is the outward manifestation in the female. If PCOS is suspected on history and examination, the diagnosis should be confirmed by specific investigation, including measurement of circulating LH, FSH and testosterone concentrations and ultrasound assessment of the ovaries. Typically, the concentrations of LH and testosterone are increased, and ovarian ultrasound (**Fig. 2.14**) shows a gonad of increased volume containing more than 10 follicles of 4–8 mm diameter, often arranged in a peripheral rosette. Treatment of PCOS depends on the presenting complaint, be it hirsutism, cycle irregularity or infertility.

The endocrine profile of a 32-year-old woman with oligomenorrhoea and hirsutism	
Follicle-stimulating hormone	6.5 mU/L
Luteinizing hormone	11 mU/L
Prolactin	380 mU/L
Thyroid-stimulating hormone	3 U/L
Oestradiol	450 pmol/L
Testosterone	3.5 nmol/L

Fig. 2.13 *Endocrine profile of a 32-year-old woman who presented with oligomenorrhoea and hirsutism.*

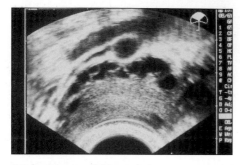

Fig. 2.14 *Ultrasonic scan of a polycystic ovary. Note the dense ovarian stroma and peripherally located follicles.*

Treatment of hirsutism

If an underlying problem has been identified, such as an androgen-secreting tumour, then specific treatment will be required. Otherwise, the aim of treatment is to offer cosmetic improvement, for example:

- Weight reduction.
- Depilatory creams, waxing, shaving and electrolysis.
- Antiandrogens (cyproterone acetate).

Weight reduction alone can be beneficial by increasing the sex hormone-binding globulin concentration which, in turn, lowers the concentration of free testosterone. Similarly, the concentration of sex hormone-binding globulin can be elevated by prescribing a low-dose combined contraceptive pill. Of the cosmetic treatments available, electrolysis offers the best results. Many women are reluctant to shave, believing that it will aggravate their condition. This is not the case. An increased density of coarse dark hair is not caused by shaving, but by the underlying change in the hair follicle that led to the hirsutism in the first place. The most commonly used antiandrogen is cyproterone acetate. Although often given in reverse sequential fashion (50mg or 100mg cyproterone acetate from day 1 to 14 of the cycle, with 20μg–30μg ethinyloestradiol from days 1 to 21), recent studies have suggested that the prescription of a combined preparation of 2mg cyproterone acetate and 35μg ethinyloestradiol is equally effective. Improvement in hirsutism is a slow process. Treatment should be continued for a minimum of 6 months.

MENORRHAGIA
Definition and aetiology

Menorrhagia can be used as a general term to describe heavy menstrual blood loss. The pathophysiology of menorrhagia is as follows:

- Organic disease.
- Dysfunctional uterine bleeding.

By definition, excessive menstrual bleeding is diagnosed when monthly menstrual loss exceeds 80ml. On the basis of large population studies, this represents the 90th centile for menstrual blood loss, and these women are at increased risk of iron deficiency anaemia. For 20% of patients, menorrhagia is the result of organic pathology such as fibroids or malignancy (endometrial or cervical), although care should be taken in distinguishing cause and association. The diagnosis of dysfunctional uterine bleeding is made by exclusion. Approximately 10% of women with dysfunctional uterine bleeding have anovulatory cycles (most often at the extremes of reproductive life). Thus, most women with menorrhagia have no organic disease and no abnormality of the hypothalamo–pituitary–ovarian axis. The problem is therefore thought to lie at the level of the endometrium. For example, prostaglandin concentrations (and particularly the vasodilatory prostaglandins PGE_2 and PGI_2) and fibrinolytic activity are elevated in the endometrium of women with menorrhagia.

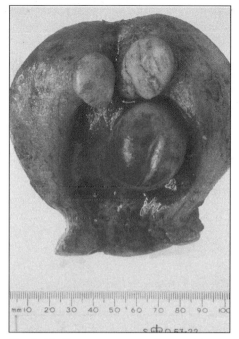

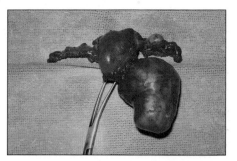

Fig. 2.16 *Subtotal hysterectomy specimen showing large fibroid which extended into the broad ligament and down into the paracervical region producing distortion of the ureteric path.*

Fig. 2.15 *Hysterectomy specimen with opened uterine cavity showing fibroids producing distortion of the uterine cavity.*

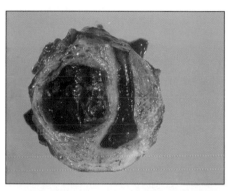

Fig. 2.17 *'Red' degeneration of a fibroid in a hysterectomy specimen.*

Fibroids

Fibroids or leiomyomata are the most common tumours in women. They are made up of whorls of smooth muscle, enclosed in a pseudocapsule. They can be located submucosally, within the myometrial wall or on the outer surface of the uterus. In some instances they are attached to the uterus by a stalk (pedunculated). The pathogenesis of these benign tumours is not fully understood, but their growth is stimulated by oestradiol and progesterone. Fibroids regress after the menopause and after treatment with GnRH analogues or the antiprogesterone mifepristone, although they grow again when drug treatment is stopped. Whereas some women with fibroids have no symptoms, others present with menorrhagia, dysmenorrhoea or a dragging discomfort in the pelvis. Large fibroids have been shown to cause miscarriage and submucous fibroids have been implicated as a cause of infertility. Caution is required, however, when linking association to cause. Hysterectomy is the surgical treatment of choice for women with symptomatic fibroids (**Figs 2.15** and **2.16**). Myomectomy (removal of fibroids while leaving the uterus) is a more complicated operation with greater morbidity (especially haemorrhage) and should be reserved for patients who wish to retain reproductive function. Fibroids can sometimes degenerate, possibly due to alterations in their blood supply, such as in pregnancy, which can cause pain (**Fig. 2.17**).

A management strategy for women with menorrhagia	
<40 years old, regular cycle	Medical treatment Consider endometrial assessment if symptoms persist
>40 years old or irregular cycle	Endometrial assessment (hysteroscopy, biopsy, dilatation and curettage)

Fig. 2.18 *Management strategy for women presenting with menorrhagia.*

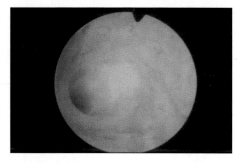

Fig. 2.19 *Hysteroscopic view of the uterine cavity.*

Management

Initial investigation should include a full blood count to detect iron deficiency anaemia. Thyroid status should be assessed (TSH concentration) if there are suggestive symptoms or signs. Bleeding diatheses are a rare cause of menorrhagia, but should be borne in mind, particularly in adolescents. The aim of investigation is to exclude an organic pathology before proceeding to specific treatment (**Fig. 2.18**). For young women (younger than 40 years old), if the cycle is regular (and there is no intermenstrual or postcoital bleeding) and examination is normal (including a recent normal cervical smear) medical treatment can be started. If treatment fails or the woman is older and/or has irregular bleeding (indicative of anovulatory cycles, unopposed oestrogen stimulation and a consequent predisposition to endometrial hyperplasia and malignancy), endometrial assessment is mandatory.

Endometrial assessment

When endometrial assessment is indicated, it is best carried out using a hysteroscope to see the uterine cavity (**Fig. 2.19**), at which time a sample of endometrium can be obtained for histological analysis. An advantage of hysteroscopy over conventional dilatation and curettage is that specific lesions such as endometrial polyps or submucous fibroids can be seen directly (although whether these lesions cause menorrhagia is debatable). Furthermore, it is possible to obtain directed biopsies of suspicious areas of endometrium. All methods of

Medical treatments for dysfunctional uterine bleeding	
Inhibitors of prostaglandin synthesis	e.g. Mefenamic acid, naproxen
Inhibitors of fibrinolysis	e.g. Tranexamic acid
Hormonal agents	Combined contraceptive pill Oral progestogens Local progestogens (medicated intrauterine system) Danazol Gonadotrophin-releasing hormone analogues

Fig. 2.20 *Medical treatments for dysfunctional uterine bleeding.*

endometrial assessment have their limitations. Lesions can be missed at hysteroscopy, particularly if the field of vision is obscured (e.g. by blood or inadequate distension of the uterine cavity). With 'blind' techniques, the sample of endometrium obtained must be representative of the remainder of the tissue. Only 60% of the endometrial surface area is sampled by dilatation and curettage or Vabra® curettage (an outpatient suction curette), and the area sampled by some of the recently introduced endometrial biopsy instruments, such as the Pipelle® curette, is even more limited.

Medical treatment
For women with anovulatory dysfunctional uterine bleeding, the prescription of cyclical progestogens such as norethisterone offers a logical therapeutic option. Taken for 7–10 days from day 19 or 16 of the cycle, they induce secretory change in the endometrium, leading to regular menstrual bleeding a few days after withdrawal of the steroid (**Fig. 2.20**). For women with ovulatory cycles, prostaglandin synthetase inhibitors and antifibrinolytic agents will reduce menstrual blood loss by 25 and 50% respectively. Both drugs are rational first line therapies. Antifibrinolytic agents are more efficacious but they are more likely to cause gastrointestinal side effects. Oral progestogens are less useful for women with ovulatory dysfunctional bleeding, unless given at high dose (10–15mg daily) for 3 out of 4 weeks. Synthetic progestogens are highly effective at reducing menstrual blood loss after local application in the form of a medicated intrauterine system (Mirena®). The synthetic steroid danazol and the GnRH analogues cause dramatic reductions in blood loss. They have significant side effects (androgenic and hypo-oestrogenic, respectively) and should be reserved for women with intractable menorrhagia for whom other treatments have been unsuccessful or are inappropriate.

Progestogen-impregnated intrauterine system (Mirena®)
Both nonmedicated and copper-containing intrauterine contraceptive devices aggravate menstrual bleeding, cause pain and predispose the user to pelvic infection. The L-norgestrel-releasing intrauterine system (Mirena®) not only provides reliable contraception, but

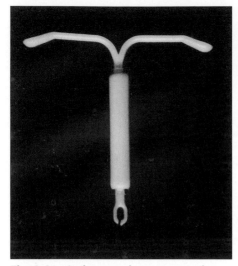

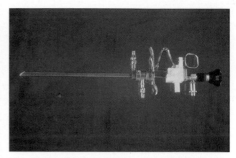

Fig. 2.22 *A resectoscope for transcervical endometrial resection.*

Fig. 2.21 *An intrauterine contraceptive system (IUS) impregnated with L-norgestrel.*

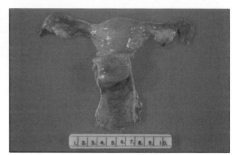

Fig. 2.23 *Hysterectomy specimen of uterus, fallopian tubes and ovaries.*

reduces menstrual blood loss, improves dysmenorrhoea and protects against pelvic sepsis (**Fig. 2.21**). Menstrual blood loss is reduced by 80–90% within 3–12 months of insertion, but this is often accompanied by troublesome intermenstrual bleeding and spotting during the first few months of treatment.

Endometrial resection

Transcervical resection of the endometrium was developed as an alternative to hysterectomy for the surgical treatment of menorrhagia. The procedure aims to remove both functional and basal endometrium, impairing endometrial regeneration and thereby reducing or abolishing menstrual bleeding. About 50% of women become amenorrhoeic after treatment. In most of the remainder, menstrual bleeding is markedly reduced, but for 10% of patients there is no improvement. The endometrium can be removed using a variety of techniques including diathermy resection (**Fig. 2.22**) and laser ablation. In comparison with hysterectomy, patients spend less time in hospital and appear to return to normal activities more quickly. The main complications of the operation are uterine perforation and fluid overload (caused by the irrigation fluid used to distend the uterine cavity). Follow-up studies have suggested that patient satisfaction is good, although 20% of individuals subsequently undergo hysterectomy.

Hysterectomy

Hysterectomy provides a definitive cure for menorrhagia. The uterus can be removed either at laparotomy (usually referred to as total abdominal hysterectomy) (**Fig. 2.23**) or vaginally (vaginal hysterectomy or laparoscopic-assisted vaginal hysterectomy). If the woman is over 45 years old or there is evidence of ovarian disease, bilateral salpingo-oophorectomy is

Forms of irregular vaginal bleeding

Intermenstrual bleeding
Postcoital bleeding
Breakthrough bleeding or spotting
Postmenopausal bleeding

Fig. 2.24 *Forms of irregular vaginal bleeding.*

often performed (and hormone replacement therapy offered) to decrease the risk of subsequent ovarian cancer. Some have advocated subtotal hysterectomy, removing the uterine fundus but leaving the cervix, arguing that removal of the cervix at the time of hysterectomy was introduced to prevent cancer in the remaining stump, before the development of cervical screening programmes. The mortality from hysterectomy is 6:10,000 procedures, excluding operations complicated by pregnancy or malignancy. Complication rates are said to be lower after vaginal hysterectomy when compared with abdominal operations, but this may be affected by case selection, the vaginal route usually being chosen for more straightforward procedures.

Irregular bleeding

Irregular vaginal bleeding (**Fig. 2.24**) should always be assessed comprehensively to exclude underlying pathology. A bimanual vaginal examination and a cervical smear (and often bacteriological swabs, including those for the detection of *Chlamydia* species) should be performed as a minimum. For women with postmenopausal bleeding and for others whose symptoms persist, the endometrial cavity should be assessed to exclude organic pathology. Intermenstrual bleeding may be caused by polyps (endocervical, endometrial or fibroid) or infection. Fluctuating ovarian steroid concentrations are said to be implicated in some cases. Postcoital bleeding may be secondary to a cervical polyp or an ectropion. Underlying

The pathophysiology of dysmenorrhoea	
Primary	Myometrial contractions (prostaglandin F2α, antidiuretic hormone, endothelins, noradrenaline)
Secondary	Extrauterine pathology (endometriosis, adhesions, infection)
	Uterine pathology (fibroids, adenomyosis, intrauterine contraceptive device)
	Outflow obstruction

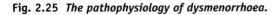

Fig. 2.25 *The pathophysiology of dysmenorrhoea.*

intraepithelial neoplasia must be considered. Breakthrough bleeding or spotting is a common problem associated with the administration of exogenous steroids for contraception or hormone replacement. The bleeding may settle if an alternative preparation is prescribed. Irregular bleeding can be particularly troublesome with exogenous progestogens (such as depot contraceptive preparations) where the problem may be a direct consequence of the action of the steroids on blood vessels in the endometrium.

DYSMENORRHOEA

Definition and aetiology

Dysmenorrhoea means painful menstruation. It can be classified as primary or secondary (**Fig. 2.25**). In primary dysmenorrhoea there is usually no underlying organic pathology and the pain is thought to result from myometrial contractions, stimulated by agents released from the endometrium at the time of menstruation. These agents include prostaglandins (especially PGF), antidiuretic hormone, endothelins and noradrenaline. Secondary dysmenorrhoea is often associated with pelvic pathology. Extrauterine pathology includes endometriosis and adhesions from pelvic inflammatory disease or previous surgery. Intrauterine causes encompass fibroids, adenomyosis or an intrauterine contraceptive device. Secondary dysmenorrhoea can also be caused by outflow obstructions, such as Müllerian duct abnormalities or cervical stenosis.

Primary dysmenorrhoea

The incidence of primary dysmenorrhoea is maximal in the late teens and twenties and decreases with age and after childbirth. The pain coincides with the onset of menstrual

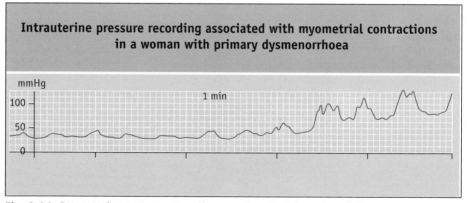

Fig. 2.26 *Intrauterine pressure recording associated with myometrial contractions in a woman with primary dysmenorrhoea.*

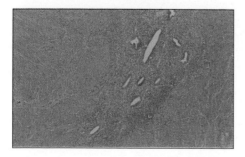

Fig. 2.27 *Low power view of histological preparation showing endometrial glandular tissue within the myometrium charactreristic of adenomyosis.*

bleeding and lasts for 12–48 hours. It is usually constant with cramping exacerbations due to uterine contractions (**Fig. 2.26**). The pain may be accompanied by headache or gastrointestinal symptoms. Diagnosis is usually made on history and examination alone. Most women with primary dysmenorrhoea gain symptomatic relief after taking nonsteroidal anti-inflammatory drugs or the combined oral contraceptive pill.

Secondary dysmenorrhoea

Secondary dysmenorrhoea is most often seen in women aged between 30 and 45 years. It can be associated with abdominal bloating, pelvic heaviness and low back pain. The pain and symptoms usually intensify during the luteal phase of the cycle and are maximal at the time of menstruation. Laparoscopy may be helpful to diagnose underlying pathology. In contrast with primary dysmenorrhoea, medical therapy is less effective for the treatment of secondary dysmenorrhoea. Surgery directed at the underlying pathology such as adenomyosis (**Fig. 2.27**) is often the preferred option.

PREMENSTRUAL SYNDROME

Definition and aetiology

Premenstrual syndrome (PMS) is a recurring cyclical disorder in the luteal phase of the menstrual cycle, involving behavioural, psychological and physical changes resulting in the loss of work or social impairment. The reported prevalence of the syndrome ranges from 1 to 90%, which reflects the wide range of criteria used to assess symptoms and the different populations sampled. Aetiological theories include oestrogen excess, progesterone deficiency, hyperprolactinaemia, hypoglycaemia, increased activity of aldosterone or renin–angiotensin and vitamin B_6 deficiency. However, many of these theories remain unsubstantiated. Current research suggests that PMS is probably multifactorial, although ovarian cyclicity seems to be a prerequisite. Alterations in 5-HT and opioid pathways in the central nervous system may also be implicated (**Fig. 2.28**).

The definition of premenstrual syndrome

Premenstrual syndrome is a recurring cyclical disorder in the luteal phase of the menstrual cycle, involving behavioural, psychological and physical changes, resulting in the loss of work or social impairment.
Reid and Yen, 1981

Fig. 2.28 *The definition of premenstrual syndrome.*

The symptoms of premenstrual syndrome	
Psychological	Emotional lability
	Irritability
	Mood swings
	Depression
	Anxiety
	Tension
Somatic	Bloating
	Myalgia
	Mastalgia
	Headaches
	Poor co-ordination

Fig. 2.29 *Premenstrual syndrome: symptoms.*

Symptoms

The symptoms of PMS are varied and nonspecific. Behavioural and emotional manifestations include emotional hypersensitivity, irritability, mood swings, depression, anxiety, tension, fear of loss of control and social withdrawal. Somatic symptoms include feelings of bloatedness, headaches, myalgia, breast tenderness and poor co-ordination. Complaints may be out of proportion to physical findings and can occur without menstrual bleeding, for example, after hysterectomy with ovarian conservation (**Fig. 2.29**).

Diagnosis

Premenstrual syndrome is often a diagnosis of exclusion. Symptoms should have been present for at least 4 of the previous 6 months. Cyclicity can be determined using simple calendars, specific questionnaires or linear visual analogue scales. Questionnaires can also be used to aid the detection of underlying psychiatric disorders. If the relationship between symptoms and ovarian cyclicity is in doubt, GnRH analogues can be used as a diagnostic tool: suppression of the hypothalamo–pituitary–ovarian axis should result in symptomatic relief (**Fig. 2.30**).

Treatment

Nonpharmacological treatment may be of benefit (reassurance, support groups, relaxation therapy and reflexology). Exercise and a balanced diet should be recommended. Restricting some dietary components such as alcohol, chocolate and dairy products has been advocated, as have dietary supplements such as vitamin B$_6$ and evening primrose oil. Pharmacological suppression of the hypothalamo–pituitary–ovarian axis should offer a rational approach to medical treatment (oestradiol implants, the combined contraceptive pill and for some women, GnRH analogues). Symptomatic relief can be achieved with diuretics or nonsteroidal anti-inflammatory drugs for women with oedema and pain. For emotional and affective symptoms, selective serotonin re-uptake inhibitors (SSRTs) (such as fluoxetine) are a good first line approach. Surgery, in the form of oophorectomy, is reserved for patients with intractable symptoms unresponsive to medical therapy.

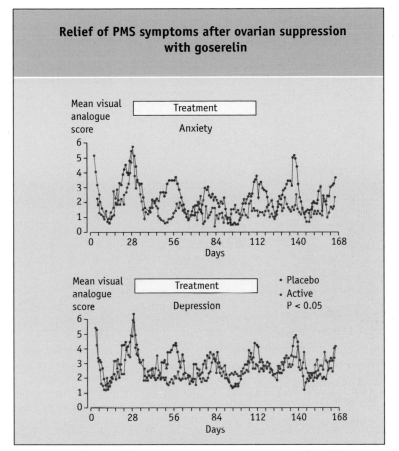

Fig. 2.30 *Relief of PMS symptoms after ovarian suppression with goserelin. Visual analogue scores for anxiety and depression before, during and after treatment. After West, C. P. and Hillier, H. 'Human Reproduction', 9: 1058–1063, 1994, with permission.*

THE MENOPAUSE

The menopause is the last menstrual period. The term, however, is widely used to describe the transition from reproductive life to the postproduction years. This period of transition is more accurately termed the climacteric and is colloquially known as 'the change of life'. Whereas the menopause itself is an isolated event, the climacteric encompasses the pre-, peri- and immediate postmenopausal years.

In the years preceding the last menstrual period, a number of events occur that are the physiological basis for the cessation of menstruation. At birth the female infant ovary has 1–2 million oocytes. During the reproductive years this supply of oocytes becomes depleted from the 300,000 that are present at puberty (**Fig. 2.31**). As a result of the decline in oocyte numbers, oestrogen production by the ovary declines and through the normal feedback mechanisms there is a consequent gradual rise in the gonadotrophins (FSH and LH). After the menopause FSH and LH are unequivocally elevated and this observation may be useful clinically.

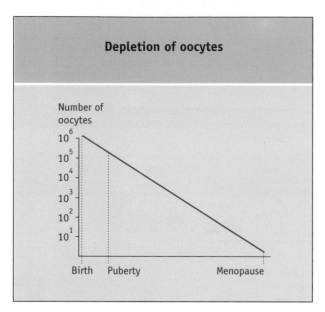

Fig. 2.31 *The ovary may have as many as 2 million oocytes at birth. By puberty this has declined to 300 000 and they are depleted by the menopause.*

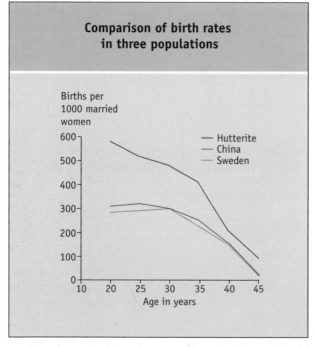

Fig. 2.32 *Birth rates in all populations, no matter their attitudes to contraception and termination, decline with increasing age.*

Associated with the decline in oocyte number is a marked decline in oocyte quality. These two events are seen clinically as a decline in fertility, an increase in chromosomal abnormalities in the conceptus and thus an increased miscarriage rate (**Fig. 2.32**).

Ultimately, there is insufficient oestrogen to stimulate endometrial proliferation and the endometrium atrophies. The menopause is the endometrial consequence of ovarian failure. There are other consequences of the hypo-oestrogenic state. The genital tract atrophies with changes to the vulva (**Fig. 2.33**), vagina, internal genitalia and the breasts. Vaginal changes are narrowing of the introitus, shortening, thinning of the epithelium and a reduction in secretions. The vaginal epithelium may become so thin and atrophic that it may be easily traumatized and give rise to postmenopausal bleeding. Although this may be a benign cause of postmenopausal bleeding, all instances should be fully evaluated to exclude more sinister causes. The internal genitalia become reduced in size with the uterine body being relatively small in comparison with the cervix and the ovaries becoming shrunken and inactive. The breasts too become reduced in size and inactive.

The effects on the genital tract are relatively short-term effects of low oestrogen. The long-term effects of low oestrogen are seen in the skeleton (**Fig. 2.34**) and cardiovascular system.

ILLUSTRATIVE CASE HISTORY

The patient presents to her general practitioner inquiring whether she may benefit from hormone replacement therapy. She is 44-year-old white woman who works in a sedentary occupation. Her last menstrual period was 6 months previously. She is currently asymptomatic and presents because her mother has recently fractured the neck of her femur. There is no other relevant history or any findings on examination except that she has a low body mass index (BMI = 18).

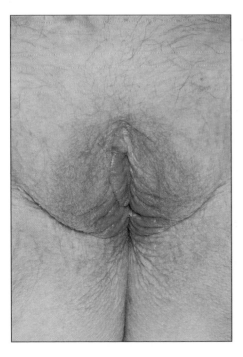

Fig. 2.33 *Postmenopausally the external genitalia undergo change. The skin becomes thin and atrophic, the labia diminish in size and there is a sparsity of pubic hair.*

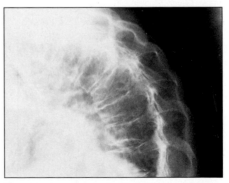

Fig. 2.34 *Osteoporosis of the spine leads to fractures in the vertebral bodies and curvature of the spine.*

Should an asymptomatic patient be treated?

Hormone replacement therapy may be prescribed as prophylaxis. For this patient, the indication would be prophylaxis against the development of osteoporosis (**Fig. 2.35**). After the menopause, bone density declines. Osteoporotic fractures are a significant healthcare problem. For a 50-year-old white women in the UK, the risk of having a fracture in the remainder of her life varies between 11% for spinal fractures and 14% for hip fractures. Approximately 150,000 osteoporotic fractures occur annually in the UK. Prophylaxis can be provided for people at risk in an attempt to prevent fractures occurring.

Patients can be assessed for their risk of osteoporosis by either bone densitometry (**Fig. 2.36**) or by computing risk factors (**Fig. 2.37**). Bone densitometry cannot predict who will become

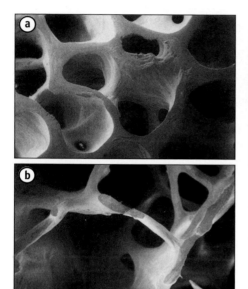

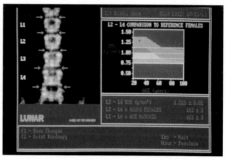

Fig. 2.37 *A bone densitometry result. This assessment of the lumbar spine in a young woman demonstrates a bone density within the normal (light blue) range. This normal range varies with age.*

Fig. 2. 35 *In normal bone (a) a lattice work of bone provides integrity and strength. In osteoporotic bone (b) the loss of crosslinks reduces the intrinsic strength of the bone. Once lost the crosslinks do not reform.*

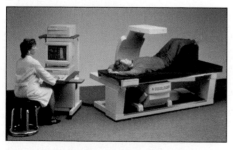

Fig. 2.36 *Densitometry examination of the lumbar spine being performed.*

Risk factors for osteoporosis

Female
White
Family history of osteoporosis
Early menopause
Low body mass index
Sedentary occupation
Smoking
High alcohol consumption
Low calcium intake
Corticosteroid therapy

Fig. 2.38 *Risk factors for osteoporosis.*

osteoporotic, however, merely detect those who are already osteoporotic. This particular patient has good indications for treatment with six risk factors for osteoporosis (**Fig. 2.38**).

There are relatively few contraindications to hormone replacement therapy and this patient has none (**Fig. 2.39**).

There are many types of hormone replacement therapy. Commonly natural oestrogens, oestradiol or conjugated oestrogens, either alone or in combination with a progestogen, are used but a synthetic alternative, tibolone is also available. Treatment is given in a variety of regimens with a progestogen required if the uterus is still present to prevent the unopposed action of oestrogen on the endometrium. Unopposed oestrogen would ultimately give rise to hyperplastic or neoplastic change within the endometrium.

Hormone replacement therapy can also be given by a variety of routes: oral, transdermal or implants (**Figs 2.40** and **2.41**). Hormone replacement can be given in a number of regimens. Cyclical regimens mimic the natural ovarian cycle with oestrogen in the first half and both oestrogen and progestogen in the second half. This pattern of administration

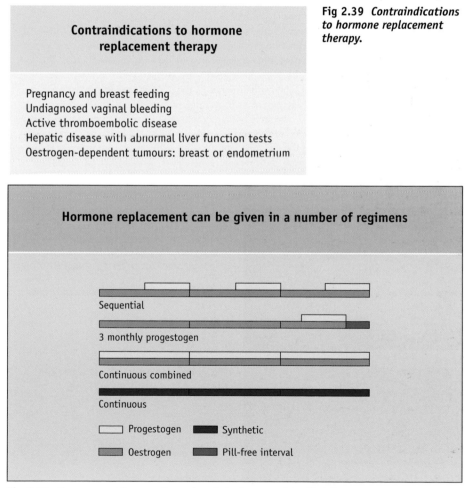

Contraindications to hormone replacement therapy

Pregnancy and breast feeding
Undiagnosed vaginal bleeding
Active thromboembolic disease
Hepatic disease with abnormal liver function tests
Oestrogen-dependent tumours: breast or endometrium

Fig 2.39 *Contraindications to hormone replacement therapy.*

Hormone replacement can be given in a number of regimens

Sequential

3 monthly progestogen

Continuous combined

Continuous

☐ Progestogen   ■ Synthetic
▨ Oestrogen   ▨ Pill-free interval

Fig 2.40 *Hormone replacement can be given in a number of regimens.*

results in monthly withdrawal bleeds. To minimise or abolish bleeding progestogens may be given once every three months or continuously. Alternatively a synthetic steroid may be given which does not give rise to endometrial stimulation.

Oestrogens are often administered by the oral route. A significant proportion of the drug administered by this route is inactivated in the gastrointestinal tract or undergoes first pass metabolism in the liver. This may result in erratic serum levels of oestradiol, a nonphysiological ratio of oestradiol to oestrone and the induction of liver proteins.

Avoiding the oral route, transdermal delivery systems and implants allow direct systemic absorption, no first pass metabolism and uniform serum oestradiol levels. There is also a reduced effect on carbohydrate, lipoprotein and hepatic protein metabolism. With implants, however, there is a small incidence of tachyphylaxis. These patients require more frequent and higher doses of oestradiol to maintain symptomatic relief and develop extremely high supraphysiological serum levels of oestradiol.

The final choice of therapy should take into account patient's views. For effective prophylaxis compliance with therapy in the long term is essential. Compliance may be affected by the route of administration and also by the return of menses. If the patient wishes to avoid regular monthly menstrual bleeding, this can be achieved by using continuous combined oestrogens and progestogen, the synthetic tibolone or the 3-monthly administration of progestogen. Hormone replacement therapy may be required for a long time: symptomatic treatment may last only 1 year but prophylactic treatment may last for between 5 and 10 years.

Before commencing hormone replacement therapy, the patient should be carefully assessed. This should include measurement of blood pressure, although controlled hypertension is not a contraindication, and breast examination and mammography (**Fig. 2.42**). If the patient is over 50 years old, a pelvic examination should also be carried out. Cervical cytology is not required if a smear is not due and endometrial sampling is required only if an abnormal bleeding pattern indicates that there may be endometrial pathology.

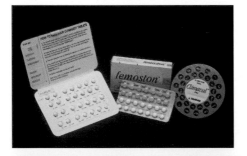

Fig. 2.41 *Hormone replacement therapies come in calendar packs to aid patient compliance. The oestrogenic and progestogenic phases of the pack are distinguished by differing coloured tablets.*

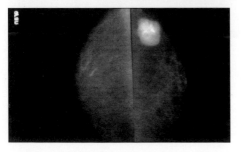

Fig 2.42 *Mammography showing the presence of a suspicious lesion.*

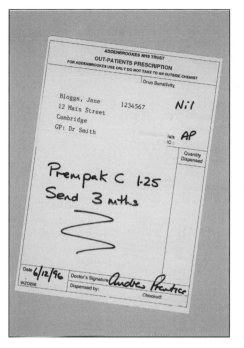

Fig. 2.43 *Compliance with hormone replacement therapy is poor.*

The benefits of hormone replacement therapy

Hormone replacement therapy is beneficial in the prevention of osteoporosis and its sequelae. It is also of value in the prevention of cardiovascular disease. After the menopause, either natural or surgically induced, there is a rise in the incidence of vascular disease in the female population. Treatment with hormone replacement therapy reduces the incidence of both ischaemic heart disease and cerebrovascular disease. Part of this effect is mediated through a beneficial effect on lipids restoring the less atherogenic premenopausal profile by raising high-density lipoproteins and reducing low-density lipoproteins. Oestrogens also have a direct effect on blood flow. Despite these benefits, compliance with hormone replacement therapy is poor (**Fig. 2.43**). Approximately only 20% of women are still on HRT at 1 year and many women do not even fill their first prescription.

The climacteric in many women is characterized not only by the menopause but also by the presence of symptoms. These symptoms can be considered to be vascular, psychological and those of the direct effects of hormomal deficiency on the urogenital tract (**Fig. 2.44**). The menopause also has a direct effect on libido and if as a consequence of vaginal dryness, the women experiences dyspareunia, that in itself may further reduce her libido.

The symptoms of the climacteric may be treated by the systemic therapies described previously. In addition, the urogenital symptoms may be amenable to local treatment. Oestrogens may be administered to the vagina as creams, pessaries, tablets or rings.

Symptoms of the climacteric	
Vascular	Hot flushes Night sweats Palpitations
Psychological	Emotional lability: anxiety and depression Irritability Poor concentration and memory Insomnia Reduced libido
Urogenital tract	Superficial dyspareunia and vaginal dryness Urinary urgency Urinary frequency Urethral syndrome

Fig. 2.44 *Symptoms of the climacteric.*

Contraception in the climacteric

Although fertility declines with advancing age, the risk of conception exists until ovulation has finally ceased. Pregnancy in women over 40 years old has higher rates of miscarriage, chromosomal abnormality and perinatal and maternal mortality. Despite these facts, many pregnancies in older women are unplanned and almost half are terminated.

Effective contraception should continue throughout the perimenopausal years and all methods may be suitable. Hormone replacement therapy, however, is not a reliable form of contraception. Natural family planning and barrier methods are more successful in the older women as a consequence of their reduced fertility. An increased incidence of anovulatory cycles may make the charting of cycles difficult and thus the identification of the safe period troublesome. An intrauterine contraceptive device normally requires changing every 5 years. After the age of 40 years, an intrauterine contraceptive device may be left *in situ* until either 12 months after the menopause or if the menopause is masked by hormone replacement therapy, until the age of 53. The oral contraceptive pill, particularly low dose 20µg preparations, may continue to be used after the age of 35 and until the age of 50 in women who are fit and healthy, normotensive and who are neither smokers, heavy drinkers nor grossly obese. Other hormonal methods, the progestogen-only pill, progestogen implants and injections are effective but irregular bleeding in these patients should not be assumed to be drug related until intrauterine pathology has been excluded.

chapter 3

Fertility Control

FERTILITY

THE OVARIAN CYCLE

The preovulatory follicle

The primordial follicle comprises a primary oocyte, surrounded by a single layer of granulosa cells, further encapsulated by a basement membrane. Follicular development is a continuum of growth and atresia. It begins with the oocyte increasing in size. The granulosa cells become cuboidal and multiply, and the primordial follicle develops into a primary follicle. The granulosa cells, which are separated from the stromal cells by a basement membrane, the basal lamina, differentiate into theca interna and theca externa. The follicle progresses to the pre-antral stage as the oocyte enlarges and is surrounded by a membrane, the zona pellucida. Follicular fluid accumulates in the intercellular spaces of the granulosa cells under the synergistic influences of oestrogen and follicle-stimulating hormone (FSH), forming a cavity as the follicle enters the antral stage. Further transition to the preovulatory follicle occurs with enlargement of the granulosa cells and their acquisition of lipid inclusions (**Fig. 3.1**).

Recruitment of the dominant follicle

With rare exceptions (demonstrated by the spontaneous multiple pregnancy rate of 1 out of 80 deliveries), a single follicle is selected to ovulate each cycle. The negative feedback of oestradiol on FSH suppresses the development of all but the dominant follicle (**Fig. 3.2**). The selected follicle however remains dependent on FSH. By day 9 of the cycle, the vasculature of the dominant follicle is such that the follicle may benefit from a preferential delivery of FSH despite declining circulating gonadotrophin concentrations. The fall in FSH leads to a decline in FSH-dependent aromatase activity, limiting oestradiol production in the less mature follicles, which become atretic.

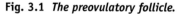

Fig. 3.1 *The preovulatory follicle.*

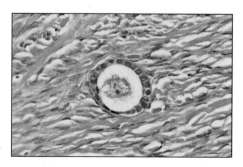

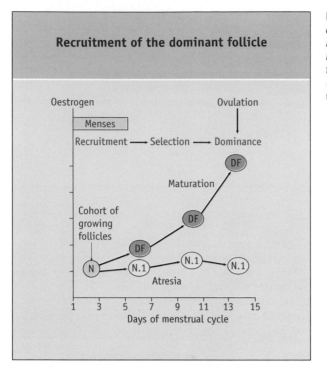

Fig. 3.2 *Recruitment of the dominant follicle. (After Hodgen, G. D. In Riddick, D. H. 'Reproductive Physiology in Clinical Practice' (Thieme, New York, 1987), with permission.)*

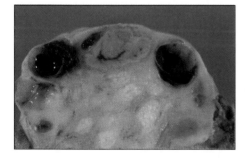

Fig. 3.3 *A cross section through the ovary showing a corpus luteum ('yellow body').*

The corpus luteum

Shortly after ovulation, profound alterations take place in the cellular organization of the ruptured follicle. The granulosa cells hypertrophy markedly, gradually filling the cystic, sometimes haemorrhagic, cavity of the early corpus luteum. The incorporation of lipid-rich vacuoles results in the granulosa becoming markedly luteinized and a new yellow body is formed (**Fig. 3.3**). This is dominated by the enlarged, lipid-rich, fully vasularized granulosa cells. However, other cells such as endothelial cells, macrophages and fibroblasts are also present. The life span of the corpus luteum is 14 days. It synthesizes and releases both oestradiol and progesterone, and is dependent on pituitary-derived luteinizing hormone. If pregnancy occurs, human chorionic gonadotrophin maintains the life of the corpus luteum, which enables it to continue to release progesterone to support the early conceptus.

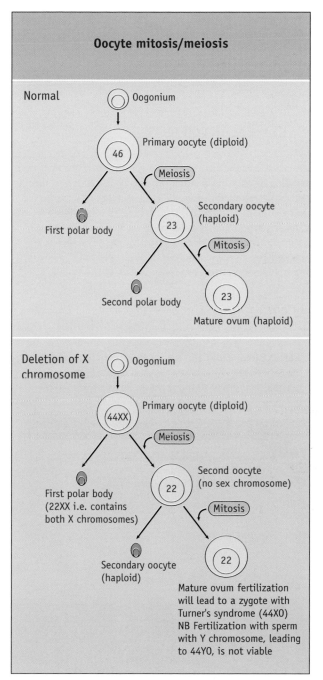

Fig. 3.4 *Oocyte mitosis/meiosis. Upper panel showing normal, lower panel showing deletion of X-chromosome.*

Oocyte mitosis and meiosis

The first signs of ovarian differentiation are seen at 6–8 weeks' gestation with the rapid mitotic proliferation of germ cells, resulting in 6–7 million oogonia by 16–20 weeks of pregnancy. The oogonia are transformed into oocytes as they enter the first meiotic division and arrest in prophase, a process which begins at 11–12 weeks' gestation. The progression of meiosis to the diplotene stage occurs throughout the rest of pregnancy and is completed by birth. At this stage, the primary oocyte contains 46 chromosomes. It remains like this until just before ovulation when the first meiotic division is completed. This results in a secondary oocyte and the first polar body, each of which contains 23 chromosomes. The second meiotic division occurs at the time of sperm penetration, leaving the mature oocyte and the second polar body (**Fig. 3.4**).

FERTILIZATION AND EARLY EMBRYOLOGY

Spermatogenesis

Spermatozoa are formed in the seminiferous tubules. Developing spermatozoa are nurtured by the Sertoli cells. Indeed, spermatozoa density in the adult appears to be related to the total volume of Sertoli cells, and this is determined during the early months of intrauterine life. Spermatozoa begin to increase in number at puberty. After several mitotic divisions, they form the primary spermatocytes. Each primary spermatocyte undergoes a reduction division to form two haploid (23 chromosomes) secondary spermatocytes. The secondary spermatocytes undergo a second meiotic division to form four haploid spermatids. The spermatids then progress through a maturation process to form mature spermatozoa (**Fig. 3.5**).

The acrosome reaction and fertilization

Capacitation is the change that sperm undergo in the female reproductive tract that enables them to penetrate the ovum. The process involves acquisition of the ability to undergo the acrosome reaction and to bind to the zona pellucida, and the acquisition of hypermotility. Capacitation changes the surface characteristics of spermatozoa and modifies their surface charge. These changes enable the plasma membrane to break down and merge with the

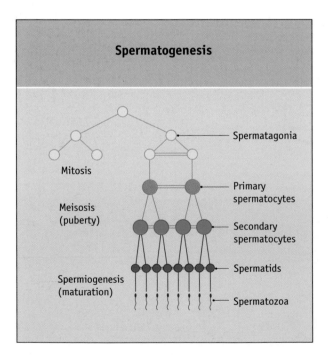

Fig. 3.5 *Spermatogenesis.*

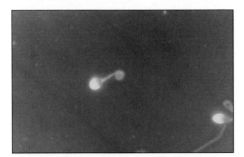

Fig. 3.6 *Acrosome reaction allows its enzyme contents to escape.*

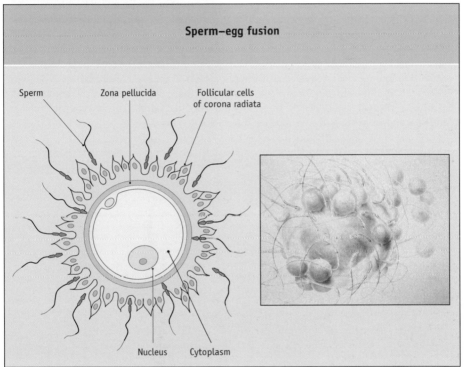

Sperm–egg fusion

Sperm   Zona pellucida   Follicular cells of corona radiata

Nucleus   Cytoplasm

Fig. 3.7 *Sperm–egg fusion. From Breckwoldt, M., Neumann, F., Brauer H. 'Exempla Endocrinologa. Pictorial Atlas of the Physiology and Morphology of the Endocrine System' (Schering A.G, Berlin, 1994), with permission.)*

membrane lying immediately beneath it, the outer acrosomal membrane. This acrosome reaction allows the enzyme contents of the acrosome to escape (**Fig. 3.6**). The enzymes, which include hyaluronidase and acrosin, are thought to play an important role in sperm penetration of the egg.

The site of fertilization

Fertilization occurs in the ampullary region of the fallopian tube. The cumulus and oocyte are found here within 2–3 minutes of ovulation. Spermatozoa have been detected in the fallopian tube 5 minutes after insemination. The outer layer of the egg, the zona pellucida, contains receptors for spermatozoa and undergoes the zona reaction during which it becomes impervious to other sperm once the fertilizing spermatozoon has penetrated. The postacrosomal region of the spermatozoal head makes contact and fuses with the egg plasma membrane (**Fig. 3.7**). The chromatin material of the sperm head then decondenses to form the male pronucleus. The male and female pronuclei migrate towards each other, their limiting membranes break down, and a spindle is formed on which the chromosomes become arranged. The first cell division then occurs.

Implantation

Implantation is defined as the process by which an embryo attaches to the uterine wall and penetrates first the epithelium and then the circulatory system of the mother to form the placenta (**Fig. 3.8**). The process begins 2–3 days after the fertilized egg enters the uterus, 3–4 days after ovulation. Thus implantation occurs 5–7 days after fertilization. The human blastocyst remains in the uterine secretions for approximately 72 hours and then hatches from the zona pellucida in preparation for attachment. Initially, implantation is marked by apposition of the blastocyst to the uterine epithelium. The uterine stromal cells undergo decidualization, a progesterone-dependent phenomenon. Early changes are seen in the last days of the normal menstrual cycle but more extensive decidualization occurs in the event of pregnancy. A dialogue between the decidual cells and the invading trophoblast may play a crucial part in regulating the implantation process. Eventually, the trophoblast invades the endothelium and muscle of the maternal spiral arterioles as the haemochorial placenta develops.

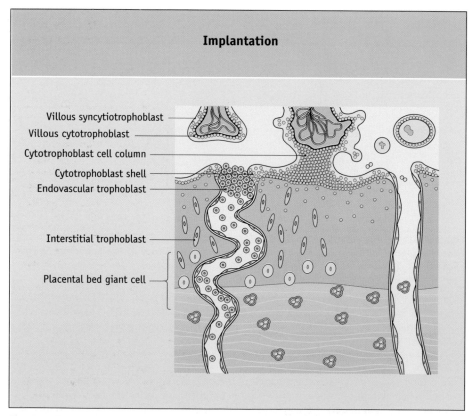

Fig. 3.8 *Implantation. After Loke, Y. W. and King, A. 'Human implantation: Cell Biology and Immunology' (Cambridge University Press, 1995), with permission.*

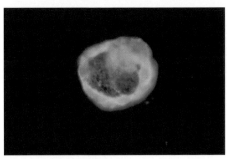

Fig. 3.9 *A blastocyst.*

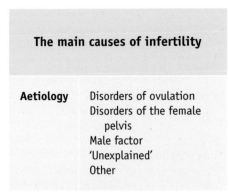

The main causes of infertility	
Aetiology	Disorders of ovulation
	Disorders of the female pelvis
	Male factor
	'Unexplained'
	Other

Fig. 3.10 *Causes of infertility.*

Formation of the blastocyst

After three or four divisions, the zygote is known as the morula. At this 12–16 cell stage, the morula consists of an inner cell mass and a surrounding layer, the outer cell mass. The former gives rise to the tissues of the embryo proper and the outer cell mass forms the trophoblast which later contributes to the placenta. When the morula enters the uterine cavity, fluid begins to penetrate through the zona pellucida into the intercellular spaces of the inner cell mass. The fluid-filled spaces coalesce to form a single cavity, the blastocoele. The conceptus is now known as a blastocyst (**Fig. 3.9**).

INFERTILITY

DEFINITION AND AETIOLOGY

Infertility is usually defined as an inability to conceive after 12 months of unprotected intercourse. This definition is based on the knowledge that about 80% of women will be pregnant within 12 months and 95% will conceive within 2 years. Disorders of ovulation, pelvic disease and male factor problems each account for about 25% of cases of infertility. In most of the remainder, a 'diagnosis' of 'unexplained' infertility is made. While couples with 'unexplained' infertility are offered a variety of treatments, 40–80% will conceive spontaneously within 3–9 years. Other causes of infertility include cervical factors, abnormalities of transport of the gametes along the fallopian tube and psychosexual problems. That the cause of infertility can reside with the woman or the man, or both (**Fig. 3.10**), highlights the importance of assessing the couple together.

INVESTIGATION

Assessment of ovulation

Ovulation is suggested by regular painful periods (menstrual interval of 21 to 35 days). Some women are aware of cyclical changes in cervical mucus, which becomes clear and stretchy ('spinnbarkeit') under the influence of oestradiol at midcycle. Others experience pain as fluid released from the ruptured follicle irritates the peritoneum ('mittelschmerz'). The mainstay of investigation is to measure the circulating concentration of progesterone. Blood must be taken in the midluteal phase of the cycle (7 days before the next period). The fact that progesterone acts centrally to increase basal body temperature led to the use of temperature charts to detect ovulation. Although these may provide supportive evidence,

The assessment of ovulation by history and investigation	
History	Menstrual cycle Cervical mucus 'Mittelschmerz'

Investigation	Basal body
	   temperature
	Serum progesterone
	   concentration
	Ovarian ultrasound
	   scan
	Laparoscopy

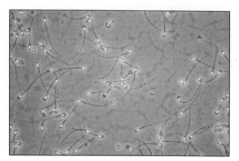

Fig. 3.12 *A normal semen analysis.*

Fig. 3.11 *The assessment of ovulation by history and investigation.*

failure to detect a temperature rise does not always indicate anovulation. Direct confirmation of ovulation can be obtained by observing the growth and collapse of the dominant follicle by ultrasound or by timing laparoscopy to inspect the ovary in the second half of the cycle (**Fig. 3.11**).

Semen analysis

Although there is no direct correlation between semen analysis and fertility, the test gives a broad indication of normality and should be performed at an early stage in the management of every couple. The normal semen analysis has a volume of 3–5ml with a sperm density of greater than 20 million/ml. Fifty per cent of the sperm should have forward motile progression and 30% should be morphologically normal (**Fig. 3.12**). The criteria for 'normality' differ from laboratory to laboratory and there is a marked variation in semen parameters from day to day. Therefore, a minimum of two specimens should be assessed before making a diagnosis. As semen characteristics can be impaired by acute insults such as systemic pyrexia, and as the maturation of undifferentiated spermatogonia to mature spermatids takes about 70 days, the second sample should be collected 2–3 months after the first specimen.

Diagnostic laparoscopy

Diagnostic laparoscopy is often used to evaluate the female pelvis. The procedure is most often performed using general anaesthesia but can be carried out with a local or regional anaesthetic. The laparoscope is usually inserted subumbilically to allow direct visualization of the uterus, fallopian tubes, ovaries, pelvic peritoneum and adjacent bladder and bowel to detect problems including adhesions or endometriosis. An injection of dilute methylene blue dye along the endocervical canal permits the assessment of tubal patency. Complications, besides those associated with the anaesthetic itself, include haemorrhage, infection, gas embolization (the peritoneal cavity is usually expanded with carbon dioxide so that the pelvic organs can be seen) and trauma, most commonly to bowel or bladder. In the absence of specific factors in the history, such as severe pelvic infection, laparoscopy is best performed after the couple have been trying to conceive for at least 12 months.

The hysterosalpingogram

A radiological assessment after an injection of opaque dye through the cervix can be used to outline the endocervical canal, uterine cavity and fallopian tubes (**Fig. 3.13**). Spillage of the dye into the peritoneal cavity confirms tubal patency. If there is a tubal blockage, the test will identify the site. Unlike laparoscopy, hysterosalpingography cannot be used to assess the rest of the pelvis. The test is usually carried out at the beginning of the cycle to avoid irradiation of an early embryo. It has been suggested that some tests of tubal patency may have a therapeutic role, by clearing away mucus plugs or debris.

INDUCTION OF OVULATION

The antioestrogen clomiphene citrate increases the release of gonadotrophin-releasing hormone (**Fig. 3.14**) and gonadotrophins from the hypothalamus and pituitary. The drug is taken orally for 5 days in the early follicular phase of the cycle (e.g. 50mg daily from day 2–6). Ovulation should be achieved in up to 90% of patients and 50% will conceive. Ten per cent of pregnancies will be multiple. Clomiphene citrate is not effective in hypo-oestrogenic women, who should receive gonadotrophins (a mixture of FSH and LH, or more purified forms of FSH). The cumulative conception rates should be the same as those of normal fertile women. Ovarian stimulation must be monitored by measuring circulating oestradiol concentrations and by serial ovarian ultrasound to limit the problems of multiple

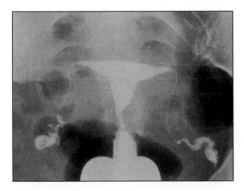

Fig. 3.13 *A normal hysterosalpingogram. The triangular outline of the uterine cavity is seen, with passage of dye along the fallopian tubes and spill into the peritoneal cavity.*

Fig. 3.14 *Induction of ovulation.*

Induction of ovulation for anovulatory women desirous of pregnancy	
General	Clomiphene citrate
	Gonadotrophins
	Pulsatile gonadotrophin-releasing hormone
Specific	Bromocriptine
	Dexamethasone
	Thyroxine

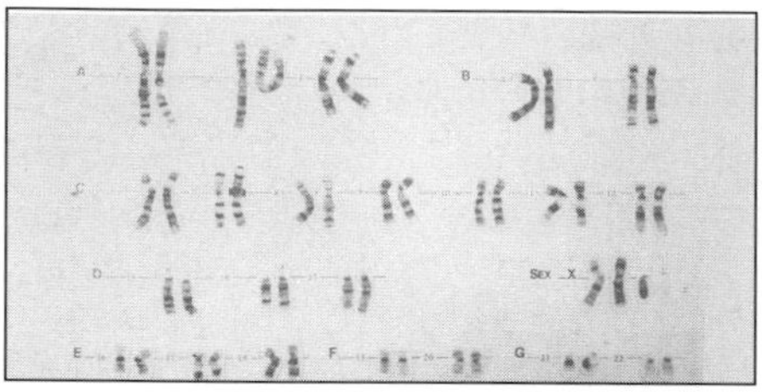

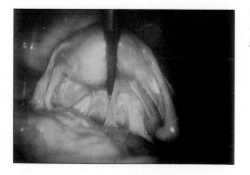

Fig. 3.15 *Karyotype of a man with Klinefelter syndrome (46XXY).*

pregnancy (30%) and ovarian hyperstimulation syndrome (4%). Excess stimulation of the ovaries is less common with pulsatile gonadotrophin-releasing hormone because the ovarian-pituitary feedback axis remains intact. When anovulation results from specific pathology, the dopaminergic agonist bromocriptine, suppression of the pituitary-adrenal axis or the correction of hypothyroidism may be indicated (**Fig. 3.14**).

MALE FACTOR INFERTILITY: AZOOSPERMIA

The management of a man with persistent azoospermia (absence of spermatozoa in the seminal fluid) depends on clinical findings and endocrine assessment. If the testes are of normal volume (15–20ml) and consistency, and gonadotrophin concentrations (particularly FSH which stimulates spermatogenesis) are within the normal range, surgical exploration should be considered to exclude blockage in the ductus deferens. The finding of small testes and elevated gonadotrophin concentrations suggests testicular failure. A low testosterone concentration indicates poor Leydig cell function and androgen replacement should be prescribed. The man's karyotype should be determined. Klinefelter syndrome (**Fig. 3.15**) occurs in 1:400–500 neonates. The disorder is characterized by small, firm testes with hyalinization of the seminiferous tubules. There is often gynaecomastia and sometimes mental retardation. Although fertility has been demonstrated in men with mosaic karyotypes containing an XY stem cell line, individuals with Klinefelter syndrome are usually sterile.

TUBAL DISEASE: PELVIC INFECTION

The formation of adhesions (**Fig. 3.16**) as a consequence of pelvic sepsis leads to infertility by preventing the spermatozoa reaching the oocyte. In the worst cases there is bilateral tubal blockage. In other situations the ovaries may be covered by filmy adhesions, hindering the release of the oocyte. Infection may be sexually transmitted or the result of pelvic disease such as a ruptured appendix. Sepsis may also follow pregnancy or complicate pelvic surgery itself. A single episode of pelvic infection can predispose to infertility in 10–15% of women. This figure increases to about 20% after two bouts of sepsis and 50% after three episodes. The extent of pelvic disease is best defined at laparoscopy. The assessment of *Chlamydia* antibodies has been used to indicate past infection but is of limited value as

Fig. 3.16 *A view through the laparoscope during investigation of infertility. Note the presence of adhesions.*

these tests are not necessarily specific for the species of *Chlamydia* implicated in the pathophysiology of pelvic disease. The treatment of choice for infertility due to pelvic adhesions is *in vitro* fertilization. Tubal surgery offers a second best option, with success rates inversely proportional to the extent of tubal damage.

UNEXPLAINED INFERTILITY: TREATMENT

The diagnosis of 'unexplained' infertility is made by exclusion. In some centres, the diagnosis will be made for couples who have not conceived after 2 years of unprotected intercourse in the face of regular ovulatory cycles, two normal semen analyses and a normal laparoscopy. Other clinics will proceed to specialized investigations (including the assessment of *in vitro* sperm–mucus interaction and the measurement of antisperm antibodies in serum and semen) before making the diagnosis. However, the results of such specialized investigations do not always alter the couple's management. For patients who have been trying to conceive for 3 years and for whom no cause has been found for their infertility, the chance of spontaneous pregnancy is 2–3% each month. A more conservative approach is appropriate when the woman is under 35 years. Therapeutic options include ovarian stimulation with gonadotrophins or assisted conception. These treatments probably work by enabling pregnancy to occur at an earlier time than it may otherwise have done so by chance. The benefits of treatment should always be weighed against the adverse risks of multiple pregnancy or ovarian hyperstimulation.

ASSISTED CONCEPTION

Classification

Assisted conception refers to artificial techniques of fertility treatment aimed at helping the apposition of the male and female gametes. Such treatments encompass donor insemination, *in vitro* fertilization (IVF), gamete intrafallopian transfer (GIFT) and the more recently introduced intracytoplasmic sperm injection (ICSI). In donor insemination, donated semen is placed at the cervical os (or inside the uterus) at midcycle. IVF and GIFT usually involve ovarian stimulation and oocyte retrieval followed by insemination *in vitro* (IVF) or *in vivo* (GIFT). Assisted conception treatments are controlled by statute in many countries. Treatment in the UK is regulated by the Human Fertilization and Embryology Authority.

In vitro fertilization

IVF was first developed as a treatment for tubal infertility; it is now also indicated for couples with unexplained infertility and some couples with male factor problems. IVF involves ovarian stimulation with gonadotrophins to achieve multiple folliculogenesis. The ovarian response is monitored by ultrasound and by measuring circulating oestradiol concentrations. When at least three follicles have reached a diameter of 17mm or more (indicating maturity), human chorionic gonadotrophin is administered to induce ovulation.

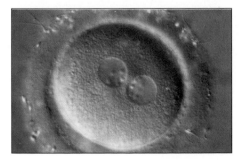

Fig. 3.17 *A fertilized human egg with two pronuclei. Spermatozoa which did not gain access to the egg can be seen outside the zona pellucida.*

Oocyte recovery is performed before the eggs are released by passing an aspirating needle through the lateral vaginal fornix (under sedation) into the ovary. The recovered eggs are inseminated and the following day they are examined for evidence of fertilization (the presence of two pronuclei, **Fig. 3.17**). Two or three embryos are transferred to the uterus transcervically 48 hours after the initial egg retrieval.

Intracytoplasmic sperm injection

After the introduction of IVF, a range of micromanipulative techniques were developed to assist access of the spermatozoa to the egg, particularly for couples with male factor infertility. These techniques included 'zona drilling', in which a hole is made in the zona pellucida, and 'subzonal insemination', in which the spermatozoa themselves are injected below the zona. The most recent development has been the direct injection of a single spermatozoon into the cytoplasm of the oocyte (**Fig. 3.18**). ICSI is now the treatment of choice when the sperm density is less than 100,000/ml or when there are significant disorders of sperm motility. In cases of obstructive azoospermia, spermatozoa can be recovered directly from the testis. About 70% of injected eggs will fertilize after ICSI, providing a realistic chance of pregnancy for couples with severe male factor defects. Follow-up studies of babies born after ICSI have failed to show an increased incidence of significant birth defects compared with babies conceived normally. However, there is an increase in sex chromosome abnormalities in ICSI-derived pregnancies (0.8% compared with 0.2% for spontaneous conception). It is not known whether this is due to the ICSI process or whether it is a reflection of chromosomal abnormalities as a cause of the underlying infertility.

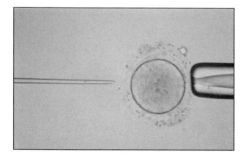

Fig. 3.18 *A human egg following the injection of a single sperm during ICSI.*

Success rates of assisted conception in the UK

Patients	Own gametes	Donated sperm	Donated eggs
Treatment cycles	24 635	1409	246
Pregnancies (%)	21	27	22
Live births (%)	18	23	18

Fig. 3.19 *Success rates following assisted conception in the UK (April 96–March 97). Results of stimulated IVF and fresh embryo transfer cycles are shown, with % pregnancies per treatment cycle.*

Success rates of *in vitro* fertilization

The 1998 annual report of the Human Fertilization and Embryology Authority quoted clinical pregnancy rates and live birth rates after IVF in the UK in 1994 of 20% and 17% per treatment cycle respectively. For women who used their own eggs (as opposed to women receiving donated oocytes), the live birth rate decreased significantly for women aged over 35 years. To put IVF success rates in perspective, they can be compared with a chance of pregnancy of 25% per cycle for couples in their first year of attempting to conceive or 2–3% per cycle for couples with 'unexplained' infertility after 3 years of trying to become pregnant. The Authority report showed a multiple pregnancy rate of nearly 30% for all IVF pregnancies. As would be expected, the chance of a multiple pregnancy and perinatal death increased as the number of embryos transferred increased (**Fig. 3.19**).

CONTRACEPTION

The need for contraception worldwide stems from at least four background problems: rapid population growth, environmental degradation, persistent poverty and unplanned pregnancy. Over 500,000 women die each year from causes related to pregnancy and childbirth. The five major causes are: haemorrhage, infection, unsafe abortion, hypertension and obstructed labour. Of these women, 500 die every day from unsafe abortion. The World Health Organization estimates that approximately 150,000 unwanted pregnancies are terminated every day (40–60 million/year) corresponding to an annual rate of 32–46 abortions per 1000 women of reproductive age. In the UK alone in 1992, there were 170,000 terminations of pregnancy, the majority of which were for unwanted pregnancy. Finally, some 12 million children under the age of 5 years old die of poverty each year.

TYPES OF CONTRACEPTION

Worldwide, from the quantitative point of view, female sterilization is the most frequently used method, followed by intrauterine devices (IUDs) and oral contraceptives. In the UK, the general household surveys in 1986, 1989 and 1991, of women aged between 16 and 49 years old, have shown that the proportion of women using at least one method of contraception remains stable (69–71%) as well as the proportion of women not using any method (20–22%). They show that approximately one quarter of couples rely on very effective methods (female and male sterilization). Another third rely on effective methods (oral contraceptive pill or IUDs) and a further one fifth rely on less effective methods (barrier methods or natural family planning). Typical pregnancy rates for various contraceptive methods are shown in **Figure 3.20**. Contraceptive failure is expressed by the Pearl Index which is defined as the number of pregnancies per 100 women years. This means the number of women out of a 100 who get pregnant using the method continuously for 1 year. Although ineffective use of contraceptives and failure of the methods account for a large fraction of unplanned pregnancies, couples who do not use contraceptives account for a higher proportion of unplanned pregnancies than couples who use them. However, even when a range of methods is available, there is a disappointing number of unplanned pregnancies related to perceived side effects and risks that adversely affect motivation.

The combined oral contraceptive pill

The 'pill' works by inhibiting ovulation, suppressing endometrial proliferation and altering cervical mucus to make it hostile to sperm. It contains one of two synthetic oestrogens: ethinyl oestradiol or mestranol. The quantity of ethinyl oestradiol has steadily reduced since the pill's first development in 1959 from 150μg to 30μg today for most preparations but

Lowest expected and typical pregnancy rates for commonly used contraceptive methods

Method	Lowest expected pregnancy rate (%)	Typical pregnancy rate (%)
Combined oral contraceptive	0.10	3.00
Depot progestogen	0.30	0.30
Progestogen implant	0.04	0.20
Intrauterine contraceptive device	<0.10	3.00
Condoms	2.00	12.00
Cap	6.00	18.00
Female sterilization	0.20	0.40
Male sterilization	0.10	0.15
Natural family planning	1–9	20.00

Fig. 3.20 *Lowest expected and typical pregnancy rates for commonly used contraceptive methods.*

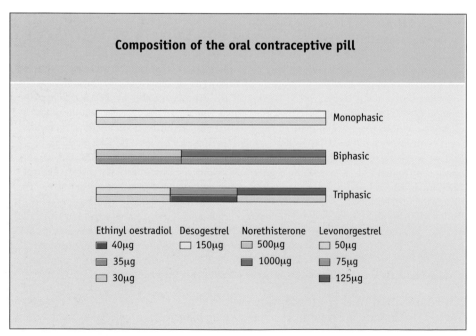

Fig. 3.21 *The combined oral contraceptive pill is a combination of synthetic oestrogen and synthetic progestogen.*

doses down to 20µg are used. For most patients these doses are adequate but for a minority, for example, women with epilepsy on medication inducing liver enzymes such as phenytoin and carbemazepine, preparations containing 50µg ethinyl oestradiol are required. The most widely used progestogens in the pill are derivatives of 19-nortestosterone: initially the estranes (norethisterone and lynestrenol) and later the gonanes (levonorgestrel, desogestrel, gestodene and norgestimate). The last three progestogens are described as 'third generation' progestogens. As a result of the association between third generation pills and thromboembolism, second generation pills are the mainstay of current practice. There are three types of pill: monophasic (same dose of oestrogen and progestogen for 21 days), biphasic or triphasic (the dose of progestogen increases as the cycle progresses and the oestrogen dose varies in order to mimic a natural cycle) (**Fig. 3.21**). A withdrawal bleed

The benefits of combined oral contraception

Prevention	Risks of pregnancy mortality, including ectopic pregnancy	90%
	Ovarian and endometrial carcinoma	40%
Reduction in the incidence of	Benign breast disease	40%
	Functional ovarian cysts	50–80%
	Pelvic inflammatory disease	40%
	Menstrual loss and iron deficiency anaemia	50%
	Dysmenorrhoea	40%

Fig. 3.22 *Benefits of combined oral contraception.*

Relative risks of combined oral contraceptive pill usage

	Risk per 100,000 woman years
Venous thromboembolism	5
Venous thromboembolism on combined pill	15
Venous thromboembolism on third generation pill	30
Myocardial infarction on pill for a nonsmoker <35 years old	10
Myocardial infarction on pill for a smoker >35 years old	50
Death on pill	1.3
Death due to pregnancy	10
Death due to driving a car	17

Fig. 3.23 *Relative risks of combined OCP usage.*

occurs during the last 7 days of the cycle and the pill is usually started on the first day of the menstrual cycle. As well as being an effective contraceptive, the pill has a number of other benefits (**Fig. 3.22**) but is also associated with an increased risk of certain complications (**Fig. 3.23**). Absolute contraindications to the combined oral contraceptive pill (OCP) summarized in **Figure 3.24**.

Progestogen-only contraception

Progestogens may be used without oestrogens as contraceptives. They can be administered orally, intramuscularly as depot preparations, subdermally as implants and also via IUDs (**Fig. 3.25**).

Progestogen-only pill – The progestogen-only pill contains no oestrogen and uses a small daily dose of progestogen (norethisterone or levonorgestrel). It suppresses endometrial proliferation and alters the cervical mucus making it hostile to sperm and also interferes with ovulation (up to 40% of cycles). It is less effective than the combined pill (**Fig. 3.20**) but is free from oestrogen-related contraindications, such as the increased risk of

Absolute contraindications to combined oral contraceptive pill	
Past or present circulatory disease	Arterial or venous thrombosis Ischaemic heart disease Transient ischaemic attacks Cerebral haemorrhage or thrombosis Pulmonary and valvular heart disease
Liver disease	Complicated diabetes Hypertension Focal or crescendo migraine
Sex steroid-dependent conditions	Acute liver disease Liver adenoma or carcinoma Gallstones Porphyria
Pregnancy	Chorea Pill-induced hypertension Pemphigoid gestationis Trophoblastic disease with raised chorionic gonadotrophin
Undiagnosed vaginal bleeding	Haemolytic–ureamic syndrome
Oestrogen-dependent neoplasms	

Fig. 3.24 *Absolute contraindications to combined OCP.*

Methods of progestogen-only contraception	
Oral	'The mini pill'
Injectables	Depo-Provera® Noristerat®
Implants	Norplant®, Norplant® 2, Norplant® 6, Implanon®
Interuterine system	Minera®

Fig. 3.25 *Methods of progestogen only-contraception.*

thromboembolic disease. Progestogen-only pills are therefore useful in older patients, smokers and also during breast-feeding as they do not inhibit lactation. The disadvantages of this method are that it requires to be taken at the same time every day, it may induce an erratic menstrual pattern and there is an increased risk of functional ovarian cysts and of ectopic pregnancy. Absolute contraindications include the suspicion of pregnancy, menstrual irregularity (unless investigated), breast cancer and acute or chronic liver disease.

Injectable progestogens – These are delivered by intramuscular injection and are mainly of two types: medroxyprogesterone acetate (Depo-Provera®) 150mg given every 12 weeks, norethisterone enanthate 200mg every 8 weeks. They have advantages in the sense that they are highly effective and do not depend on user compliance as well as the fact that they have a decreased risk of pelvic inflammatory disease, ectopic pregnancy and decreased menstrual blood loss, as well as being able to be used during lactation. The main disadvantages are menstrual irregularity including amenorrhoea, weight gain, galactorrhoea and slow reversibility (up to 9 months). The absolute contraindications are the same as those of the progestogen-only pill.

Long-acting reversible contraception – There are several long-acting, highly efficient and immediately reversible contraceptives. These include subdermal contraceptive implants (1–5 years' action), copper IUDs (5–8 year action) and the levonorgestrel-releasing intrauterine system currently licensed for 3 years but has a 5-year action.

Contraceptive implants – These are sustained released, progestogen-only systems and provide low, stable levels of synthetic progestogens over several years

These preparations employ the newer progestogens (gonanes) which are less androgenic. The advantages are freedom from oestrogen-related risks, and avoidance of the first-pass peak dose effect in the liver. These preparations also improve compliance and provide more effective, easy to use and immediately reversible contraception. Activity is mainly by reducing the cervical mucus permeability to sperm, making the endometrium hypotrophic, and by ovulatory dysfunction (ranging from anovulation to insufficient luteal phase). The main side effect is irregular menstrual bleeding caused by the erratic shedding of hypotrophic endometrium. There are three nonbiodegradable implants (Norplant® 6, Norplant® 2 and Implanon®) and biodegradable implants should be available this year.

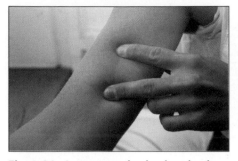

Fig. 3.26 *A contraceptive implant in situ. Its position is illustrated by the patient's fingers.*

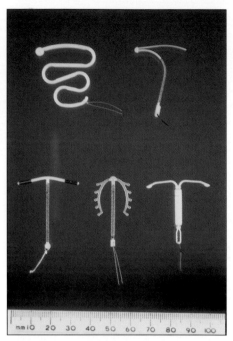

Fig. 3.27 *Intrauterine contraceptive devices. The upper row shows two devices no longer available in the UK: the inert Lippes loop and the copper containing Copper 7. In the lower row is a 'Copper T', a copper containing Multiload® and the progestogen releasing Mirena®.*

In practice, the 5-year implants (Norplant® 6) have been shown to be effective with a first-year pregnancy rate of 0.2% increasing to a maximum of 1.6% in the fourth year, and the five-year cumulative pregnancy rate of 3.9%. Insertion by trained practitioners (**Fig. 3.26**) takes an average of 5–10 minutes, and removal approximately 20–30 minutes. An acceptability study of users in the USA showed that, although 40% were anxious about insertion and removal of the implant, 87% of users experienced no pain or only slight discomfort at insertion, and 74% reported little or no pain at removal. A return to fertility after removal was not impaired, that is, a pregnancy rate of 90% at 24 months was achieved, which is the same as that of fertile women not using contraception. The median duration of use is 3.6 years. The main reason for discontinuation was disruption of the menstrual cycle; this affects 60–80% of users in the first year. Other side effects include headaches, weight gain, mood swings, acne and functional ovarian cysts, which affect less than 10% of users. In spite of these drawbacks, with effective counselling this method has the best continuation rate compared with any reversible method of contraception.

Intrauterine contraceptive devices

The intrauterine contraceptive device (IUD or coil) is usually inserted through the cervix during menstruation and placed inside the uterine cavity. It works by creating a sterile inflammatory reaction in the endometrium which prevents implantation and also by a

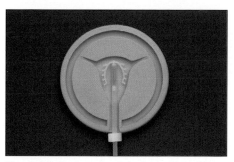

Fig. 3.28 *Correct fundal placement of IUD is important.*

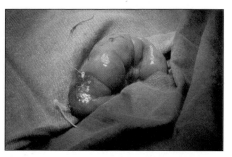

Fig. 3.29 *Copper 7 IUD having perforated the uterus and bowel being retrieved at laparotomy.*

direct toxic action on sperm (copper IUDs). Initially IUDs were 'inert' or nonmedicated and made of plastic (polythene) but this led to a high incidence of heavy periods and dysmenorrhoea. Then followed three generations of copper IUDs. The Cu T 200 and Cu 7 (first generation; duration of action 3 years), the Nova-T®/Novagard® and the Multiload® Cu 250 (second generation; duration of action 5 years) and finally the Cu T 380 S and the Multiload® Cu 375 (third generation Cu IUDs with more than 350mm² surface area of copper; duration of action 10 years and 8 years respectively) (**Fig. 3.27**).

IUDs require fundal placement (**Fig. 3.28**) for their effectiveness. After placement the woman should be asked to check the threads regularly and seek advice if the threads cannot be felt. Screening, at least for *Chlamydia* infection, should ideally be undertaken before insertion. If threads cannot be felt and there is doubt as to a device's situation, radiography and ultrasound can help localization. Spontaneous expulsion occurs with about 10% of insertions and is most likely during the first 6 weeks after insertion. Occasionally, IUDs may perforate through the uterus either due to inadequate placement when partial perforation can occur at the time of insertion or by subsequent 'migration' through the uterine wall, particularly postpartum when involution is occurring. Insertion therefore requires training in order to reduce the risk of perforation of the uterus (the perforation rate is 0.62–1.3 per 1000 insertions). Copper-containing devices in the abdominal cavity will promote adhesions by peritoneal irritation. Occasionally, they can perforate other structures (**Fig. 3.29**) such as bowel. Generally, copper-containing devices should be removed if possible. Approximately 25% of IUDs are removed because of pelvic pain or bleeding. Comparative studies have shown a very low incidence of ectopic pregnancy, ranging from 1.1 in 100 (Nova T®) to 1 in 1000 women years (Cu T 380, which is significantly lower than the background rate for ectopic pregnancy in the noncontraceptive user but significantly higher than in pregnant controls. Therefore, in general, IUDs protect against both intrauterine and ectopic pregnancy, but in the rare circumstance that they fail, there is a relative risk of ectopic pregnancy. Similarly, studies of the incidence of pelvic inflammatory disease have shown a remarkably low incidence ranging from 0.2–1.49 in 100 women years. In part, this must be caused by the exclusion of potential users who are at high risk of STDs.

In the event of an intrauterine pregnancy with an IUD *in situ*, the incidence of miscarriage is greater if the IUD is not removed. Thus the device should be localized with ultrasound and if it is in a location where removal is possible this should be done with gentle traction on the threads. If removal is not easy, the attempt should be abandoned and the device recovered at delivery. Problems associated with a device being *in situ* during pregnancy include increased risk of miscarriage, membrane rupture and infection. Copper

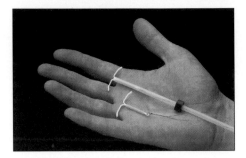

Fig. 3.30 *The Mirena® intrauterine system. The system is shown on its own and within its introducer, the diameter of which is slightly greater than similar copper-containing IUDs.*

IUDs can be inserted at the time of termination of pregnancy, caesarean section, 6 weeks' postpartum as well as for emergency contraception. Although they are better suited to multiparous women, some nulliparous women request their use which is satisfactory after full counselling about the risks and benefits. For these women additional local anaesthesia (2% lignocaine gel, glycerol trinitrate spray or a paracervical block) may be necessary to allow placement with minimal discomfort.

Levonorgestrel intrauterine system – This device uses the frame of a Nova-T® Cu IUD but the copper is replaced by a silastic chamber releasing levonorgestrel at the rate of 20μg daily (**Fig. 3.30**). The inserter is therefore slightly wider (1.1mm) than other coil inserters. The levonorgestrel intrauterine system has significantly lower rates of pregnancy and removals for pain and bleeding than copper coils. However, the rates of removal for amenorrhoea using this device have been significantly higher making counselling before insertion absolutely essential. In fact, recent studies have shown a reduction in menstrual blood loss by 75% on average at the end of 12 months of use (leading to amenorrhoea in 20% of users) (**Fig. 3.31**). The incidence of ectopic pregnancy is also very low (0.2 in 1000 women years) as well as the rate of pelvic infection (0.4 in 100 women years compared with 3.4 in 100 women years for the Nova T® after 5 years of use). In comparison with third generation

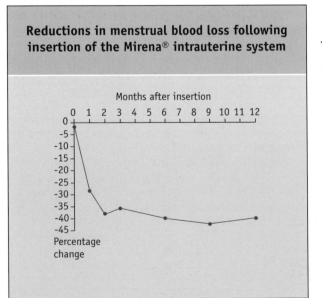

Reductions in menstrual blood loss following insertion of the Mirena® intrauterine system

Months after insertion

Percentage change

Fig. 3.31 *Reductions in menstrual blood loss following insertion of the Mirena® intrauterine system.*

copper IUDs (Cu T 380), continuation rates are similar. It is therefore a question of targeting the IUD to each woman's requirements and preferences and this requires full counselling about the advantages and disadvantages. The absolute and relative contraindications to the use of the IUD are summarized in **Figure 3.32**.

Barrier methods

The main barrier methods that are commonly used are the condom (male and female), the diaphragm, the cervical cap and the contraceptive sponge (**Fig. 3.33**). Pregnancy rates with these methods vary greatly (**Fig. 3.20**) depending on the motivation of the couple. They all have benefits apart from contraception, including the prevention of transmission of sexually transmitted diseases, pelvic inflammatory disease and possibly against cervical carcinoma. Barrier contraceptives prevent sperm from entering the cervical canal either by mechanical occlusion (condoms and caps) or by direct toxic action on sperm (spermicides).

Condoms – Currently available condoms are generally of a very high standard latex (vulcanized rubber) available in prelubricated packs. In some, the lubricant contains spermicide. 'Nonallergenic' condoms are available for those who may be allergic to the standard products. Concern over HIV transmission has led to renewed interest in the condom by consumers as well as by the medical profession. This has led to the 'double Dutch' approach, that is, when the risk of sexually transmitted diseases is considered significant, a dual method is recommended (prevention of pregnancy and prevention of STD), for example, the pill and the condom. Condoms may be accused of decreasing sensitivity but they are easily available and can be used with spermicides for extra protection. A female condom is available but it is not widely used.

Diaphragm – The vaginal diaphragm (**Fig. 3.33**) is the most popular female barrier method of contraception. It comes in sizes from 55–100mm in 5mm intervals. It consists of a thin latex rubber hemisphere with a flexible metal spring. It is fitted across the vaginal vault and thus prevents sperm from getting to the cervix. It is left in place for 6–12 hours after intercourse while most sperm are killed by the acidity of the vagina. As with condoms,

Absolute and relative contraindications to intrauterine contraceptive use

Previous tubal pregnancy or tubal surgery
Uterine cavity distortion
Current pelvic infection
Exposure to a high risk of sexually transmitted diseases
HIV or AIDS
Immunosuppression
History of bacterial endocarditis
Pelvic infection in women with cardiac lesions or
   prosthetic valves
Undiagnosed vaginal bleeding
Suspicion of pregnancy
Nulliparity or young age
Menorrhagia
Severe primary dysmenorrhoea

Fig. 3.32 *Absolute and relative contraindications to IUD use.*

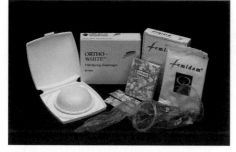

Fig. 3.33 *Different barrier methods of contraception. From left to right: the diaphragm, male condom and female condom. These should be used in conjunction with spermicidal agents.*

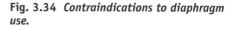

Contraindications to diaphragm use

Uterovaginal prolapse

Vaginal abnormalities

Rubber allergy

History of toxic shock syndrome

Recurrent cystitis

Cultural or personal aversion to
    genital touching

Fig. 3.34 *Contraindications to diaphragm use.*

associating spermicide provides extra protection. Women need guidance with regard to the fitting of diaphragms and they need time to learn the technique of comfortable fitting and removal. The skill, confidence and support of approach of the teacher are therefore of major importance. Occasional problems arise in some users due to a greater frequency of urinary tract infection and very rarely vaginal irritation. There are very few contraindications but these are listed in **Figure 3.34**.

Cervical caps – These are less often used and are particularly useful for women who find it difficult to use a diaphragm. Unlike the diaphragm these are held in place over the cervix by suction. They have slightly higher failure rates compared with the diaphragm because they can be dislodged more easily during intercourse. The cervical cap is indicated when the cervix is long, parallel-sided and not pointing backwards, hence accessible to the woman's examining fingers. It should be used to cover only a healthy cervix. The vault cap is a shallow, bowl-shaped cap suitable for covering a short, wide cervix. The vimule combines the characteristics of both the cervical and the vault cap. It can therefore be used for the irregular cone-shaped cervix. As with all barrier methods, these caps will have increased efficacy when used with spermicide.

Contraceptive sponge – This is made of polyurethane foam impregnated with spermicide. It is inserted high into the vagina and has a loop for ease of removal. It is effective for 24 hours to cover multiple acts of intercourse during that period. It must not be removed until 6 hours after intercourse. Compared with other barrier methods, it is less effective and should be reserved for women whose natural fertility is reduced (lactational or perimenopausal period).

Spermicides – Spermicides alone should not be relied on. They are available in a variety of forms: creams, gels, pessaries, foams and films. One dose of spermicide needs to be applied for each act of intercourse. There is evidence to suggest that spermicides protect against some sexually transmitted diseases and pelvic inflammatory disease. *In vitro* studies indicate that the nonoxinol 9 (the most commonly used spermicide) also inactivates the HIV virus. Occasionally, spermicides may cause local irritation.

Sterilization

Sterilization is the permanent prevention of pregnancy. It can be achieved either by male vasectomy or female tubal occlusion. Careful counselling of both partners before the procedure is essential and should provide all the information relating to various procedures including the methods and the complications, the irreversibility and the finality of the procedure and the small failure rate. It may be necessary to consider features such as age, medical conditions, economic circumstances and the stability of the relationship. The timing must be suitable, that is, not usually at the time of termination of pregnancy or immediately postpartum as judgement may be impaired and failure rates are increased.

Vasectomy – This is a simple procedure often performed under local anaesthetic as an outpatient procedure. It involves division and ligation of the vas deferens on each side. Three months are usually necessary postoperatively before ejaculates are free of sperm and consccutive semen analyses with negative count should be obtained before assuming effective contraception. Possible rare complications include haematoma or bruising of the scrotum as well as a tender sperm granuloma.

Female sterilization – Female sterilization is usually performed by laparoscopy with a tubal occlusion. Laparotomy may be needed if the patient is unsuitable for laparoscopy (e.g. because of multiple adhesions due to previous abdominal surgery) or when sterilization is performed as part of another operative procedure (caesarean section, hysterectomy). When laparoscopy is performed, the fallopian tubes are occluded by clips (Filshie or Hulka) or by a fallope ring (**Figs 3.35–40**). Unipolar or bipolar diathermy has also be used but this has become unpopular because of the possibility of burns to other pelvic organs such as the

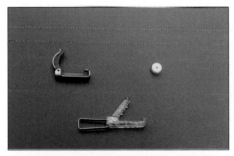

Fig. 3.35 *Hulka clip (top), Falope ring and Filshie clip (bottom).*

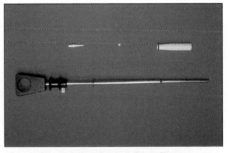

Fig. 3.37 *Falope ring and applicator including the loading system to place the ring on to the applicator.*

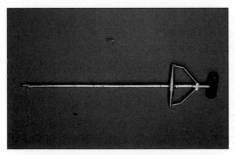

Fig. 3.36 *Filshie clip and applicator.*

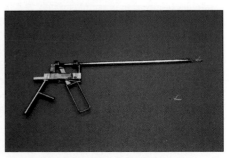

Fig. 3.38 *Hulka clip and applicator.*

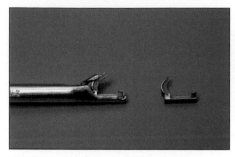

Fig. 3.39 *Close up of Filshie clip and applicator showing placement of clip in 'jaws' of applicator.*

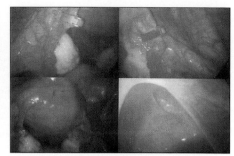

Fig. 3.40 *Laparoscopic sterilization with Filshie clips. The upper panel demonstrates placement across both tubes. The lower left panel shows that placement is across the tubes and not on other structures such as the round ligament which can be mistaken for the tube. In the lower right panel a peritoneal pocket which may contain endometriosis is demonstrated; unexpected pathology may be found at the time of sterilization.*

bowel or bladder. Failure rates (1 in 200–300) of the mechanical methods are similar. Preoperative counselling is essential and the patient must be aware of the nature of the procedure, the risk of failure, the limited possibility of reversibility requiring tubal micosurgery, the possibility of a laparotomy if a laparoscopy is not feasible, the risk of inadvertent damage to the bladder, bowel or major pelvic blood vessel (up to 1 in 100) and the relative risk of ectopic pregnancy in the event of failure. This counselling must be documented in the medical records. Many apparent 'failures' are caused by the patient being pregnant at the time of the procedure. Thus sterilization should ideally be performed in the first half of the menstrual cycle and other contraception must be continued until the sterilization is completed. If the patient is on the pill, then this should be continued until the end of the cycle.

Emergency contraception

This is most commonly provided by the combined oral contraceptive pill (Yuzpe regimen) and improperly referred to as the 'morning-after pill' or 'postcoital contraception'. In fact, it may be used up to 72 hours after the earliest unprotected intercourse episode in that cycle. Its failure rate is approximately 2–4%. Two preparations exist in the UK (Ovran® 50, Schering PC4®) containing 100µg of ethinyl oestradiol and 500µg levonorgestrel given as two tablets immediately and repeated after 12 hours. Nausea is a common side effect and if vomiting occurs within 3 hours of taking a dose, another dose should be taken.

An intrauterine contraceptive device can also be fitted for emergency contraception up to 5 days after the earliest unprotected episode of sexual intercourse in that cycle. Its failure rate is 100 times lower than that of the Yuzpe regimen but it should not be inserted in women at high risk of sexually transmitted diseases.

Termination of pregnancy

Within the terms of the Abortion Act of 1967, a pregnancy may be terminated in the UK but excluding Northern Ireland if two registered medical practitioners are of the opinion

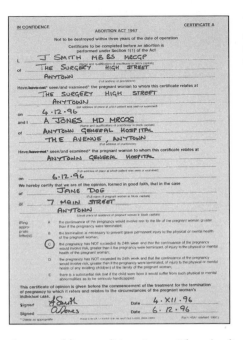

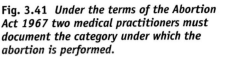

Fig. 3.41 *Under the terms of the Abortion Act 1967 two medical practitioners must document the category under which the abortion is performed.*

that one of five conditions is met. These are listed on the form that has to be signed before the termination takes place (**Fig. 3.41**). Following termination a further form is completed specifying the indication, the gestation, the method of termination and any complications. A single practitioner may give an emergency certificate before termination, or if not reasonably practical within 24 hours of termination, if it is necessary to save the life of the pregnant woman or to prevent grave injury to her physical or mental health. Such certification is rare.

As a result of the Abortion Act there has been a marked reduction in the number of septic abortions admitted to hospital but this must be balanced against the fact the rate of induced abortion has steadily increased. There has also been a reduction in the number of mortalities associated with abortion and this has been clearly documented in the Confidential Enquiries into Maternal Mortality (**Fig. 3.42**).

Counselling and preparation – Pretermination counselling is important and should focus on several areas: the reason for the request, discussion of the implications, informing the patient of the process, discussion of the risks and benefits to her, the provision of emotional support and contraceptive advice. The services of a counsellor not involved with the medical aspects of the process can be extremely beneficial in the assessment and support of many patients.

An accurate assessment of gestation must be made to guide the type of process suited to the patient and ultrasound is valuable for this, although clinical bimanual examination will provide an approximate guide. The opportunity to perform a cervical smear should not be missed if a smear is due. In addition, screening for infection, particularly *Chlamydia*, with high vaginal and endocervical swabs can prevent subsequent problems with infection by pre- or perioperative antibiotic treatment. Depending on the nature of infection, contact tracing may be required and this is best done through the genitourinary medicine service. Infection is important because it is associated not only with the acute morbidity of pelvic infection but also tubal damage and subsequent infertility. The blood group must be assessed to determine the need for anti-D prophylaxis.

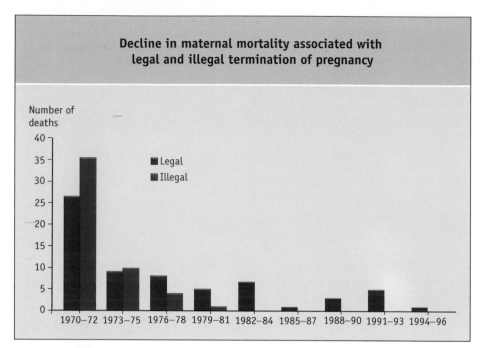

Fig. 3.42 *Decline in maternal mortality associated with legal and illegal termination of pregnancy (Source of data: Reports on Confidential Enquiries into Maternal Deaths in the UK).*

Medical termination – This is provided by the antiprogestogen mifepristone (RU486) at the dose of 600mg orally 48 hours before a vaginal prostaglandin pessary (gemeprost, a synthetic prostaglandin is usually employed in a dose of 1mg, although other preparations such as misoprostol are also effective). This regimen is 95% efficacious at inducing a complete abortion before 9 weeks' gestation. In medical termination after 12 weeks' gestation, a prostaglandin preparation such as gemeprost vaginal pessaries is used. Gemeprost 1mg pessaries are given every 3 hours (five doses maximum), which is usually followed by the spontaneous onset of labour and vaginal delivery. This may be combined with pre-treatment with mifepristone as above. Very rarely extra-amniotic prostaglandin (prostaglandin E$_2$) infusions through transcervical catheters are used for the induction of medical abortion in the second trimester. When late terminations are being performed, administration of intracardiac potassium chloride may be given to the fetus, under ultrasound guidance, to induce cardiac arrest before termination.

Surgical abortion – This is usually performed by suction curettage (**Fig. 3.43**) and up to 12 weeks' gestation, the cervix can be dilated with metal dilators and a suction curette inserted to empty the contents of the uterus. Beyond 12 weeks' gestation, termination may be effected surgically by dilatation of the cervix and evacuation of the uterus surgically involving grasping and crushing of fetal parts to effect removal, but this has largely been superceded by the safer procedure of medical termination in the second trimester. Prostaglandin preparations such as gemeprost (1mg pessary) or misoprostol are also used to 'ripen' the cervix before surgical termination, particularly in nulliparous patients, to minimize the risk of surgical trauma during dilatation of the cervix. Such pretreatment will also significantly reduce blood loss at termination. Complications of this procedure include

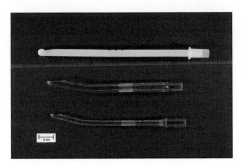

Fig. 3.43 *Suction curettes used for first trimester termination. Top: flexible curette. Middle and bottom: rigid curettes of differing sizes*

primary or secondary haemorrhage, infection and uterine perforation. Very rarely, abdominal hysterotomy is used when medical termination is contraindicated and has the subsequent risk in future pregnancy of uterine scar rupture.

Other aspects of care relevant to the termination of pregnancy are the administration of anti-D immunoglobulin to all Rhesus negative women to prevent isoimmunization, and contraceptive advice which should be given before discharge with appropriate arrangements for contraceptive follow-up made. In view of the risk of infection and retained products, women should be advised to seek medical advice should bleeding or vaginal discharge persist. Normally some vaginal staining and cramping pains will persist for a few days after termination. The emotional support of the patient must also be considered. Although many women express relief because their immediate problem is solved, others suffer feelings of guilt, depression and grief, particularly if the pregnancy has been a wanted one with termination performed for fetal abnormality. Counselling by an experienced worker may be of value to these women and such a service is important to complement the medical aspects of termination.

Natural family planning

Natural family planning is based on observation of the natural signs and symptoms of the fertile and infertile phases of the menstrual cycle. The major and minor indicators of

Methods of natural family planning	
Single index methods	Cervical mucous Cervical changes Basal body temperature Lactational amenorrhoea
Multiple index methods	Double check Mucal–thermal method (cervical mucous and basal body temperature) Calculothermal method (calendar calculation and basal body temperature)

Fig. 3.44 *Methods of natural family planning.*

fertility can be used individually or in combination to detect the fertile phase of the menstrual cycle. The methods employed are indicated in **Figure 3.44**.

With the cervical mucus method, the fertile phase is the earliest day in the cycle on which mucus is perceived at the vulva either by sensation or appearance. The end of the fertile phase is the evening on the fourth day after the peak, that is the last day of watery, stretchy mucus before it reverts to a thick plug. With the cervix method, the fertile phase is detected by the first discovery of any degree of softness, openness or upward movement of the cervix. The end of the fertile phase is the fourth day after the peak cervix day, that is the day on which the softness, openness or upward movement are maximal.

For the basal body temperature method, temperature is usually taken in the morning after a night's sleep. The increased progesterone after ovulation causes a sudden upward shift in the basal body temperature. This remains at a higher level during the luteal phase and returns to baseline levels towards the end of the cycle. The basal body temperature does not detect the onset of the fertile phase. It merely indicates the postovulatory infertile phase.

Patients can plot these observations on special charts to determine their most fertile time (**Fig. 3.45**). Plotting changes in temperature and mucous may be affected by other events as demonstrated here by the temperature change associated with a late night and the mucous change associated with intercourse. The Unipath personal contraceptive system combines the principles of natural family planning with the measurement of oestradiol in urine samples. The meter employs a predictive algorithm to interpret results. In this case the yellow light indicates the need for a urine test. Urine testing is acheived by holding the test strip in the urine stream before inserting it into the meter. A red light would indicate fertile days and a green light indicates that intercourse should be safe.

These methods can of course be used to enhance fertility as well as for contraception.

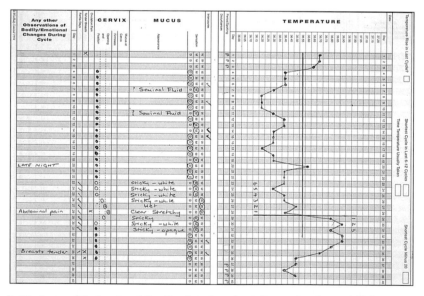

Fig. 3.45 *A completed natural family planning chart demonstrating a definite temperature change together with changes in cervical mucous and cervical position.*

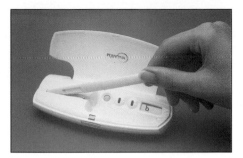

Fig. 3.46 *The Unipath personal contraceptive system.*

Lactational amenorrhoea is an efficient interim contraceptive method in the fully or almost fully breast-feeding women in the first 6 months postpartum provided that she remains amenorrhoeic. To be successful it requires that the mother is virtually fully breast-feeding both day and night with no long intervals between feeds, that menstruation has not returned and that the infant is not receiving regular food supplement breast milk.

It has long been recognized that some form of immunochemical urine test could offer an alternative to natural methods for an accurate prediction of the fertile phase, particularly if it were combined with an electronic device to record and process the daily signal. This is the basis of the Unipath personal contraceptive system which measures hormones in the early morning urine to identify the fertile days in the cycle. It defines the beginning of the fertile phase by pinpointing the oestradiol rise and the end of this phase by allowing for a few days of ovum release and survival following detection of the luteinizing hormone surge. A battery-operated, hand-held electronic monitor reads the test stick and uses a predictive algorithm to interpret the results in terms of fertility status. The fertility status is indicated by a red light for fertile days, green for nonfertile days and yellow denoting that a urine test is required (8 days per cycle). With use the system adapts to the individual woman. As a result of accurate monitoring of the hormones involved in fertility, the number of potentially fertile days is considerably reduced compared with other natural methods: 8 days for the system as opposed to 12–14 days for modern, natural methods (**Fig. 3.46**).

chapter 4

Early Pregnancy Problems

BASIC EMBRYOLOGY AND PLACENTAL DEVELOPMENT

THE EMBRYO
Four weeks from last menstrual period (14 days from fertilization)
Gestation sac approximately 3mm in diameter.
Ectoderm, mesoderm and endoderm formed.

Six weeks
Yolk sac present at 6 weeks.
Gestational sac approximately 20mm in diameter.
Embryo less than 10mm long (**Fig. 4.1a**).
Ultrasound visualization possible from this time (**Figs 4.2** and **4.3**).
Embryo has cylindrical form with head and tail end present.
Fetal heart pulsations present. Umbilical cord formed.

Eight weeks
Gestational sac 30–50mm in diameter, fetus approximately 25mm in length.
Limbs well formed, toes and fingers present, ossification centres present.

Twelve weeks
Gestational sac 100mm in diameter, fetus approximately 90mm long, primary development of all organ systems has occurred.

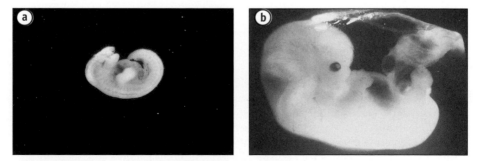

Fig. 4.1 *Embryos at different stages of development. (a) Human embryo at approximately 6 weeks' gestation by menstrual dates. Crown–rump length 3–5mm. (b) Human embryo at approximately 9 weeks' gestation by menstrual dates. Crown–rump length around 18mm.*

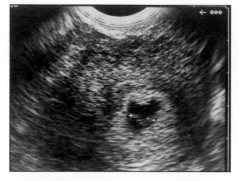

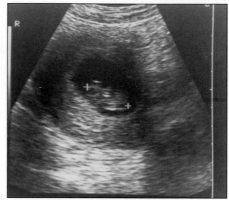

Fig. 4.2 *Transvaginal ultrasound scan showing a gestation sac and singleton fetal pole with crown–rump length of 6.9mm equivalent to 6 weeks and 5 days' gestation. A fetal heartbeat was seen in the course of the scan confirming viability.*

Fig. 4.3 *Transabdominal scan showing a crown–rump length of 26mm equivalent to 9+3 weeks gestation in a singleton pregnancy.*

Fig. 4.4 *Fetal membranes.*

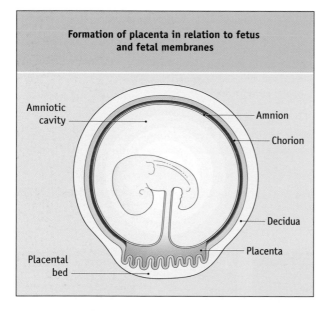

EARLY PLACENTAL DEVELOPMENT

The gestational sac containing the embryo is made up of two membranous tissues: the amnion forms the innermost area and the chorion the outermost layer (**Fig. 4.4**). After initial implantation, the placental tissue proper will develop from the chorion where it comes into contact with the decidua. Thus, the chorion is continuous with the placenta proper and the amnion covers the embryonic or fetal side of the placenta and can easily be separated from it.

Placental villi bud out from the chorionic plate, the villi initially are formed from only cytotrophoblast tissue. A mesodermal core develops within each villus and blood vessels within this core form capillary loops (**Fig. 4.5**). A functioning fetal circulation has

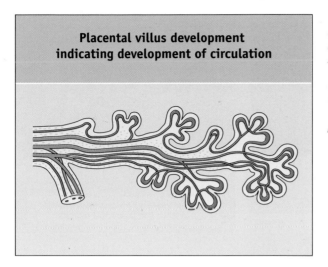

Placental villus development indicating development of circulation

Fig. 4.5 *Placental villus development indicating development of circulation. After Kaufmann, P. 'Contributions to Gynaecology and Obstetrics', 1985; 13: 5–17 (Karger, AG, Basel) with permission.*

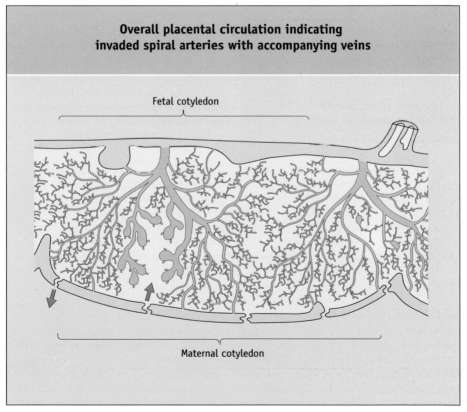

Overall placental circulation indicating invaded spiral arteries with accompanying veins

Fetal cotyledon

Maternal cotyledon

Fig. 4.6 *Overall placental circulation indicating invaded spiral arteries with accompanying veins. After Benirschke, K. and Kaufmann, P. 'Pathology of the Human Placenta' (Springer Verlag GMBH and Co., KG, 1995) with permission.*

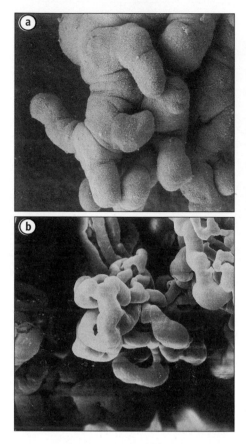

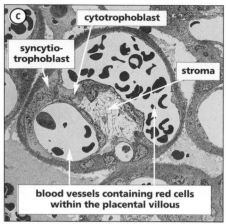

Fig. 4.7 *(a) Electron microscopy of the placental surface showing the terminal villi which are bathed in the maternal blood surrounding the placental villi. (b) Electron micrograph of vascular cast of the blood vessels contained within the placental villi shown in Figure 4(a). Note the coiled capillary loops. (c) Transmission electron micrograph of a terminal villus within the placenta. Within the villus there are vessels containing fetal red cells and some cytotrophoblast and syncytiotrophoblast are labelled.*

developed by 22 days. At 8 weeks' gestation, the villi have a well-organized circulatory system. They have a double layer of trophoblast, the innermost layer being the cytotrophoblast, consisting of single trophoblast cells, and the outer layer is syncytiotrophoblast which results from the cytotrophoblasts forming a syncitium. Cytotrophoblast columns will also invade the decidua basalis helping to anchor the placenta to the mother. The placenta develops further by branching of the villi which become longer and larger with the thinning of the trophoblast. The trophoblast cells also invade the maternal circulation converting the high-resistance spiral arteries to low resistance channels by destroying the maternal vascular endothelium and muscular coat of the spiral artery (see **Fig. 3.8**). This allows maternal blood being delivered from the mother to bathe the placental villus tree. The trophoblast layer of the fetal placenta will thin out further such that there is a very narrow distance between the maternal blood and the fetal capillaries to allow oxygen and nutrients to transfer across the trophoblast while keeping the maternal and fetal circulations separate (**Fig. 4.7**). These placental villi generated by trophoblast proliferation with repeated branching provide a large surface area to facilitate feto-maternal exchange of oxygen and nutrients. In addition, trophoblast also grows down into the placental bed of the uterus so anchoring the placenta to the mother. It also invades the maternal circulation transforming the spinal arteries from high pressure low flow vessels to low pressure high flow vessels by eroding the endothelium muscular layer and elastic layer of the vessel replacing it with trophoblast. The trophoblast itself differentiates into two layers – the outer layer, termed syncytotrophoblast, is in contact with maternal blood and is a multinuclear syncitium with no distinct cell boundaries, while the inner layer or cytotrophoblast forms a single layer of cells.

BLEEDING IN EARLY PREGNANCY

The main diagnostic problem in early pregnancy is the differentiation of miscarriage in its various forms and ectopic pregnancy. The classification of miscarriage in all its varieties and the differentiation from ectopic pregnancy is based on features present on the history and examination and on ultrasound findings supported by the presence of a positive pregnancy test. The potential causes of miscarriage are shown in **Figure 4.8**.

Technically, a miscarriage is the spontaneous termination of a pregnancy before the 24th week of gestation. The aim of taking a history (**Fig. 4.9**), examination (**Fig. 4.10**) and investigation of patients complaining of bleeding and/or pain in early pregnancy are:

- To confirm that a pregnancy is present.
- To determine whether it is intrauterine or ectopic.
- To determine whether the pregnancy is viable.

It is also useful to have a past obstetric and gynaecological history to identify patients with recurrent miscarriage. Women with recurrent miscarriage will require investigations to exclude the causes shown in **Figure 4.8**. It is worth noting that in cervical incompetence, miscarriage is often associated with minimal pain and may initially be in the midtrimester with subsequent miscarriages occurring at earlier gestations.

An examination of the patient will assess her general status and some assessment should be made of cardiovascular status, particularly if bleeding is heavy, but it is usually obvious if shock is present from severe intra-abdominal haemorrhage as may occur with an ectopic

Aetiology of spontaneous miscarriage

Chromosomal or genetic factors, e.g. autosomal trisomies, 45X and triploidy.

Endocrine abnormalities, e.g. luteal phase defect, thyroid disease.

Reproductive tract abnormalities, e.g. cervical incompetence, congenital abnormality of the uterus such as bicornuate or unicornuate, submucous fibroids.

Infection, e.g. listeria, mycoplasma, toxoplasmosis.

Systemic disease, e.g. chronic renal disease, systemic lupus erythematosus, anticardiolipin antibody syndrome.

Fig. 4.8 *Aetiology of spontaneous miscarriage which may occur in 25% of all pregnancies.*

Fig. 4.9 *Features to be elucidated on history.*

Features to be elucidated on history

Date of last menstrual period?

Use of contraception?

Whether pregnancy is possible?

Whether pregnancy test was positive?

When bleeding occurred and how heavy it was?

Whether bleeding was accompanied by pain?

If pain was present, what was its localization and how severe was it?

Has any tissue been passed?

Fig. 4.9 *Features to be elucidated on history.*

Fig. 4.10 *Features on examination.*

Features on examination

Degree of bleeding?

Is the cervix open?

What size is the uterus?

Is there any adnexal mass or tenderness?

Fig. 4.10 *Features on examination.*

pregnancy. The abdomen will be examined for any area of localized tenderness. Most bleeding in early pregnancy occurs before 12 weeks' gestation and the uterus will not usually be palpable abdominally. A vaginal examination should include an inspection to assess the degree of bleeding with note being taken of evidence of heavy bleeding, not only by large amounts of blood in the vagina, but also by blood stains on the legs or feet of the patient. A speculum examination should be performed to assess whether blood and/or products are present in the vagina. The cervix should be visualized and note taken of any incidental cause that could explain minor degrees of bleeding in early pregnancy such as a cervical polyp or ectropion. Bimanual examination should assess whether the cervix is open, whether the uterus is enlarged and whether there is any adnexal mass or tenderness (Fig. 4.10).

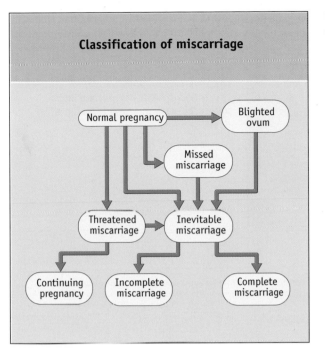

Fig. 4.11 *Classification of miscarriage.*

INVESTIGATIONS AND DIAGNOSIS

The fundamental investigations are a pregnancy test and an ultrasound scan. The pregnancy test should confirm whether a pregnancy is present and an ultrasound scan will identify whether or not the pregnancy is intrauterine. The diagnosis of ectopic pregnancy is made if the pregnancy test is positive and the uterine cavity is empty. If an intrauterine pregnancy is present, it should be assessed for viability. If it is nonviable, the size of the gestational sac should be noted and the extent of any retained products. It should be noted that transvaginal scanning allows diagnosis of an intrauterine pregnancy at an earlier stage gestation than transabdominal scanning and may also allow direct visualization of an ectopic pregnancy in the tube.

A traditional clinical diagnosis of spontaneous miscarriage is divided into three categories (**Fig. 4.11**):

- Threatened miscarriage. Painless vaginal bleeding, which may settle spontaneously with a continuing pregnancy or progress to an inevitable miscarriage, results from bleeding from the placental site which is not of sufficient severity to terminate the pregnancy.
- Inevitable miscarriage. In this situation bleeding may be of variable quantity, the cervical os is usually open due to uterine contractions attempting to expel the conceptus and there is usually pain accompanying this cervical dilatation.
- (In)complete miscarriage. Incomplete miscarriage is associated with the passage of part of the products of conception and complete miscarriage occurs when all of the products have been expelled through the cervical os. The cervix is usually open in incomplete miscarriage but may be closed in a complete miscarriage.

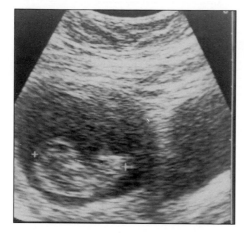

Fig. 4.12 *Ultrasound scan of threatened miscarriage showing normal features with crown–rump length of 36mm compatible with 10+3 weeks' gestation. The fetal heart was seen pulsating in the course of the scan and on physical examination the cervix was closed. The patient had presented with painless bleeding after 9 weeks' amenorrhoea.*

An ultrasound examination will result in an alternative or additional classification for spontaneous miscarriage. These are:

- Blighted ovum (anembryonic pregnancy).
- Missed miscarriage.
- Live miscarriage.

A blighted ovum is when placental tissue develops but no embryo or fetus develops in the gestation sac.

Missed miscarriage is diagnosed when the embryo or fetus is seen but the fetal heart is absent. This would be visualized on ultrasound before the development of any clinical symptoms or signs such as pain or bleeding, although the patient may have ceased to feel pregnant.

Live miscarriage is when the fetal heart can still be identified *in utero* before expulsion of the products of conception, implying that the fetal loss is a consequence, rather a direct cause of the process.

Ultrasound will also confirm a viable pregnancy with a threatened miscarriage or incomplete or complete miscarriage.

Thus, threatened miscarriage can be diagnosed by painless bleeding in early pregnancy with a viable intrauterine pregnancy seen on ultrasound scan and with a closed cervix on clinical examination (**Fig. 4.12**). Treatment is reassurance. Traditionally, bed rest has been used but there is no evidence that this is of any benefit over reassurance and demonstration to the mother of a viable pregnancy with ultrasound.

An inevitable miscarriage is diagnosed when the cervix is open and there is continued bleeding associated with pain. The pregnancy has usually perished by this stage and the treatment is to proceed to evacuation of the uterus.

An incomplete miscarriage can be diagnosed when the cervix is open; tissue may be found within the cervix or vagina and products of conception can also be seen on ultrasound scan (**Fig. 4.13**). The treatment for this is usually surgical evacuation of the uterus.

A complete miscarriage can be diagnosed when there is good evidence of a pregnancy having been present such as a positive pregnancy test, often on more than one occasion, with ultrasound showing an empty uterus. Care must be taken at this stage to exclude an

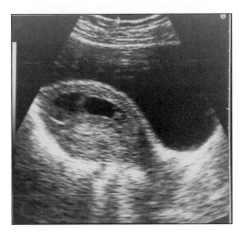

Fig. 4.13 *Transabdominal ultrasound scan of incomplete miscarriage showing a gestational sac distending the uterus but with no fetal pole and small areas of retained products of conception in the uterus. The patient had presented with vaginal bleeding and cramping abdominal pain after 8 weeks' amenorrhoea in her first pregnancy. On examination the cervix was open. Surgical evacuation of the uterus was performed and retained products confirmed histologically.*

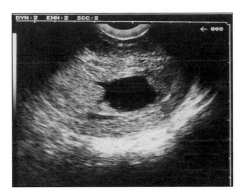

Fig. 4.14 *Ultrasound scan showing intrauterine sac but no fetal pole after 8 weeks' amenorrhoea. There had also been an episode of slight vaginal bleeding 1 week earlier when ultrasound had shown a small sac and no fetal pole in the uterus. A diagnosis of blighted ovum was made and surgical evacuation performed.*

ectopic pregnancy in which the uterus would be empty but a continuing pregnancy is present. An ectopic pregnancy is usually associated with continued pain and persistently elevated human chorionic gonadotrophin (hCG) measurements. If an ectopic pregnancy is excluded, the treatment is reassurance and explanation.

A blighted ovum should be diagnosed on serial ultrasound scan confirming no development of an embryonic or fetal pole with at least 1 week between ultrasound scans (**Fig. 4.14**). It is imperative that serial scans are carried out as the possibility of the dates being wrong should be considered. If the stage of the pregnancy is earlier than thought, the ultrasound findings may be misinterpreted because the size of the gestational sac may not be compatible with dates and the pregnancy may not have reached a stage in which the fetal pole will be visible on ultrasound. Transvaginal ultrasound may allow visualization of a fetal pole at an earlier stage than transabdominal scanning. Eventually, a blighted ovum will progress to an inevitable miscarriage.

Missed miscarriage is usually a diagnosis made on ultrasound scan in which the fetal pole is seen with no fetal heart (**Fig. 4.15**). Inevitably this will progress to a complete or incomplete miscarriage if left because the embryo or fetus has perished. Should the size of the fetal pole indicate a fairly early stage in gestation, it is usual that the scan is repeated to

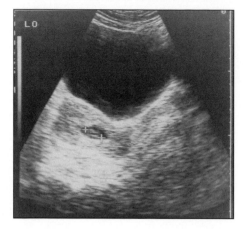

Fig. 4.15 *Ultrasound scan of missed miscarriage. An intrauterine sac containing a fetal pole is present. The crown–rump length was 15mm which was not consistent with her estimated gestation. No fetal heartbeat was seen. The diagnosis was made following booking scan at 10 weeks' gestation by certain dates. The patient had noted early resolution of her morning sickness some three weeks earlier.*

confirm that no change has occurred as a differential diagnosis is that the dates are wrong. The treatment for missed miscarriage and blighted ovum is usually surgical or medical evacuation of the uterus.

SURGICAL EVACUATION OF UTERUS

This is usually carried out under general anaesthesia. Intravenous oxytocin may be given to contract the uterine muscle. The cervix is often sufficiently dilated to allow access to the uterus, if not, it is dilated using serial dilators. Ovum forceps or sponge-holding forceps are introduced into the uterus and fragments of products of conception removed. This may also be carried out digitally. The wall of the uterus is usually curetted to ensure all significant portions of tissue have been removed. An alternative to surgical evacuation for situations such as missed miscarriage or incomplete miscarriage is medical miscarriage using prostaglandins such as gemeprost administered vaginally.

The complications of a spontaneous miscarriage can include: severe haemorrhage, which can on occasion be life-threatening, disseminated intravascular coagulation and infection, which is reduced by prompt evacuation of the uterus and/or treatment with antibiotics, particularly when the retained products of conception are found as necrotic tissue and may predispose to infection. Occasionally, when products are stuck in the cervical os, intense vagal stimulation can result in hypotension and bradycardia which can be treated by digital extraction of the products in the cervical os. In cases of severe haemorrhage, oxytocin or ergometrine can be given intravenously to reduce the bleeding while awaiting surgical evacuation. An infection will be associated with fever, pain, tenderness and often a purulent discharge. Common organisms are *E. Coli*, *Streptococci* and bacteroides. Appropriate broad-spectrum antibiotics should be given while culture and sensitivity are awaited and evacuation of retained products performed once antibiotic therapy is underway.

ECTOPIC PREGNANCY

Ectopic pregnancy is a continuing cause of maternal morbidity and mortality with haemorrhage being the most common problem. There is a rising incidence of ectopic pregnancy in the Western world with a several-fold increase over the past 20 years (**Fig. 4.16**).

Fig. 4.16 *Increase in incidence and aetiology of ectopic pregnancy.*

Increase in incidence and aetiology of ectopic pregnancy

Tubal damage caused by pelvic inflammatory disease which is increasing in incidence.

Tubal surgery including sterilization and its reversal.

Intrauterine contraceptive devices. Although the overall risk of pregnancy, including ectopic pregnancy is reduced, the relative risk of ectopic pregnancy relative to intrauterine pregnancy is increased by the use of intrauterine devices.

In addition, the rising incidence may reflect, at least in part, improvements in diagnosis due to the increased use of laparoscopy, high-quality ultrasound examination and the use of sensitive assays of hCG or its β subunit. These may have allowed the identification of ectopic pregnancies which in the past may have resolved spontaneously before becoming a significant clinical problem. Such improvements in diagnosis along with greater clinical awareness have contributed to the improvement in mortality. In addition, the fertility prognosis is poor in this patient group. Approximately two thirds will never subsequently bear a live child and 12–18% will have a further ectopic pregnancy. The most common implantation site for ectopic pregnancy is the fallopian tube where over 95% occur. Less than 1% will occur in the ovary and it can rarely occur in the cervix or abdominal cavity (**Fig. 4.17**). Pathologically, the villus trophoblast rapidly invades tubal mucosa with most of the growth occurring in the connective tissue between the endosalpinx and the serosa. As the pregnancy grows, a haematoma may form at the site and eventually the tube may rupture and cause a substantial intraperitoneal haemorrhage. In some instances, the pregnancy will perish and will be absorbed spontaneously or may be aborted through the fimbrial end of the tube, thus resolving spontaneously. Histologically, chorionic villi are

Fig. 4.17 *Site of implantation of ectopic pregnancy.*

Site of implantation of ectopic pregnancy

Fallopian tube

Cornua of uterus

Ovary

Abdomen

Cervix

seen within the tube (**Fig. 4.18**). Decidualization of the endometrium also occurs and the typical histological Arias–Stella reaction will be seen (**Fig. 4.19**). This consists of cellular enlargement, hyperchromatosis pleomorphism and mitotic activity. In addition to bleeding resulting from the ectopic pregnancy and bleeding in the tube, bleeding can also occur if the ectopic pregnancy perishes because of a loss of hormonal support for the decidua which will manifest itself as vaginal bleeding.

The diagnosis of ectopic pregnancy is discussed above. In severe intra-abdominal haemorrhage, the patient may be shocked or have severe abdominal pain. She may also complain of shoulder tip pain, due to diaphragmatic irritation. It may be misdiagnosed as pelvic infection as well as the various presentations of miscarriage discussed. A ruptured ovarian cyst or corpus luteum may also enter the differential diagnosis. It is imperative that a high degree of suspicion is required for all women presenting with gynaecological symptoms which could be associated with an ectopic pregnancy.

The absence of chorionic villi in the presence of an Arias–Stella decidual reaction in 'products of conception' obtained from women having uterine evacuation for presumed incomplete or complete miscarriage also suggest a possible diagnosis of ectopic pregnancy.

Modern assays for hCG or its β subunit in the plasma and urine provide a sensitive pregnancy test and can confirm the presence of trophoblast in the body. With biochemical confirmation, the pregnancy differential is between intrauterine and extrauterine pregnancy and this can usually be discriminated with ultrasound scanning. Thus, a positive pregnancy test coupled with an empty uterus implies ectopic pregnancy. Occasionally, a pseudosac formed from the decidualization of the endometrium may be misleading on ultrasound but a mass of free fluid in the pelvis or pouch of Douglas is highly suspicious. Transvaginal ultrasound provides a better image and the potential for early detection of ectopic pregnancy. The patient in **Figure 4.18** presented with 7 weeks' amenorrhoea followed by

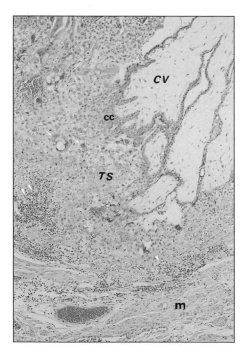

Fig. 4.18 Tubal or ectopic pregnancy. Chorionic villi (CV) with mesenchymal cores are attached to the muscular wall (m) of the fallopian tube via the trophoblastic shell (TS). The chorionic villi are covered by an outer layer of syncytiotrophoblast which faces the tubal lumen and an underlying proliferative cytotrophoblastic layer. Invasive extravillous cytotrophoblast forms cell columns (cc) at the tips of the placental villi, that invade the trophoblastic shell, which is mainly composed of syncytiotrophoblast. Note the syncytial giant cells (arrows) in the trophoblastic shell. The surrounding muscular layer of the fallopian tube shows marked inflammation (arrowheads) adjacent to the implantation site.

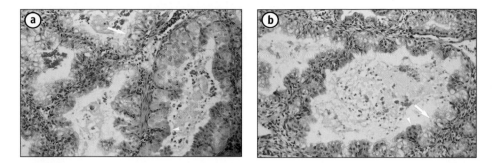

Fig. 4.19 *Gestational hyperplasia and Arias-Stella reaction of endometrium occurring in early pregnancy. Tightly packed endometrial glands show extreme coiling and the lining epithelium shows papillary folds. The epithelial cells exhibit marked nuclear pleomorphism and hyperchromatism. The cytoplasm may be strikingly vacuolated and cleared (clear cells, arrow) or eosinophilic (dark cells, arrowhead). Ultrastructurally the clear cells may contain abundant glycogen. Normal and abnormal mitotic figures may be present. The Arias-Stella phenomenon is almost always focal. It may be present in the cervix and occur in a variety if clinical settings including endocervical polyps, adenomyosis, and endometriosis. The changes are more often seen in post abortion currettings but they are also seen in normal orthotopic pregnancy, hydatidiform mole, choriocarcinoma and following the administration of exogenous hormones. Arias-Stella reaction is therefore not specific for pregnancy. The most important differential diagnosis is endometrial clear cell adenocarcinoma.*

slight vaginal bleeding and right iliac fossa pain, where she was also tender on examination. Serum hCG measured 6430IU/L. The diagnosis was confirmed by laparoscopy and salpingectomy was performed. An early ultrasound was advised in any future pregnancy.

The clinically stable woman at early gestation may, with a combination of ultrasound and serial assay of hCG, be managed conservatively rather than proceeding directly to laparoscopy to confirm the diagnosis. The individual variation of hCG levels in pregnancy and the uncertainty about the exact gestational age with these patients makes a single estimation of hCG of limited value. However, a discriminatory hCG level for an intrauterine pregnancy which should be visible on ultrasound is approximately 6000–6500 IU/L. The doubling time of hCG in early pregnancy is also of value because hormone synthesis by the trophoblast is depressed in ectopic pregnancy. In normal pregnancy, the rate of doubling of hCG in plasma is 1.4–2.1 days and it is not influenced by the initial concentration of hCG. When this fails to occur, there is an increased risk of an ectopic pregnancy, particularly when the uterus is empty on an ultrasound scan.

Conservative management may have a place in unruptured ectopic pregnancy but has no place when serious haemorrhage is present. When significant pain and the risk of intra-abdominal bleeding occurs, the patient should be anaesthetized as required and taken for immediate surgery. In the presence of shock, diagnostic tests are not required and laparotomy will be necessary as an emergency. The first objective is the arrest of the haemorrhage to prevent the patient rapidly deteriorating as the bleeding can be overwhelming from a ruptured ectopic pregnancy.

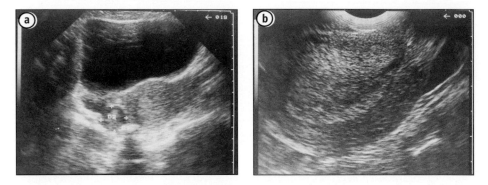

Fig. 4.20 *Ultrasound scan showing ectopic pregnancy: (a) Transabdominal scan showing empty uterus with a complex mass in the right adnexa measuring 21 x 22 mm. (b) Transvaginal scan showing absence of gestational sac in the uterus and decidual reaction with marked endometrial thickening. There is free fluid in the pouch of Douglas (blood will be found there in ruptured ectopic pregnancy).*

The classic treatment of an ectopic pregnancy, ruptured or unruptured, is laparotomy and salpingectomy to arrest or to prevent haemorrhage. There is, however, an increasing use of less aggressive treatment and this can often be carried out laparoscopically with salpingotomy, opening of the tube and evacuation of the ectopic pregnancy, or laparoscopic salpingectomy; the former will preserve the tube. This may be important to maintain fertility. It is imperative to assess the state of the contralateral tube because this will have a bearing on the procedure carried out.

If the tube is badly damaged, the loss of the other tube would present a serious fertility problem for the patient. Other conservative approaches include direct injection of prostaglandins into the ectopic pregnancy, the use of chemotherapy with methotrexate to destroy the trophoblast and it is also possible that antigestagens may have a role.

A summary of early pregnancy problems is shown in **Fig. 4.21**.

Early pregnancy problems

Type of miscarriage	Vaginal bleeding	Pain	Cervical dilatation	Pregnancy test	Ultrasound findings	Treatment
Threatened	+	Occasionally	–	+	Continuing pregnancy	Reassurance
Inevitable	+	+	+	Usually +ve	Products of conception in uterus	Evacuation of retained products of conception
Incomplete	+	+	+	Usually +ve	Products of conception in uterus	Evacuation of retained products of conception
Complete	Minimal or –ve	Settled	–	+/–	Empty uterus	Reassurance and explanation
Missed	–ve, no dark vaginal staining	–	–	Maybe –ve	Fetal pole seen within gestation sac, no fetal heart, no change on serial scanning	Medical or surgical evacuation
Anembryonic pregnancy	–ve until miscarriage occurs	–	–	+	No fetal pole, no fetal heart seen, only gestation sac present, no embryo develops over 1–2 weeks	Medical or surgical evacuation
Ectopic pregnancy	+/–	Usually +ve	–	+	Empty uterus, adnexal mass sometimes seen, particularly on transvaginal scan	Laparoscopic assessment proceeding to laparoscopic treatment of ectopic pregnancy or laparotomy to deal with intra-abdominal bleeding

Fig. 4.21 *Early pregnancy problems.*

HYDATIDIFORM MOLE

An hydatidiform mole is a peculiar condition of the placenta showing degenerative changes in the stroma or villi combined with neoplastic activity in the chorionic endothelium. The incidence varies geographically and is relatively uncommon in the UK with an incidence of approximately 1 in 2000 pregnancies. It is more common in the Orient. A complete hydatidiform mole includes abnormal proliferation of the trophoblast and replacement of normal placental trophoblastic tissue by hydropic placental villi. Complete moles do not include the formation of a fetus and the fetal membranes are characteristically absent. Partial moles are characterized by focal trophoblastic proliferation and degeneration of the placenta and are associated with a chromosomally abnormal fetus. The genetic features of these two types of molar pregnancies are different. Complete moles are entirely of paternal origin as a result of the fertilization of a blighted ovum by a haploid sperm, thus, the karyotype of a complete mole is 46XX. The partial mole is usually triploid, the most common being 69XXY. The triploidy is comprised of one haploid set of maternal chromosomes and two haploid sets of paternal chromosomes which arise from dispermic fertilization. The complete mole is more common. Malignant transformation to choriocarcinoma can occur and it is more common in complete moles, although both types have to be followed serially for evidence of malignancy developing (**Figs 4.22–24**).

A laboratory assessment of a possible hydatidiform mole will show a very high level of hCG which, coupled with ultrasound and the clinical picture, should provide a diagnosis

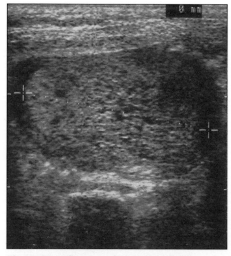

Fig. 4.22 *Ultrasound showing classic 'snowstorm' appearance of hydatidiform mole.*

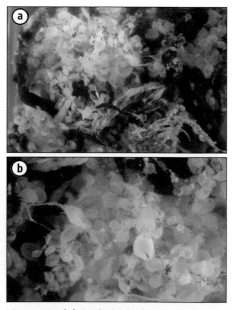

Fig. 4.23 *(a) Pathological appearance of hydatidiform mole following evacuation. (b) Note the multiple grape like vesicles.*

Clinical presentation of hydatidiform mole	Treatment of molar pregnancy
Vaginal bleeding Passage of tissue Exaggerated pregnancy symptoms, e.g. severe nausea and vomiting, hyperthyroidism due to excessive chorionic gonadotrophin stimulating the thyroid, risk of early-onset pre-eclampsia	Uterine evacuation, usually by suction curettage. Medical evacuation can be performed. Follow-up with regular urinary chorionic gonadotrophin measurements to exclude persistent molar disease.

Fig. 4.25 *Treatment of molar pregnancy.*

Fig. 4.24 *Clinical presentation of hydatidiform mole.*

that should be confirmed pathologically with the products of conception. Treatment is by uterine evacuation (**Fig. 4.25**).

Choriocarcinoma is a rare condition, particularly in the Western world. The majority arise from hydatidiform moles. The carcinoma can arise many months after the mole has been evacuated, thus, extended follow-up is needed for moles. This includes warning the patient of the possibility of persistent molar disease, regular monitoring of urinary hCG levels until these become normal, and early ultrasound examination and quantitative hCG assessments in future pregnancies. In the UK, all patients with moles are registered through the Royal College of Obstetricians and Gynaecologists at designated centres and followed for 2 years.

The malignant complications from an hydatidiform mole such as choriocarcinoma are usually treated with chemotherapy drugs such as methotrexate, actinomycin D and vinca alkaloids. A response to treatment can be judged by monitoring hCG levels. The treatment of such conditions is highly specialized and requires referral to specialist units.

HYPEREMESIS GRAVIDARUM

A further common complication during early pregnancy is hyperemesis gravidarum. The majority of women experience some degree of nausea and vomiting in the first trimester of pregnancy, classically known as 'morning sickness', although it may occur throughout the day and even in the evening. The aetiology of this condition is unclear but it may be related to hCG levels which peak at approximately 12 weeks' gestation in line with the time when the problem of hyperemesis may be worst. There is no evidence that hyperemesis gravidarum is associated with an adverse outcome for the fetus. The patient should be reassured and she should try frequent small meals. Prenatal iron supplementation may aggravate the condition and may need to be withheld. Simple antiemetics are needed on occasion and the first line drugs are antihistamines. Major tranquillizers, such as chlorpromazine, and corticosteroid therapy may have a role for more severe cases. With such patients, intravenous fluid replacement will also be required and this would require hospitalization. The use of antiemetics, intravenous fluids and 'resting' the gastrointestinal tract may, along with reassurance, be sufficient to alleviate the condition. These women are also at risk of thrombosis and thromboprophylaxis should be considered.

OVARIAN CYSTS IN EARLY PREGNANCY

Ovarian cysts may be found incidentally on ultrasound examination during pregnancy. Most are functional cysts, corpus luteum cysts that appear simple on ultrasound (**Fig. 4.26**) or dermoid cysts (**Figs 4.27**). Simple, small, asymptomatic cysts often resolve spontaneously. A repeat ultrasound examination will be required to confirm resolution. If they are symptomatic causing pain, large (greater than 5cm) or solid then they should be removed as there is a risk of complications such as torsion which could precipitate not only severe pain and emergency laparotomy, but also miscarraige or preterm labour. Laparotomy will be required. This is usually performed in the second trimester between 15 and 20 weeks to minimize risk of postoperative miscarriage; it also allows sufficient time for the scar to heal before labour. Tocolytic therapy (e.g. indomethacin or nifedipine) may be given after surgery to suppress uterine activity.

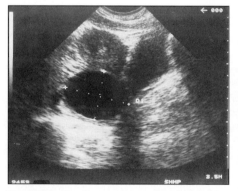

Fig. 4.26 *Ovarian cyst complicating a 12-week pregnancy as seen on ultrasound. The patient presented with abdominal pain. The cyst measured 55 x 42 x 50mm and cystectomy was performed at laparotomy.*

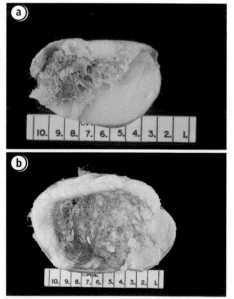

Fig. 4.27 *(a) Dermoid cyst (benign teratoma) removed at laparotomy in a woman at 16 weeks' gestation with lower abdominal pain. The cyst was identified with ultrasound. These cysts are lined with stratified squamous epithelium. (b) Note the presence of hair and sebaceous material within the cyst. Teeth, cartilage and even thyroid tissue can also be found.*

chapter 5

Antenatal Care

Pregnancy should not be viewed as an illness. Rather, pregnancy, for the vast majority of women, can be considered an alternative physiological state of good health. Although pregnant women can suffer from pre-existing medical problems that may influence pregnancy, from complications of pregnancy or coincidental illness, most women remain healthy. Nonetheless, pregnancy is treated to varying degrees as a medical condition with care provided by obstetricians (other hospital specialists, e.g. physicians), general practitioners and midwives. The aim of this input of medical resources is the end result of a healthy infant delivered from a healthy mother.

Antenatal care serves a number of different functions (**Fig. 5.1**):

- It is a well-developed screening programme aimed at identifying pre-existing and new problems in pregnancy (although its effectiveness has never been formally tested).
- It provides a vehicle for health education.
- It allows the so-called minor ailments of pregnancy to be treated.

ANTENATAL CARE AS A SCREENING PROGRAMME

Formalized antenatal care provides the framework within which a series of clinical and laboratory-based investigations can be performed. Initially, screening aims to identify on the basis of history and examination pregnancies that should be considered to be high risk. Secondly, by applying a series of routine clinical and laboratory investigations it aims to identify either that the pregnancy continues to be low risk or to identify at an early stage pregnancies in which adverse events have occurred to allow prompt and efficient

Fig. 5.1 *The objectives of antenatal care.*

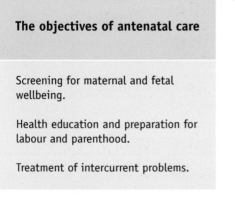

The objectives of antenatal care

Screening for maternal and fetal wellbeing.

Health education and preparation for labour and parenthood.

Treatment of intercurrent problems.

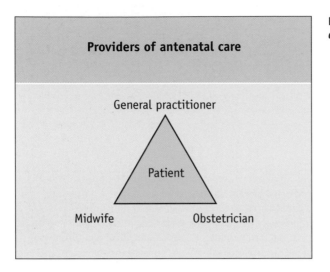

Fig. 5.2 *Providers of antenatal care.*

management to minimize the effect of the adverse event. Finally, the antenatal clinic provides a forum where other screening can be carried out, for example, cervical smears.

ANTENATAL CARE AS A VEHICLE FOR HEALTH EDUCATION

For a significant proportion of women, pregnancy is a novel and often a frightening or anxiety-provoking life event. As part of the process of antenatal care, women, and their partners, can be prepared for the forthcoming events. It is important that their concerns and anxieties are voiced and dealt with. Much of this education is provided through one-to-one contact with GP, midwife and obstetrician, but the vehicle of parentcraft classes is also useful. The preparation for labour and parenthood is not the only educational role of antenatal care. The antenatal clinic provides a suitable forum for advice on other matters, for example, smoking, diet and lifestyle. Overall, the woman should be reassured and her fears allayed.

THE TREATMENT OF INTERCURRENT PROBLEMS DURING THE ANTENATAL PERIOD

Although for the majority of women pregnancy is not associated with any serious illness, many suffer from minor ailments. These problems vary from leg cramps, carpal tunnel syndrome through to gastrointestinal problems such as dyspepsia and constipation. In addition to these so-called minor ailments, more serious intercurrent illnesses may need to be identified, treated or monitored during the antenatal period.

THE PROVISION OF ANTENATAL CARE

Antenatal care is provided by a number of different professionals (**Fig. 5.2**) in a number of different settings. Care can be considered to be community-based, hospital-based or shared between the two environments. In the community, care is provide by community midwives and GPs. In the hospital, care is provided by obstetricians and midwives, but in addition, care may be provided by physicians, dieticians, specialist nurses (e.g. diabetic nurses), physiotherapists, radiographers and ultrasonographers. Occasionally, high-risk pregnancies will be referred to tertiary centres for antenatal management.

Ideally, the pattern of antenatal care should be unique for each patient but in reality, standard patterns of care develop locally that match the patient's needs and level of risk. Low-risk women can be looked after entirely by midwives and/or GPs with obstetric support if problems develop. Clearly, such care can be provided almost exclusively in the community. A common pattern is for the patient to attend for booking at the hospital where an ultrasound examination can be performed and an assessment of risk made. The low-risk woman will return to community-based care with further hospital-based assessment in the third trimester. Intermediate-risk women should have at least a proportion of their care provided by the obstetrician. Usually this will mean attending a hospital clinic but increasingly consultant clinics are appearing in the community. High-risk women will usually have a substantial amount of their care in a hospital-based setting but the GP should still be involved to allow continuity of care. Each member of the team of midwife, GP and obstetrician, should be allowed to make full use of their skills which are complementary. The woman should also be involved in the decision about the type of care she wishes in the low-risk situation, for example, only midwife care, GP and midwife care, traditional obstetrician, midwife and GP shared care.

Traditionally, pregnant women are seen monthly from the diagnosis of pregnancy until 28 weeks' gestation, fortnightly until 36 weeks' gestation and weekly thereafter until delivery. This traditional pattern is widely followed despite the fact that it has little scientific validity. It is increasingly being questioned and for the low-risk woman with an uncomplicated pregnancy is almost certainly too high a frequency.

ANTENATAL MANAGEMENT

DIAGNOSIS OF PREGNANCY

Like any medical condition the diagnosis of pregnancy can be suspected from the clinical history and examination and confirmed by investigation.

The symptoms of early pregnancy include amenorrhoea, nausea, frequency of micturition and breast swelling and tenderness. During clinical examination, it may be possible to detect an enlargement of the uterus, changes in the breast and pigment changes which may affect the nipples (**Fig. 5.3**), the abdominal wall (linea nigra) or the face (the so-called mask of pregnancy or chloasma, **Fig. 5.4**).

The diagnosis is usually confirmed by detecting the presence of the β subunit of human chorionic gonadotrophin (βhCG) in the urine. βhCG may be detected even before the first missed period and rises rapidly in the first trimester of pregnancy. For the diagnosis of pregnancy, a qualitative measurement is all that is required (**Fig. 5.5**). Quantitative measurements may be used in the management of suspected ectopic pregnancy, as part of a battery of analytes measured in screening programmes for Down syndrome and as a tumour marker in gestational trophoblastic disease.

Further confirmation of the presence of a viable intrauterine pregnancy is achieved by ultrasound scanning.

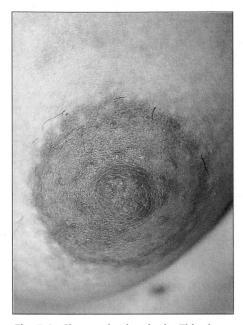

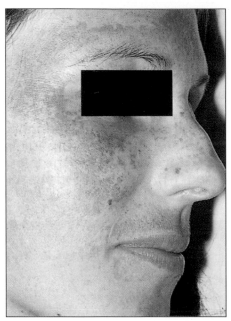

Fig. 5.3 *Changes in the nipple. This shows increased pigmentation and the development of raised sebaceous glands known as Montgomery's tubercles. (From Symonds, E. Malcolm and Macpherson, Marion B. A. 'Diagnosis in Color: Obstetrics and Gynecology' (Mosby-Wolfe, 1997) with permission).*

Fig. 5.4 *Chloasma: the 'mask' of pregnancy. Pigmentation occurs across the forehead and the cheeks in some women during pregnancy and later disappears. (From Symonds, E. Malcolm and Macpherson, Marion B. A. 'Diagnosis in Color: Obstetrics and Gynecology' (Mosby-Wolfe, 1997) with permission).*

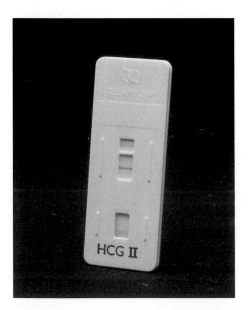

Fig. 5.5 *Pregnancy testing assessing the presence of hCG in urine.*

ANTENATAL BOOKING

The concept that antenatal care is a screening programme is best embodied in the antenatal booking visit. After the diagnosis of pregnancy, it is usual for the patient to 'book' for confinement. Whereas booking for confinement relates to the place of delivery, the concept of booking has now been extended to describe the first antenatal visit, usually at the obstetric unit.

The booking visit comprises a number of components. It is normal to take a full medical and past obstetric history (**Figs 5.6 and 5.7**). The past medical history covers events in this pregnancy, relevant past gynaecological history, significant past general medical and surgical history, and a family history. Previous obstetric performance is important in predicting the outcome of subsequent pregnancies. The details are recorded with respect to the antenatal period of previous pregnancies, the labour and delivery, and the fetal outcome. When abnormalities have occurred, it is valuable to review previous records or obtain details from other obstetric units.

History-taking in the antenatal setting is not confined to the purely medical and obstetric aspects. It is important also to enquire about social circumstances and lifestyle as these may be of importance to the outcome of the pregnancy and the wellbeing of the child. Routinely at further antenatal visits, there are checks of blood pressure and urinalysis to screen for pre-eclampsia. Urinalysis also allows screening for urinary tract infection and glycosuria (see below). Later in the pregnancy a clinical assessment of fetal growth by measuring the symphysial fundal height and an assessment of the fetal lie, presentation and engagement are made.

ANTENATAL INVESTIGATIONS AND SCREENING FOR FETAL ABNORMALITIES

In addition to obtaining a full medical and obstetric history at the booking visit, a number of investigations are undertaken. Between different units there will be some differences in the precise nature of the tests undertaken but the general principle is consistent. **Figure 5.8** demonstrates the tests undertaken in one teaching hospital centre (as the medical records are held by the patient an explanation of the need for each test is given).

In most units routine investigations will include screening for anaemia and in selected ethnic groups for the presence of sickle cell trait or disease and haemoglobinopathies (screening of the partner is also required to assess the risk to the fetus, e.g. if both parents are carriers for sickle cell trait, the baby has a 1:4 chance of having sickle cell disease). Screening for anaemia enables detection of patients who would benefit from iron supplements during pregnancy. Certain women, such as those with multiple gestation, should receive iron supplements. All women should receive folic acid supplements in the first trimester to reduce the risk of neural tube defects. As the neural tube closes at 7 weeks, folic acid administration should ideally begin preconceptually. It is usual that a full blood count is repeated routinely early in the third trimester.

All antenatal patients have their blood group established and the serum is screened for the presence of antibodies to red cell antigens. Important in this respect is a history of previous blood transfusion. Screening is usually repeated at 28 and 36 weeks' gestation in women who are rhesus negative. More frequent testing and close monitoring of pregnancies is required when red cell antibodies are detected. Problems potentially arise when the fetal blood group differs from the maternal blood group. Maternal antibodies against the fetal antigen may be raised and maternal IgG may cross the placenta and cause fetal anaemia and compromise. In severe cases the fetus can be become oedematous with ascites, associated with cardiac failure, so-called hydopic. The placenta also becomes large and oedematous in an attempt to compensate for the severe anaemia. This rarely happens with

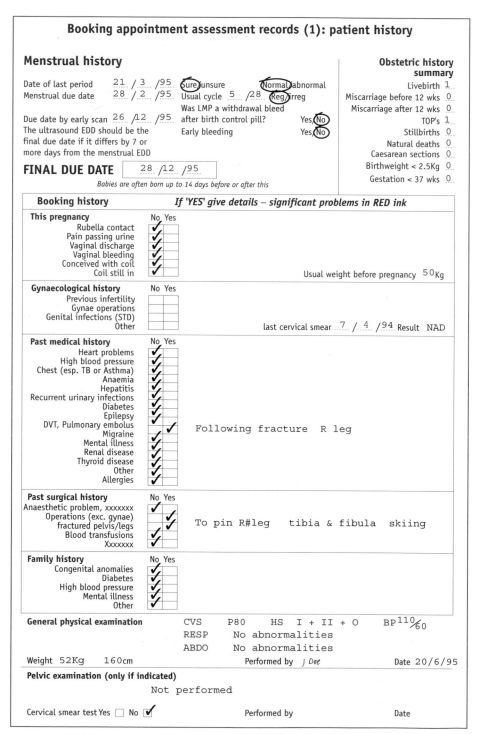

Booking appointment assessment records (1): patient history

Menstrual history

Date of last period   21 / 3 /95   (Sure) unsure   (Normal) abnormal
Menstrual due date   28 / 2 /95   Usual cycle 5 /28 (Reg)/ irreg
                                   Was LMP a withdrawal bleed
Due date by early scan 26 /12 /95   after birth control pill?   Yes (No)
The ultrasound EDD should be the   Early bleeding   Yes (No)
final due date if it differs by 7 or
more days from the menstrual EDD

FINAL DUE DATE   28 /12 /95

Babies are often born up to 14 days before or after this

Obstetric history summary

Livebirth 1
Miscarriage before 12 wks 0
Miscarriage after 12 wks 0
TOP's 1
Stillbirths 0
Natural deaths 0
Caesarean sections 0
Birthweight < 2.5Kg 0
Gestation < 37 wks 0

Booking history	If 'YES' give details – significant problems in RED ink
This pregnancy	No Yes
Rubella contact	✓
Pain passing urine	✓
Vaginal discharge	✓
Vaginal bleeding	✓
Conceived with coil	✓
Coil still in	✓ Usual weight before pregnancy 50 Kg

Gynaecological history	No Yes
Previous infertility	
Gynae operations	
Genital infections (STD)	
Other	last cervical smear 7 / 4 /94 Result NAD

Past medical history	No Yes
Heart problems	✓
High blood pressure	✓
Chest (esp. TB or Asthma)	✓
Anaemia	✓
Hepatitis	✓
Recurrent urinary infections	✓
Diabetes	✓
Epilepsy	✓
DVT, Pulmonary embolus	✓ Following fracture R leg
Migraine	✓
Mental illness	✓
Renal disease	✓
Thyroid disease	✓
Other	✓
Allergies	✓

Past surgical history	No Yes
Anaesthetic problem, xxxxxxx	✓
Operations (exc. gynae)	✓ To pin R#leg tibia & fibula skiing
fractured pelvis/legs	✓
Blood transfusions	✓
Xxxxxxx	✓

Family history	No Yes
Congenital anomalies	✓
Diabetes	✓
High blood pressure	✓
Mental illness	✓
Other	✓

General physical examination   CVS   P80   HS   I + II + O   BP 110/60
                                    RESP   No abnormalities
                                    ABDO   No abnormalities

Weight 52Kg   160cm   Performed by J Doe   Date 20/6/95

Pelvic examination (only if indicated)
                          Not performed

Cervical smear test Yes ☐ No ☑   Performed by   Date

Fig. 5.6 *Booking appointment assessment records (1): patient history.*

Booking appointment assessment records(2): lifestyle

Health Promotion/Lifestyle Discussion

Cigarettes

				28 Week Visit
Smoker   Yes/**No** _____ /Day

Partner   **Yes**/No   10   /Day

Still smoking	☐ _____ /Day
Cut down to	☐ _____ /Day
Given up	☐

Advice given   Advised partner to stop

Alcohol   Yes/**No** _____ Units/Weeks

Advice given _____

Exercise/Recommendations   Continue moderate exercise

Diet

Any specific requirements: e.g. Vegetarian, Vegan   None

Any advice given _____

Discussion/Advice on:

Listeria: Precautions to follow   ☑   Vitamin A: Precautions to follow   ☑

Toxoplasmosis: Precautions to follow   ☑   Other reasons discussed   Yes/No

                        At risk   Yes/**No**

                        Requests screening   Yes/**No**

Linkworker   Yes/**No**   Name _____

Social Worker	☐
Interpreter	☐
Physiotherapist	☐
Dietitian	☐

Referred to Linkworker by

Parentcraft Classes discussed   **Yes**/No   Booked   ☑

Antenatal Record explained   ☑

Bloods discussed   ☑

Booking history completed by (name)   J Smith

Designation: Midwife (community)

Date 20/12/96

Fig. 5.7 *Booking appointment assessment records (2): lifestyle.*

Laboratory test checklist			
Test	Date Taken	Result	Reason for test
Full blood count (inc. Hb)			Mainly to test for anaemia to see if you need iron tablets or further tests.
ABO Group			Blood Group in case an emergency blood transfusion is necessary.
Rhesus Factor			If Negative, baby is sometimes at risk of jaundice. Extra tests are needed.
Rubella Status			To see if you need immunisation against German Measles after delivery.
BTS antibodies			Blood Transfusion Service check for antibodies in addition to Rhesus.
Syphilis check			This rare but easily treated infection can damage babies if missed.
Hepatitis check			Check for blood-born Hepatitis virus if at risk.
Sickle/ Thalassaemia check			These conditions can cause problems in particular groups of people.
Mid stream urine			Check for urine infection.
Plasma Glucose (RBS)			
Glucose Tolerance Test			
Toxoplasmosis Screening			If considered high risk
16-20 weeks Triple Screen Test Other			Screening tests for some problems affecting babies Test discussed by 1 2
24 weeks BTS antibodies if requested			
28 weeks BTS antibodies if requested Full Blood Count Glucose Challenge Test			**GLUCOSE CHALLENGE TEST** At your 28 week visit, a special blood test is necessary to get an accurate measurement of your blood sugar levels at this stage of pregnancy. You need to drink a 250ml bottle of Lucozade (any flavour) made by Smith, Kline and Beecham. You can drink this at home before attending surgery depending on how far away you live. Exactly one hour later have your routine 28 week bloods taken. Please note the time yourself and tell the receptionist on arrival at the doctor's surgery. DO NOT eat or drink during this hour.
34-36 weeks Full Blood Count if required BTS antibodies if requested			Copies of results should be filed in the notes or written in the appropriate places. Significant or important results (such as Rhesus Negative should be noted under special features on central pages.

Fig. 5.8 *Antenatal tests performed in one teaching hospital.*

the ABO system. It is most frequently seen against the rhesus blood group (**Fig. 5.9**) but is also seen, usually in mild forms, with other blood groups such as Kell and Duffy sensitization which can occur after transfusion.

The introduction of passive immunization of rhesus negative mothers with anti-D immunoglobulin has seen a dramatic reduction in the proportion of affected pregnancies. Anti-D immunoglobulin is given to all rhesus-negative mothers by intramuscular injection after any event in which there is a risk of exposure to fetal cells. This allows a rapid clearance of rhesus-positive fetal cells from the maternal circulation before a maternal

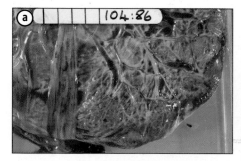
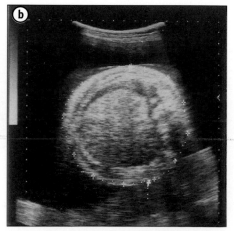

Fig. 5.9 *(a) Odematous hypertrophic placenta in severe rhesus disease. (b) Ultrasound scan showing enlarged abdominal circumferance and ascites.*

antibody response can be raised. Potential sensitizing events are miscarriage, ectopic pregnancy, termination of pregnancy, amniocentesis, antepartum haemorrhage, external cephalic version and delivery. After delivery it is usual to check the maternal blood for fetal cells by a Kleihauer test (**Fig. 5.10**). The volume of fetal blood entering the maternal circulation can be estimated from the Kleihauer test and an appropriate dose of anti-D immunoglobulin given. If a large fetal–maternal haemorrhage is diagnosed, then additional anti-D can be given. The usual doses of anti-D are 250IU before 20 weeks and 500IU thereafter. Prophylactic anti-D administration is also under assessment. This consists of administering anti-D to all rhesus-negative women at the end of the second and during the third trimester to prevent sensitization.

Pregnancies affected by rising titres of red cell antibodies are monitored closely with serial measures of antibody levels and serial scans of fetal wellbeing. In rhesus isoimmunization, antibody levels can be used to determine whether intervention is required. Depending on gestation, delivery or intrauterine infusion can be undertaken. When the delivery is performed, the affected infant may require an exchange transfusion.

Another important component of the booking visit is the ultrasound scan. When performed it is used to confirm viability and gestational age (**Fig. 5.11**). An early diagnosis of multiple pregnancy (**Fig. 5.12**) can also be made and, importantly in multiple pregnancies, the presence or the absence and thickness of any membrane between gestational sacs can be used to determine the zygosity of the pregnancy. Ultrasound is also routinely performed in many units at approximately 19–20 weeks' gestation to detect gross

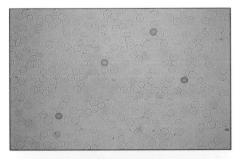

Fig. 5.10 *A positive Kleihauer test with fetal cells seen in a background of 'ghost' maternal cells from which haemoglobin has been eluted by acidification. As the fetal cells contain HbF they resist acidic environments in contrast to the maternal cells containing HbA.*

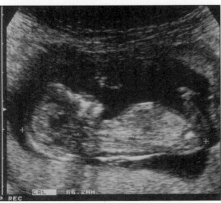

Fig. 5.11 *Ultrasound scan confirming singleton pregnancy with crown–rump length being measured.*

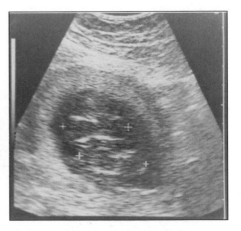

Fig. 5.12 *Ultrasound showing twin amniotic sacs at 10 weeks' gestation.*

structural abnormalities (**Fig. 5.13** and **5.14**). Abnormalities detected by ultrasound include neural tube defects (e.g. spina bifida [**Fig. 5.15**] and anencephaly), cardiac defects, anterior abdominal wall defects, facial and palatal clefts and structural abnormalities that would be considered markers for chromosomal abnormalities such as a thickened nuchal fat pad.

In later pregnancy, ultrasound may be routinely used to assess growth in multiple pregnancies or to determine the placental site in patients for whom early scans have demonstrated a low-lying placenta.

Screening for abnormality is not confined to ultrasound. Biochemical investigations can be used to screen for both chromosomal and structural abnormalities. Screening programmes most commonly assess patients at high risk of Down syndrome. This test is usually offered between 15 and 20 weeks' gestation. The principle behind the test is that in pregnancies that have chromosomal abnormalities there is either an elevation or reduction in a number of factors in maternal serum. In Down syndrome there is a reduction of both serum α fetoprotein and unconjugated oestriol whereas βhCG is elevated. None of these analytes on their own is specific or sensitive enough to be employed as a screening test and therefore they are used in combination. The levels of all analytes vary with gestation and are not normally distributed. For this reason, the results are expressed as multiples of the median (MoMs) before individual risk is calculated from a nomogram (**Fig. 5.16**). Patients identified as being at increased risk

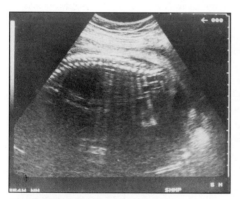

Fig. 5.13 *Normal fetal spine on ultrasound.*

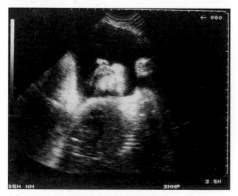

Fig. 5.14 *Normal facial view on ultrasound showing absence of clefting.*

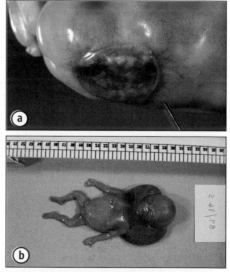

Fig. 5.15 *(a) and (b) show neural tube defects in fetuses following termination. Both were identified by ultrasound showing absence of clefting.*

are offered amniocentesis to enable a definitive diagnosis to be made. Amniocentesis involves the insertion of a fine needle into the amniotic sac under ultrasound control (**Fig. 5.17**). Amniotic fluid (10–15ml) is withdrawn and from this fetal cells are obtained and cultured. From these cell cultures, a fetal karyotype can be established (**Fig. 5.18**).

Not all patients undergoing amniocentesis will have a biochemical screening test. Patients at increased risk of chromosomal abnormality either on the basis of having a previously affected child, family history or maternal age may elect to have a diagnostic procedure without prior screening. This may allow the diagnostic procedure to be undertaken at a slightly earlier gestation. Amniocentesis is not the only diagnostic procedure that is used to diagnose chromosomal abnormality. Chorionic villous sampling, in which a sample of chorionic villous is aspirated under ultrasound control, either

Results from 'triple tests' to screen for Down syndrome			
Age alone (35 years)		**Result in multiples of the median**	**Risk** 1:384
Test 1	Maternal serum α-fetoprotein	0.4	1:16
	Oestriol	0.4	
	Chorionic gonadotrophin	2.0	
Test 2	Maternal serum α-fetoprotein	2.5	1:52,000
	Oestriol	1.5	
	Chorionic gonadotrophin	0.5	

Fig. 5.16 *How different triple test results affect the risk of Down syndrome.*

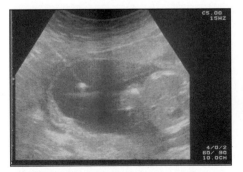

Fig. 5.17 *Amniocentesis being performed under ultrasound guidance to locate the needle in a pool of liquor and avoid trauma to the fetus. The needle can be seen within the amniotic sac.*

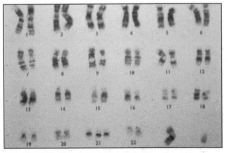

Fig. 5.18 *Fetal karyotype obtained following amniocentesis precipitated by abnormal 'triple test'. The karyotype is 47XY with an additional chromosome 21. The fetus has Down syndrome.*

Fig. 5.19 *Screening for gestational diabetes. Note that glycosuria is common in pregnancy as the renal threshold for glucose may be reduced.*

Screening for gestational diabetes
Family history (affected first degree relative)
Past obstetric history (previously affected pregnancy, previous large infant, i.e. >4 kg)
Urine testing for glycosuria
Random or fasting blood glucose
Modified glucose tolerance test
Formal glucose tolerance test

transabdominally or transcervically, may be undertaken between 9 and 12 weeks' gestation. The pregnancy loss rate associated with chorionic villous sampling is between 1 and 2%, whereas the rate associated with amniocentesis is between 0.5 and 1%.

Diabetes mellitus and gestational diabetes are important causes of maternal and fetal morbidity and fetal mortality. Screening for diabetes, and impaired glucose tolerance, is initiated at the booking. The exact mechanism of screening varies from obstetric unit to obstetric unit. Methods of screening are listed in **Figure 5.19**.

Other investigations routinely performed include screening for infections of the urinary tract and for evidence of infection with, or immunity to, viral or bacterial infections that can give rise to congenital damage. In some units testing for HIV is offered.

INFECTIONS IN PREGNANCY

SCREENING FOR BACTERIURIA

Asymptomatic bacteriuria is much more common in women than in men. It affects between 3 and 8% of pregnant women and between 15 and 45% will develop a symptomatic infection giving rise to the complications of acute cystitis and pyelonephritis. A variety of screening techniques are used. In some units all women have a culture of a midstream urine sample whereas other units rely on dipstick testing for the presence of urinary nitrites or protein (**Fig. 5.20**).

URINARY TRACT INFECTION

The pregnant woman is prone to urinary tract infection because there is an increased urinary stasis with dilatation of the collecting systems, a physiological hydronephrosis and hydroureter; this is thought to be due to the influence of progesterone. There is also increased glycosuria due to an alteration in the renal threshold for glucose. The most common organisms are *E. coli*, and other Gram-negative organisms such as *Klebsiella* and *Streptococcus faecalis*. The symptoms are similar to the those of patients infected while not

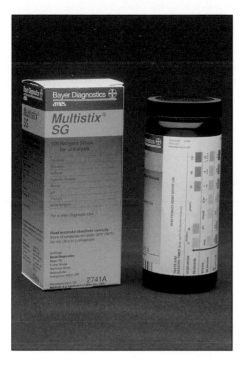

Fig. 5.20 *Screening of urine for protein and blood with Multistix.*

pregnant: cystitis, frequency, dysuria, urgency and possibly haematuria without serious systemic upset. Whereas pyelonephritis is associated with fever, shivering, rigors, loin pain and tenderness, nausea and vomiting. It may also precipitate preterm labour. A mid-stream specimen of urine (MSSU) and culture and sensitivity of organisms are required for diagnosis with associated blood cultures in pyelonephritis.

Treatment is usually by a broad spectrum antibiotic such as a cephalosporin in the first instance (*E. coli* is now frequently resistant to ampicillin). With pyelonephritis the woman should be hospitalized, placed on intravenous fluids and antibiotics, receive analgesia and antipyretic therapy, and be carefully monitored to assess hydration and renal function, white cell count and response to infection as well as any additional complications. Prophylactic antibiotics, usually given at night when bladder-emptying is reduced, are used for patients with chronic pyelonephritis, a past history of infections or recurrent infection in pregnancy, urological abnormalities or complications.

SCREENING FOR SYPHILIS

Although syphilis is now a rare infection in the UK, all women continue to be screened at booking for evidence of infection. Screening by a variety of serological tests, VDRL, FTA-ABS or MHA-TP, is important because patients are usually asymptomatic and also because treatment of the mother before 16 weeks' gestation prevents congenital disease.

Neonates affected by syphilis may present with fulminating disease including secondary bacterial infection, hepatitis and pulmonary haemorrhage. Alternatively, the presentation may be less dramatic with nonspecific symptoms such as a rash. The late sequelae of infection include meningoencephalitis, Hutchinson's teeth and interstitial keratitis. These may occur throughout childhood.

INFECTION WITH *LISTERIA MONOCYTOGENES*

Infection with *Listeria moncytogenes* usually occurs by the oral route as the organism is present in many foods, particlarly soft cheeses made from unpasteurized milk and can multiply at low temperature. It is destroyed by cooking. It is a Gram-positive bacillus and infection during pregnancy may result in miscarriage or intrauterine death. Infection may also present as preterm labour with rupture of the membranes. The liquor in this scenario is often stained with meconium. For infected neonates who survive *in utero*, approximately half will subsequently die as a result of the infection. Diagnosis of this pyrexial and 'flu-like' illness is difficult but is most reliably achieved by a maternal blood culture. A high degree of suspicion must be exercised towards women presenting with a possible infection which can often mimic a urinary tract infection in its initial presentation. When the diagnosis is made, treatment is with intravenous amoxicillin. The best strategy to prevent the consequences of infection is to advise women to alter their lifestyle to minimize risk. Dietary advice, that is, the avoidance of soft cheeses and patés, is usually given to pregnant women at time of booking. Increased public awareness and health education has substantially reduced the problem.

VIRAL INFECTION DURING PREGNANCY

A number of viral infections can give rise to congenital damage. These infections include German measles (rubella), slapped cheek syndrome (parvovirus B19), chickenpox (varicella zoster) and cytomegalovirus (CMV).

German measles is usually a mild infectious disease characterized by a transient erythematous maculopapular rash, lymphadenopathy characteristically affecting the postauricular and suboccipital nodes, and more rarely arthritis and arthralgia. It is an RNA virus spread by respiratory droplet exposure. As a consequence of the transient and fleeting nature of the disease, the clinical diagnosis of the disease is difficult and poses particular problems in pregnancy (see case history). The importance of infection in pregnancy is the resultant congenital infection and congenital rubella syndrome (**Fig. 5.21**).

To reduce the incidence of the congenital rubella syndrome an immunization programme was introduced in the UK in 1970 to immunize prepubertal girls and nonimmune women. This immunization programme was extended in 1988 with the advent of the combined measles–mumps–rubella vaccine. It is hoped that the immunization of all young children will interrupt the circulation of the rubella virus and prevent the exposure of nonimmune women to the risk of infection. This policy has largely been successful with a reduction from 164 laboratory confirmed cases of rubella in pregnant women in 1987 to 15 in 1992 (**Figs 5.22 and 23**).

Fig. 5.21 *Congenital rubella syndrome.*

Congenital rubella syndrome

Microcephaly
Meningoencephalitis
Deafness
Mental handicap
Cataract, retinopathy
Anaemia, thrombocytopaenia, purpura
Hepatosplenomegaly and jaundice
Cardiac anomalies
Intrauterine growth retardation

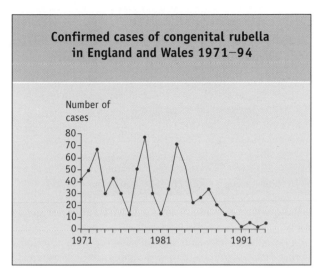

Confirmed cases of congenital rubella in England and Wales 1971−94

Number of cases

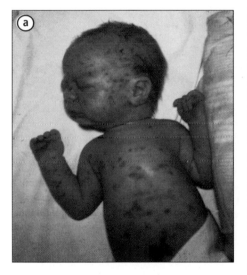

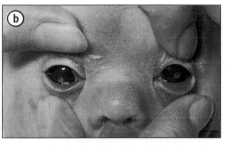

Fig. 5.23 *(a) Congenital rubella presenting as a small-for-dates baby with a pupuric rash caused by thrombocytopaenia. Children born with congenital rubella are a potential source of infection to others, and it is important that appropriate steps are taken to protect other patients and staff. (b) Cataracts causing blindness in this newborn baby with congenital rubella. (From Milner A. D. and Herber S. M. 'Colour Atlas of the Newborn' (Wolfe 1983) with permission.)*

CASE HISTORY

The patient is a 26-year-old woman in her first pregnancy. She is currently at 8 weeks' gestation and has not yet attended the surgery in this pregnancy. She has within the last few days been in contact with her 5-year-old nephew who has had an erythematous rash. She wonders whether she should be particularly concerned as she thinks she may have had rubella as a child, although she cannot remember if she was immunized.

The question the patient is posing is has she been in contact with an individual with rubella and what risk is there to her unborn child. Rubella infection is common in children between the ages of 4 and 9 years but the clinical diagnosis is notoriously difficult, particularly as the symptoms and signs may be transient. The differential diagnosis would also include parvovirus B19 infection. It is not possible to assume from the history that the patient is not at risk. Neither history of previous immunization or infection is a guarantee of immunity to infection.

How should this patient be investigated? The diagnosis of acute infection can easily be made by serologically detecting IgM specific for rubella or a fourfold rise in serum IgG. More than one sample may be required to demonstrate rising titres.

The patient returns to your surgery for the results which indicate she has been infected. She enquires what risk there is to her baby as she has heard that not all pregnancies are affected.

Fetal damage is common in the first 8–10 weeks of pregnancy affecting up to 90% of pregnancies. By 16 weeks, the risk declines to approximately 10% and in the second half of pregnancy the risk is negligible.

The patient is distressed at the thought that her unborn child may be handicapped and asks if termination would be possible.

Termination for abnormality is allowed in the UK under the terms of the 1967 abortion act when there is a significant risk that the child will be born with significant handicap. As this is a possibility in this case termination could be undertaken.

What if your patient were found to be nonimmune and not infected? What would your subsequent management be?

All women identified as being nonimmune should be immunized in the postpartum period. Other women who may be identified as being at risk of infection are those attending family planning and infertility clinics. They should also be offered immunization. Although there appears to be little or no risk of the vaccine causing the congenital rubella syndrome, all immunized women should be advised not to become pregnant within a month of immunization.

Infection with the human parvovirus B19, erythema infectiosum, presents with a clinical picture very similar to rubella (**Fig. 5.24**), but the clinical consequences are very different. Parvovirus B19 does not cause congenital damage. Infection in early pregnancy may give rise to miscarriage and later in pregnancy, infection may give rise to nonimmune hydrops fetalis associated with fetal haemolytic anaemia which if severe, may require intrauterine transfusion. Fetal demise may occur and fetal wellbeing should be monitored by ultrasound. When fetal recovery occurs, there are no long-term sequelae. Suspected infection can be confirmed serologically.

Whereas rubella and parvovirus B19 infections are usually relatively benign diseases in the mother, chicken pox or varicella zoster infection (a DNA virus of the herpes family) during pregnancy gives rise to a significant morbidity. The primary infection consists of fever, malaise and pruritic rash which progresses to the characteristic vesicles that crust over before healing. The incubation period is 10–20 days and the condition is contagious, spread by respiratory droplets, the infectious period is 2 days before the rash appears until the vesicles crust over. Most of the adult population is immune, thus, although contact with chicken pox is common in pregnancy, infection is not. When infection does occur in the mother, it can be severe. Approximately 10% of women develop varicella pneumonia. Among these women, the mortality may be as high as 40% and treatment with systemic antiviral agents such as acyclovir is indicated and assisted ventilation may be required. The incidence of the congenital varicella syndrome is low (1–2%) and the risk is only in the first 20 weeks of pregnancy. The syndrome is characterized by eye defects such as cataracts, skin scarring in a dermatome distribution, limb hypoplasia, skin lesions and neurological abnormalities such as microcephaly and mental retardation. Infection of the fetus or infant within one week of delivery may be associated with severe complications of clinical

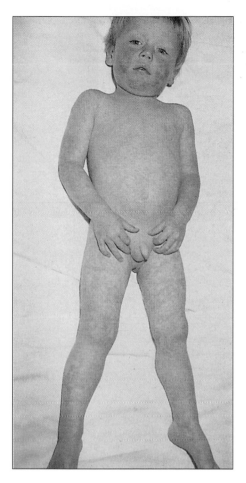

Fig. 5.24 *Erythemia infectiosum. This boy's erythematous rash appeared 24 hours after the onset of a mild fever and sore throat. Note the 'slapped cheek' appearance of the face. (From Forbes, C. D. and Jackson, W. F. 'Color Atlas and Text of Clinical Medicine' (Mosby-Wolfe, 1997), with permission.)*

varicella for the neonate. Infection occurs most commonly when the mother is infected in the 4 weeks before delivery. Treatment is usually with zoster immune globulin which is administered within 3 days of exposure. A vaccine is not yet available (**Fig. 5.25**).

The herpes simplex virus is from the same viral family as herpes zoster. Herpes simplex infection of the newborn is acquired from the mother in between 1 in 2500 and 1 in 10,000 births and is fatal in between 15 and 50% of patients. Infants at most risk are those with potentially prolonged exposure to the virus, for example, prolonged ruptured membranes. Caesarean section to avoid infection during delivery is only recommended when there is clinical evidence of active disease and a high likelihood of viral shedding from the genital tract. Most obstetricians would now restrict caesarean section to patients with a primary genital herpes infection. Acyclovir can be employed for severe or disseminated infections

CMV infection is a problem because it is frequently asymptomatic with 1% of at-risk mothers acquiring infection during pregnancy. Transmission of this DNA virus of the herpes family to the fetus will occur in approximately one-third of patients independent of gestation. Infection will be fatal in 1% of fetuses and between 10 and 30% of infected babies will display symptoms and signs of congenital infection. The more severe effects are

The management of suspected contact and infection with chickenpox

Assessment of contact and previous infection (indicating likely immunity).

Check for varicella zoster IgG in the maternal blood (if present, reassure the mother that she is immune).

If the mother is not immune and contact is before 20 weeks, give zoster immunoglobulin.

If serology shows infection (positive IgM), discuss the 2% risk of congenital infection and arrange a detailed ultrasound assessment.

If the pregnancy is continued, neonatal assessment at birth.

When chickenpox occurs during pregnancy, the mother should be isolated from other mothers and babies, acyclovir may have a role, particularly for neonatal infection.

seen with primary infection in pregnancy. These features are similar to congenital rubella. Nonimmune hydrops can also occur. Confirmation of infection can be made by detection of CMV-specific IgM antibody. No vaccine is currently available.

TOXOPLASMA GONDII INFECTION

Although it is a protozoan rather than a virus, *Toxoplasma* infection has many features in common with congenital rubella and CMV infection. Infection with *Toxoplasma* during pregnancy may result in congenital damage at any stage of a pregnancy. In mothers with an acute infection, the risk is 25–65%, with the risk being greater at later gestations. One fifth of infected infants will display symptoms at birth. Deafness and retinal disease may develop later in childhood. Like CMV infection, the maternal disease is frequently asymptomatic. Infection should be suspected in pregnant women who present with a mild, viral-type illness. The fetus should be assessed for the stigmata of congenital infection such as intracranial calcification, microcephaly and hydrocephaly. The infection can be treated with a sulphonamide or spiramycin. Screening these women is by serological testing for *Toxoplasma*-specific IgM. The only other patients that justify screening are those whose lifestyle exposes them to risk: contact with cat faeces or eating of undercooked meat.

HIV INFECTION AND PREGNANCY

HIV infection is becoming an increasingly important consideration in the management of pregnant women. In some parts of the country (London) as many as 1 in 600 women may be infected, but in the remainder of the UK the prevalence is closer to 1 in 10,000. HIV infection is important both for the risk to attendants, particularly during labour and delivery, but also because the risk of a poor pregnancy outcome is greater with infected individuals. Poor pregnancy outcomes associated with HIV infection include prematurity, low birth weight and stillbirth as well as potential fetal infection.

Care attendants are not the only ones at risk of infection. Vertical transmission of infection can occur from mother to fetus and to infant. The rate of infection is about 20%. Transmission is more likely in a mother with full-blown AIDS and low CD4 lymphocyte counts, in whom the viral load is likely to be high. Infants at particular risk are those born prematurely, after prolonged rupture of membranes and vaginal delivery.

Careful prepregnancy counselling is required for women with infection who may chose to avoid pregnancy. Counselling and screening of (high-risk) women may also be offered. The usual preventive measures to avoid infection should be in place but these should probably be applied to every pregnancy as unidentified infection will clearly pose as much risk as identified. Screening for other infections may be of value. The CD4 lymphocyte count should be monitored and opportunistic infection treated. The prevention of vertical transmission may be achieved by elective caesarean section, treatment with antiviral agents and avoidance of breast-feeding.

HEPATITIS B AND C INFECTION

Perhaps a greater risk to healthcare workers than HIV infection is hepatitis B (and C) infection from contaminated body fluids. Patients suspected of being at risk of being carriers should be offered screening. These groups include known or past intravenous drug abusers, patients with tattoos (especially amateur tattoos) and individuals from areas where there is a high incidence of hepatitis B infection, for example, China and Southeast Asia. Screening programmes have been undertaken to establish the incidence of viral carrier status in populations (both hepatitis B and HIV) but are surrounded by significant ethical problems. The implications of a positive screening result are such that patients should be fully informed before they consent to screening; this is both labour and cost intensive. Anonymous screening (to establish population statistics) raises the dilemma of whether to inform the patient of a positive result. The baby should be immunized against hepatitis B after delivery and receive concomitant HB immune globulin.

The group most likely to be carriers of either hepatitis or HIV are intravenous drug abusers. Infants of these patients are more likely to be premature and growth retarded and these pregnancies should be considered to be high risk. The infants of mothers who continue to abuse drugs throughout their pregnancies are at particular risk and may experience withdrawal after delivery. Paediatric staff should be alerted to the problem.

chapter 6

Common Medical Conditions During Pregnancy

It is important when dealing with medical disorders during pregnancy to address the effects of the disorder and the drugs taken for it on the pregnancy, and also the effects of the pregnancy on the disorder and its drug therapy. When considering these principles, a knowledge of the physiological changes of pregnancy is required in the context of the medical condition and its therapy. As many medical disorders have serious implications for pregnancy and vice versa, the treatment and assessment should start before pregnancy with prepregnancy counselling. This will allow the patient to consider whether or not she wishes to conceive, delay conception until her medical condition has improved or avoid pregnancy altogether. She will also be guided to the way the pregnancy will be managed and the risks and hazards associated with it.

VENOUS THROMBOSIS

PREGNANCY-RELATED CHANGES IN THE VENOUS SYSTEM

During pregnancy there is a dramatic reduction in the venous flow from the legs which is evident by the end of the first trimester and is maximal at term. The haemostatic system is altered with increased coagulation factors such as fibrinogen, factor VIII and von Willebrand factor, and suppressed fibrinolysis. These changes in the coagulation system which may be designed to deal with the haemostatic challenge of delivery are associated with an enhanced thrombotic risk during pregnancy. Trauma to the pelvic veins in the course of delivery, particularly if it is instrumental or abdominal, will also add to the risk. Thus, during pregnancy all features of Virchow's triad for the pathophysiology of venous thrombosis are present: hypercoagulability, venous stasis and trauma to the vessel wall. In view of these changes, pregnancy must be considered a particular time of risk for venous thromboembolism. Pulmonary embolism is a leading cause of maternal death in the UK with many thromboses going unnoticed until the fatal event occurs. It is therefore important to identify risk factors and provide prophylaxis for women at increased risk, as well as being vigilant to the possibility of deep venous thrombosis (DVT) or pulmonary thromboembolism (PTE).

Other risk factors for venous thrombosis are shown in **Figure 6.1**.

THROMBOPHILIA

The body has natural anticoagulant systems. These take the form of the antithrombin system and the activated protein C/protein S. Antithrombin inhibits many activated coagulation factors such as factor Xa and IIa. Its action is enhanced by binding with heparin and this is the mechanism by which heparin has its anticoagulant effect. When the coagulation system is activated, thrombin binds to thrombomodulin on the endothelial cell surface. This, in turn, activates protein C which, along with its cofactor, protein S, will

**Risk factors for venous thrombosis
in pregnancy**

Fig. 6.1 *Risk factors for
venous thrombosis in
pregnancy.*

Age >35 years old

Immobility

Obesity

Operative delivery

Pre-eclampsia

Parity >4

Surgical procedure in pregnancy or puerperium, e.g.
    postpartum sterilization

Previous deep venous thrombosis

Thrombophilia
        Congenital
                Antithrombin deficiency
                Protein C deficiency
                Protein S deficiency
                Factor V Leiden
                Prothrombin gene variant
                Hyperhomocysteinaemia
        Acquired
                Lupus anticoagulant
                Anticardiolipin antibodies

Excessive blood loss

Paraplegia

Sickle cell disease

Inflammatory disorders and infection, e.g.
    inflammatory bowel disease and urinary tract
    infection

Dehydration

Fig. 6.1 *Risk factors for venous thrombosis in pregnancy.*

inhibit coagulation, providing negative feedback to any thrombotic challenge. The activated protein C inhibits factor VIIIa and factor Va by proteolytic cleavage. Clearly, a deficiency of antithrombin, protein C or protein S will result in an increased risk of thrombosis (**Fig. 6.2**).

Many deep venous thromboses occurring in young women during the course of pregnancy are the first manifestion of underlying thrombophilic problems, the most

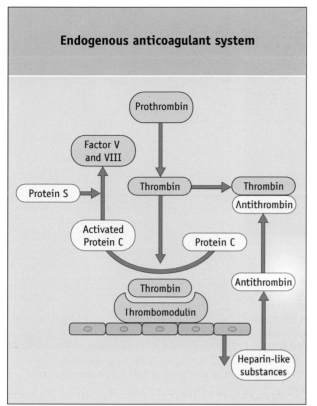

Fig. 6.2 *Endogenous anticoagulant system.*

common problem being that of factor V Leiden. This is the most common congenital thrombophilia with a gene frequency of between 3 and 10% in Western populations. Investigations of DVTs during pregnancy may find factor V Leiden in over 20% of patients. Factor V Leiden is an abnormal form of factor V which has a normal coagulation function but which is resistant to breakdown by the inhibitor of coagulation, activated protein C, resulting in an increase in thrombotic risk. It has also been associated with a large number of thrombotic problems while taking the oral contraceptive pill.

Deficiencies of the endogenous anticoagulants antithrombin, protein C and protein S are much less common than factor V Leiden and taken together they will be found in approximately only 5% of women with a DVT during pregnancy. Antithrombin deficiency carries a very high risk of venous thrombosis during pregnancy. Thrombosis that occurs in association with protein C and protein S deficiency usually occurs postpartum. More recently, a variation has been found in a prothrombin gene with individuals being heterozygous for the prothrombin gene variant having higher levels of prothrombin and enhanced risk of thrombosis. The problems of acquired thrombophilia are described in the section on cardiolipin antibody syndrome and lupus anticoagulant.

Clearly, any patient presenting with a DVT or PTE during pregnancy should be screened for underlying congenital or acquired thrombophilia and such screening may have to be delayed until after anticoagulant therapy is complete because anticoagulants will interfere with some of the tests used for the assessment of these abnormalities. Any patient with a past history or significant family history of thrombosis should also be screened.

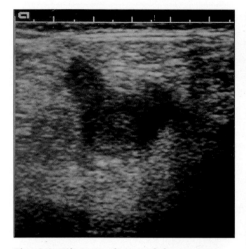

Fig. 6.3 *Ultrasound scan of deep venous thrombosis in pregnancy. The scan is taken at the top of the thigh in the transverse plane. The common femoral vein is in the centre of the picture with the saphenous vein to one side and the femoral artery on the other side. Echoes can be seen within the lumen of the vein representing the clot. If the leg is compressed by pressure on the ultrasound probe, then because of the clot the vein will fail to collapse. In the absence of a clot the vein will collapse under gentle pressure. Doppler ultrasound can be coupled to realtime ultrasound to help the diagnosis by showing absent blood flow in an occluded vein.*

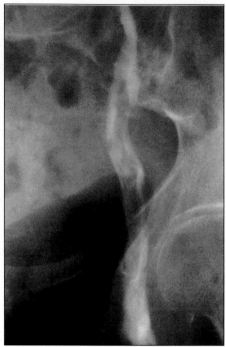

Fig. 6.4 *X-ray venogram showing a clot in the ileofemoral section of the venous system.*

THE PATIENT WITH SUSPECTED DVT OR PTE

Swelling of the lower limbs is common during pregnancy with over two thirds of women having significant oedema. However, any patients with symptoms suggestive of DVTs must be carefully assessed. Most DVTs during pregnancy arise on the left and in contrast to the normal situation are ileofemoral as opposed to popliteofemoral. This is important because ileofemoral thrombi are more likely to break off and become pulmonary thromboemboli. Thus, the disorder is somewhat different during pregnancy from the normal state. The diagnosis of DVT is critical during pregnancy because failure will place the patient at risk of fatal PTE, which is one of the leading causes of maternal death, whereas unwarranted anticoagulation will place her at risk of haemostatic problems.

The patient with suspected DVT should be assessed clinically, in particular, a past and family history of thrombotic problems should be elucidated, and also an assessment should be performed of any risk factors or other problems that may mimic the presentation, such as a ruptured Baker's cyst or soft tissue injury. Questions should also elicit any symptoms of possible PTE. A clinical assessment of the legs will include an assessment of any leg swelling and, in particular, calf and thigh girth measurement. Observation of the colour and temperature of the leg can be helpful but as oedema is a common feature of pregnancy and temperature can be difficult to gauge, they are unreliable signs. Homan's sign is entirely unreliable and should not be used in the clinical assessment of DVT.

The clinical diagnosis of DVT is unreliable during pregnancy just as it is in the normal state. Objective assessment is essential. This can be carried out, either with real time or Duplex ultrasound or venography. Radiographic venography is possible during pregnancy and should not be withheld when there are compelling indications. When it is used, shielding of the fetus should be employed to minimize X-ray exposure. Ultrasound assessment of DVT has largely replaced venography. It is noninvasive and has high levels of sensitivity and specificity. Where this is available, it is usually the first line assessment of underlying DVT. It is however limited in its ability to delineate major thrombosis in the iliac vessels above the level of the inguinal ligament and to gain comprehensive visualization of the calf vein. Nonetheless, it would be unusual for a large iliac vein thrombosis not to produce either an extension to the femoral vein or an alteration in the flow that would be apparent on ultrasound examination. If there is significant doubt, a venogram should be performed. If pulmonary embolism is suspected, a ventilation–perfusion lung scan should be performed, the radiation dose is extremely small and given the risks of pulmonary embolism, it should not be withheld from a patient with a suspected problem during pregnancy in view of the need to make an accurate diagnosis (Figs 6.3–5).

In the diagnosis of PTE, it should be noted that although electrocardiograph, chest radiography and blood gases are often employed, their value essentially is in diagnosing other conditions such as chest infection or myocardial infarction which may mimic PTE. Thus, PTE should not be excluded simply on the basis of these tests. When PTE is suspected in the first instance, rather than DVT, a ventilation–perfusion lung scan should be performed. If the result is equivocal, then ultrasound assessment of the leg veins is useful as the diagnosis of DVT would lead to therapeutic anticoagulation whether or not a pulmonary embolism was present.

The treatment of DVT and PTE during pregnancy

The treatment of DVT during pregnancy is, in principle, no different from usual. Once an objective diagnosis is confirmed, the patient should be started on therapeutic doses of heparin, either given by continuous intravenous infusion, by syringe pump or by subcutaneous injection given twice daily. By subcutaneous injection, the dose of unfractionated (UF) heparin is likely to be in the order of 20,000IU twice daily to begin with and a similar dose would be required intravenously with approximately 1600IU/hour being infused in the first instance. Therapy should be monitored and adjusted by measuring the activated partial thromboplastin time. This should be maintained at a ratio of 1.5–2 times the normal control value. Occasionally during pregnancy, particularly if there is an extensive thrombus combined with the changes to the coagulation system during pregnancy that increase factor V, factor VIII and fibrinogen, the activated partial thromboplastin time may not provide an accurate assessment

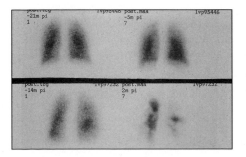

Fig. 6.5 Normal ventilation–perfusion lung scan. Top panel: the image from the ventilation scan (left) matches that of the perfusion scan (right). In pulmonary embolism (bottom panel) the occlusion of the vessels by a clot results in a normal ventilation scan but a perfusion scan showing defects in the areas supplied by the occluded vessels, the so called mismatch is compatible with a high probability of pulmonary thromboembolism.

of heparin dose and the patient may appear refractory to heparin based on the activated partial thromboplastin time. In this situation the use of specific heparin levels may be of value.

Normally, the initial course of heparin would be followed by rapid warfarinization. However, there are particular concerns with warfarin during pregnancy because it freely crosses the placenta. In the first trimester, it is associated with fetal abnormality and in particular with warfarin embryopathy. In addition, as the fetal liver is immature, therapeutic anticoagulation in the mother will result in overanticoagulation of the fetus with a subsequent risk of fetal haemorrhage. The risks are greatest close to the time of delivery when abruption and intracranial haemorrhage can occur in the course of labour and delivery. As a result of this, for a patient developing a DVT antenatally, it is usual to continue with heparin throughout the antenatal course, switching to warfarin after delivery (**Fig. 6.6**).

Heparin itself is not without hazard during pregnancy, although as it does not cross the placenta, there is no direct risk to the fetus. With long-term use, however, there is a risk of heparin-induced osteopaenia, the risk of which relates poorly to the dose and duration, with problems being seen at doses as low as 15,000IU/day and after periods of treatment as short as 7 weeks. It usually manifests clinically as vertebral crush fractures which will occur in approximately 2% of women on long-term heparin therapy during pregnancy. Other complications are heparin-induced thrombocytopaenia (**Figs 6.8** and **6.9**) and heparin allergy. Heparin allergy normally manifests itself as raised erythematous plaques at heparin injection sites (**Fig. 6.7**).

The side effects and risks of anticoagulants during pregnancy	

Warfarin	Warfarin embryopathy
	          Midface hypoplasia
	          Frontal bossing
	          Stippled chondral
	          calcification
	Fetal haemorrhage
	Maternal haemorrhage

Heparin	Heparin allergy Heparin-induced osteoporosis Heparin-induced thrombocytopaenia

Fig. 6.6 *The side effects and risks of anticoagulants during pregnancy.*

Fig. 6.7 *Heparin allergy in a pregnant patient on unfractionated heparin. Note the erythematous patches at the injection sites. The patient was allergic to different types of heparin and low molecular weight heparin and was eventually managed with thromboembolic deterrent stockings and low dose aspirin (anti-platelet therapy) in view of her past history of deep venous thrombosis.*

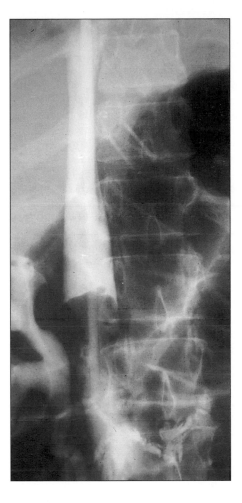

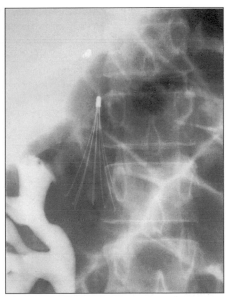

Fig. 6.8 *Venogram showing an extensive clot in the vena cava in a patient with DVT in pregnancy. She developed heparin-induced thrombocytopaenia with extension of the DVT into the vena cava and renal veins. Note the upper limit of the clot above the level of the renal veins with the upper part of the cava containing radio-opaque contrast medium which had been injected through a catheter inserted via the neck veins.*

Fig. 6.9 *Caval filter inserted in the patient described in Fig. 6.8 to prevent pulmonary thromboembolism.*

Heparin allergy can sometimes be dealt with by switching between different heparins or from unfractionated to low molecular weight heparin. Heparin-induced thrombocytopaenia can be a serious problem of long-term heparin use occurring in 2–3% of patients. In this situation, thrombotic problems can arise due to platelet activation. This is due to an antibody directed against a platelet–antibody complex. In view of this, the platelet count should be checked regularly in all patients on heparin during pregnancy.

Heparin should be reduced to prophylactic doses at the time of labour and delivery. In the immediate postpartum period the patient should continue on heparin but can be switched to warfarin with the heparin discontinued once the heparin is in the therapeutic range with an INR of 2–2.5. Neither warfarin nor heparin cross into breast milk, thus, there is no significant problem with breast-feeding.

Low molecular weight heparin given subcutaneously is now being used in the treatment of DVT during pregnancy. Experience is limited, nonetheless these agents are likely to play a major role in therapy in the future, particularly as they have a reduced level of side effects such as heparin-induced thrombocytopaenia. They are being used increasingly for thromboprophylaxis during pregnancy.

THE PATIENT WITH PREVIOUS DVT

It is important in the antenatal assessment of any patient to enquire about their past medical history for venous thromboembolic disease and any family history of such an event. If a patient has had a previous DVT, her risk will be increased during pregnancy. It is also important that she is screened for congenital or acquired thrombophilia. Ideally, these patients should be seen for prepregnancy assessment and counselling so that they are aware of the risk of recurrence of venous thromboembolism during pregnancy and the problems of anticoagulants both for the mother and the fetus. In patients with multiple previous venous thromboembolic problems, it would be usual to initiate thromboprophylaxis 4–6 weeks in advance of the gestation at which the previous thrombosis occurred or, if not associated with pregnancy, in the latter part of the second trimester. The timing of such therapy may be influenced if the patient has a congenital or acquired thrombophilia and a history of a previous DVT, particularly with antithrombin deficiency. Such patients require specialist care from centres experienced in the management of thrombophilia during pregnancy.

For a patient with a single previous DVT, either within or without pregnancy, and with no underlying thrombophilia, there is controversy as to whether antenatal prophylaxis is required in view of the risks of long-term heparin therapy. Each case has to be judged on its merits. However, there is no doubt that postpartum thromboprophylaxis is essential. Thromboprophylaxis during pregnancy can be carried out by way of unfractionated or low molecular weight heparin. Unfractionated heparin should be given in a dose of 10,000IU/twice daily after 20 weeks' gestation. Low molecular weight heparins such as enoxaparin should be administered in a dose of 40mg/once a day, or dalteparin 5000IU/once a day. The low molecular weight heparins have the advantage of a once-daily administration and less risk of heparin-induced thrombocytopaenia. It is not yet clear whether they carry less risk of heparin-induced osteoporosis but there is some evidence to suggest that they do.

Postpartum patients with a history of DVT should not take the combined oral contraceptive pill and alternative forms of contraception should be found in view of the association between the oestrogen-containing pills and venous thrombosis.

DIABETES

The first effect of diabetes during pregnancy is that it increases fetal problems (**Fig. 6.10**). There is an increased risk of congenital abnormality, particularly cardiac, renal and neural

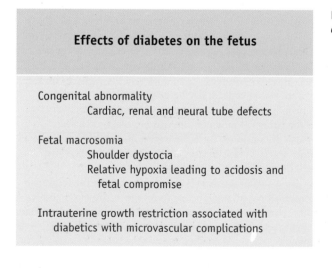

Effects of diabetes on the fetus

Congenital abnormality
    Cardiac, renal and neural tube defects

Fetal macrosomia
    Shoulder dystocia
    Relative hypoxia leading to acidosis and
        fetal compromise

Intrauterine growth restriction associated with
    diabetics with microvascular complications

Fig. 6.10 *Effects of diabetes on the fetus.*

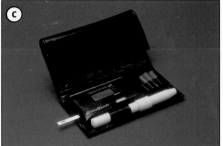

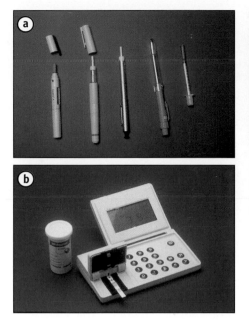

Fig. 6.11 *(a) Insulin syringe and 'pens' used to help obtain optimal glycaemic control. (b) and (c) Blood glucose monitoring devices.*

tube defects. This increased risk is thought to be related to maternal hyperglycaemia during embryogenesis. This clearly emphasizes how critical diabetic control is in the early weeks of pregnancy. Although the risk of fetal abnormality in a diabetic woman who is well controlled is reduced, all patients should be offered detailed assessment and screening for abnormality. In addition, as disturbance in fetal growth can occur (particularly macrosomia), growth should be monitored throughout the pregnancy for women with diabetes, and assessment of fetal wellbeing undertaken in the latter part of pregnancy, particularly when growth disturbances occur.

Diabetes will also place the mother at increased risk of antenatal problems such as pre-eclampsia.

Pregnancy influences diabetes by increasing the dose of insulin required because of the physiology of pregnancy, during which a high level of insulin antagonism occurs; this may be related largely to human placental lactogen. During pregnancy insulin requirements increase dramatically as gestation advances, however, after delivery of the placenta they return to the prepregnancy values. In patients with microvascular disease, pregnancy can lead to a worsening of microvascular complications particularly retinopathy and nephropathy (**Figs 6.14–6.17**) and careful assessment of the eye and of the renal function must be made during any diabetic pregnancy.

THE MANAGEMENT OF A DIABETIC PREGNANCY

Ideally, management should start before the pregnancy when the patient should receive advice about the importance of good glycaemic control before and during the early weeks of pregnancy to avoid or minimize the risk of fetal abnormality. Folic acid supplements may also be of value in preventing neural tube defects. The patient should be aware of the problems that can occur during pregnancy and the need for increased vigilance both in maternal and fetal interests. The patient should report early for care when she becomes pregnant and an early ultrasound to confirm dates and viability is helpful. Prenatal diagnosis should be discussed. A screen for urinary tract infection by mid-stream specimen of urine (MSSU) and a

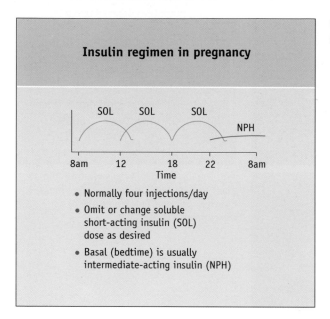

Fig 6.12 *Insulin regimen in pregnancy.*

check of thyroid function is important (thyroid disease often coexists with diabetes). During pregnancy, an assessment should be made of the overall condition of the patient and, in particular, a fundoscopy should be performed to assess for any problems with retinopathy.

The patient should aim for optimal glycaemic control throughout the pregnancy with a target blood sugar concentration of 4–6mmol/L before meals. Glycosylated haemoglobin (usually HbA1c) is a useful assessment of glucose control over the preceding 4–6 weeks. A target of HbA1c of less than 6% before conception (as fetal abnormality is related to hyperglycemia) and during pregnancy is usually given. Insulin therapy needs to be adjusted and careful records kept of blood glucose and insulin dosage. It is often useful to provide the patient with a home glucose meter facility for regular and frequent monitoring of blood sugar, including intermittent nocturnal measurement (**Fig. 6.11**). The management of such patients is most effective at a combined specialized obstetric–diabetic clinic, where the obstetric and diabetic problems that are interlinked can be reviewed. The insulin therapy will require to be adjusted, usually switching from twice daily insulin to four times daily (**Fig. 6.12**). This usually takes the form of short-acting insulin before breakfast, lunch and dinner with an intermediate-acting insulin at night. Hypoglycaemia is a relatively common occurrence when the patient attempts to maintain optimal blood sugar control and it is important that both she and her partner are aware of this risk and how to remedy the situation by way of local supplements and the use of intramuscular glucagon injections (**Fig. 6.13**). By the end of pregnancy, the insulin requirements may be two to three times that of the prepregnancy requirements.

As well as carefully reviewing the mother, her diabetic control and screening for hypertensive, eye (**Figs 6.14–16**) and renal problems (**Fig. 6.17**), an ultrasound scan should be performed at 18–20 weeks' gestation to screen for fetal abnormalities. In the latter half of pregnancy ultrasound scans should be performed on a regular basis to assess fetal growth, looking particularly for macrosomia or intrauterine growth restriction. Liquor volume should also be assessed. When there is any evidence of growth disturbance, an assessment of fetal wellbeing should be carried out by way of cardiotocography or biophysical profiles. A regular assessment of blood pressure is particularly important during

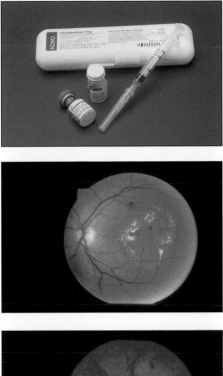

Fig. 6.13 *Glucagon for treatment of hypoglycemia.*

Fig. 6.14 *Diabetic background retinopathy.*

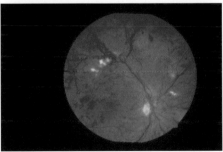

Fig. 6.15 *Proliferative diabetic retinopathy.*

a diabetic pregnancy because of the increased risk of pre-eclampsia. Should there be any evidence of fetal compromise, delivery should be carried out. As there is an increased risk to the fetus during diabetic pregnancy, it is unusual to allow the pregnancy to go beyond its estimated date of delivery; earlier delivery may even be indicated, particularly when problems are present .

The mode of delivery should be considered in the context of each particular case. Clearly, if there is gross macrosomia or any evidence of fetal compromise, then caesarean section would be best. When a vaginal delivery is anticipated, the main risks to the fetus lie in asphyxia and trauma from shoulder dystocia. As a result of these problems, continuous monitoring of the fetal heart rate should take place during a diabetic pregnancy, and progress in labour should be carefully assessed in view of the increased risk of cephalopelvic disproportion and shoulder dystocia. If slow progress is made during labour or there is evidence of cephalopelvic dysproportion, then a caesarean section should be performed. Glycaemic control during labour is usually obtained by way of a regimen involving an intravenous infusion of 5–10% glucose and saline administered at an initial rate of 100ml/hour in conjunction with an intravenous infusion of soluble insulin at an initial dose

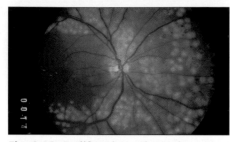

Fig. 6.16 *Proliferative retinopathy following laser therapy.*

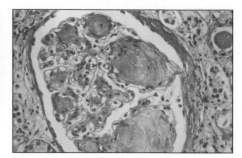

Fig. 6.17 *Diabetic nephropathy.*

Fig. 6.18 *Indications for a glucose tolerance test.*

Indications for a glucose tolerance test

Glycosuria ×2 on fasting specimens
Strong family history of diabetes
Previous macrosomic baby
Previous gestational diabetes
Previous unexplained stillbirth
Polyhydramnios
Maternal obesity
Macrosomic fetus or fetus large for date

of 1IU/hour, titrating this against hourly blood glucose measurements. If a caesarean section is performed because of the risk of infection due to diabetes during pregnancy (particularly urinary tract infection and wound infection), then prophylactic antibiotics should be given. After delivery, the insulin dose should be reduced to the prepregnancy values.

The neonate will be at increased risk of problems such as respiratory distress syndrome, hypoglycaemia, polycythaemia and neonatal jaundice.

GESTATIONAL DIABETES AND IMPAIRED GLUCOSE TOLERANCE

Carbohydrate intolerance during pregnancy is not unusual. Clearly, diabetes can present for the first time during pregnancy but more often this is a gestationally related phenomenon. During a normal pregnancy, there is a degree of insulin resistance. A woman who can not compensate sufficiently for this will develop impaired glucose tolerance.

Gestational diabetes should be considered during pregnancy for women with a significant glycosuria on fasting specimens on two occasions, or when there is a strong family history, a history of previous macrosomic babies, a history of previous gestational diabetes, previous unexplained stillbirth, polyhydramnios or macrosomia complicated with pregnancy or maternal obesity (**Fig. 6.18**).

Although some clinics perform a routine screening for all pregnant women, such as a random blood sugar, others select on the criteria above. An oral glucose tolerance test (75g

Oral glucose (75g) tolerance test results during pregnancy		
	Fasting value	2-h value
Impaired glucose tolerance	<8 mmol/L	8–11 mmol/L
Gestational diabetes	>8 mmol/L	>11 mmol/L

Fig. 6.19 *75g oral glucose tolerance test results in pregnancy.*

Glucose tolerance test result	
Time (min)	Plasma glucose (mmol/L)
Fasting	8.8
30	12.9
60	15.7
90	17
120	15.2

Fig. 6.20 *Glucose tolerance test result showing a frankly diabetic picture in a woman who had recurrent fasting glycosuria. She required treatment with insulin during pregnancy. The fetus was macrosomic.*

glucose) can be used to make a diagnosis of such problems. Gestational diabetes can be diagnosed if fasting glucose is greater than 8mmol/L or the 2-hour level is greater than 11mmol/L, whereas impaired glucose tolerance is diagnosed if the fasting glucose is less than 8mmol/L and the 2-hour level is between 8 and 11mmol/L (**Figs 6.19** and **6.20**).

Women with impaired glucose tolerance should usually receive some dietary advice. Women with gestational diabetes should in the first instance be started on a diet that will exclude simple carbohydrates. Careful blood glucose monitoring should occur as with pre-existing insulin-dependent diabetes and if control is unsatisfactory on that diet, then insulin should be introduced. Clearly, problems such as macrosomia may exist before the gestational diabetes being diagnosed, thus, the role of insulin in preventing such complications is limited. As with pre-existing insulin-dependent diabetes, careful fetal monitoring should be carried out along with an assessment for additional complications. A decision about the delivery is similar to that of pre-existing insulin-dependent diabetes. An appreciation of the risk of problems related to macrosomia, such as shoulder dystocia, is required for labour. After the delivery, reassessment should be made on the need for insulin and usually this will be able to be stopped. It should also be appreciated that these women are at risk of noninsulin-dependent diabetes in later life.

ANAEMIA

The most common form of anaemia during pregnancy is iron deficiency anaemia. A deficiency of folic acid may coexist along with iron deficiency, particularly as both can be associated with a poor diet. If folic acid and iron are both deficient, the effects of folic acid deficiency are masked by the iron deficiency. Vitamin B_{12} deficiency is extremely rare during pregnancy. The diagnosis of anaemia is altered during pregnancy because of changes in the plasma and blood volume. Plasma volume increases by approximately 50% with a concomitant increase in red cell mass of the order of 25%. Therefore, in view of the relatively greater increase in plasma volume, haemoglobin concentrations will fall due to dilution. This effect is progressive through pregnancy reaching its peak at approximately 32 weeks' gestation. Normally, the haemoglobin should not fall below 10.5–11g/dl at any time during pregnancy.

THE DIAGNOSIS OF ANAEMIA

The main diagnostic criteria are on the full blood count: mean corpuscular haemoglobin, mean corpuscular volume and mean corpuscular haemoglobin concentration. All of these parameters are reduced in iron deficiency anaemia. Consideration should be given to the differential diagnosis of thalassaemia, which shows a reduced mean corpuscular volume and mean corpuscular haemoglobin, but normal or only slightly reduced mean corpuscular haemoglobin concentration. The blood film in classic iron deficiency anaemia shows hypochromic microcytic red cells just as it does when not pregnant. However, this characteristic red cell morphology occurs relatively late in the development of the anaemia and will be preceded by a reduction in the mean corpuscular volume and, subsequently, a reduction in the mean corpurscular haemoglobin concentration. When red cell indices are not diagnostic of iron deficiency anaemia, serum ferritin and total iron binding capacity are useful measures of iron status with a concentration of serum ferritin of less than 12μg/L being compatible with iron deficiency. In the normal situation, serum ferritin falls over the course of a pregnancy and needs to be taken into account in the interpretation of serum ferritin results. Serum iron and the percentage saturation of the total iron binding capacity may also be helpful but as these measurements can fluctuate widely during pregnancy and are affected by iron ingestion, they are less helpful in the diagnosis than serum ferritin. Nonetheless, if total iron binding capacity saturation is reduced along with serum iron this would be compatible with iron deficiency anaemia. An assessment of folic acid status is also useful. Anaemia during pregnancy is usually picked up on routine screening of the full blood

Severe iron deficiency anaemia in pregnancy		
	Normal range	Patient value
Haemoglobin (g/dl)	10.5–15	6.2
Mean cell volume (fl)	76–99	60.8
Mean cell haemoglobin (pg)	27–32	17.8

Fig. 6.21 *Severe iron deficiency anaemia in pregnancy. Serum ferritin was <1 μg/mL (normal 6–81 μg/mL).*

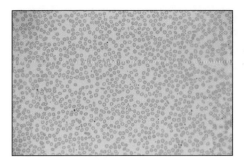

Fig. 6.22 *Hypochromic microcytes characteristic of iron deficiency anaemia.*

count that occurs at booking and in the third trimester. Clearly, such checks should also occur if the patient presents with any symptoms compatible with anaemia such as tiredness, although such symptoms are commonplace in normal pregnancy (**Figs 6.21** and **6.22**).

The usual treatment of iron deficiency anaemia is oral iron supplements which should be combined with folic acid supplements. Vitamin C is commonly prescribed along with the iron as this enhances absorption. Parenteral iron therapy is rarely required and should only be used when there is a degree of urgency in attempting to restore the haemoglobin concentration, such as impending delivery or when there is serious intolerance of oral iron. With the appropriate correction of iron deficiency, the haemoglobin should increase by between 0.8 and 1g/dl/week. A common prescription for iron deficiency anaemia would be 200mg ferrous sulphate two-three times a day, with 50mg vitamin C and 5mg folic acid on a daily basis.

CASE HISTORY

A woman who is para 4+0 at 31 weeks' gestation complains of excessive tiredness; her previous pregnancy had been only 1 year earlier. You perform a full blood count which shows the haemoglobin to be 8.5g/dl, mean corpuscular haemoglobin and mean corpuscular haemoglobin concentration are low and the blood film is compatible with iron deficiency anaemia. The findings suggest iron deficiency anaemia and the patient should be prescribed iron, folic acid and vitamin C supplements as previously described. In addition, patients such as this should be considered at particular risk of iron deficiency anaemia. Women entering pregnancy with grossly depleted iron stores, resulting from several pregnancies in which the iron stores have not been allowed to recover fully, may rapidly develop anaemia during pregnancy with clear evidence of iron deficiency in the red cell indices. In view of the gestation, it would be anticipated that with appropriate haematinic therapy, the projected rate of increase to normal levels of haemoglobin should be obtained by term.

THYROID DISEASE

THYROID PHYSIOLOGY

The normal physiology of pregnancy can mimic many thyroid symptoms as pregnancy itself causes alterations in the structure and function of the thyroid gland. This can cause diagnostic confusion in the interpretation of thyroid function tests. However, the overall control of the thyroid gland is unaltered in normal pregnancy. The thyroid gland increases in size early on in normal pregnancy and indeed this was used by ancient civilizations as a way of diagnosing pregnancy. The thyroid hormones T_3 and T_4 increase dramatically during pregnancy, predominantly because of the increased binding of these active thyroid hormones to thyroid-binding globulin which increases in concentration substantially from the first trimester. These alterations in thyroid-binding globulin are likely to be oestrogen dependent. Thus, total T_3 and T_4 will increase during pregnancy, although the concentrations of free T_3 and T_4 show no change. Similarly, thyroid-stimulating hormone shows no change during pregnancy. Thus, when interpreting thyroid function tests during pregnancy, it is important to derive an index of free thyroxine either directly or via the free thyroxine index which is calculated from the total T_4 and the T_3 resin uptake. Most clinical chemistry laboratories now offer free thyroxine measurements as this is the best guide to thyroid function.

HYPERTHYROIDISM

Hyperthyroidism is a relatively common medical condition that may occur in approximately 1 in 500 pregnancies. Most are secondary to Grave's disease, an autoimmune disorder with circulating thyroid-stimulating antibodies being present. Some improvement can occur during pregnancy, although a worsening of the condition may occur postpartum. Women with a history of hyperthyroidism should have their thyroid function monitored regularly through pregnancy. The frequency will be governed by the particular circumstances and various symptoms that the patient may have, and usually not be any less than once in each trimester of pregnancy. It is often difficult to gauge hyperthyroidism during pregnancy as many of the signs and symptoms of hyperthyroidism such as tachycardia, heat intolerance and an ejection systolic murmur are similar to those seen in the normal hyperdynamic cardiovascular state of pregnancy. This emphasizes the need for biochemical as opposed to clinical assessment of thyroid status. Patients with good thyroid control rarely have problems during pregnancy, however, if problems do occur, the main worry is uncontrolled disease which may even manifest itself as a 'thyroid storm'. Such problems can be precipitated by infection or stress, and are characterized by tachycardia and hyperpyrexia. High-output cardiac failure can occur and this may be associated with atrial fibrillation. There is gastrointestinal upset with vomiting, diarrhoea and central nervous system dysfunction.

Hyperthyroidism is usually controlled during pregnancy with drugs, in particular carbimazole, propylthiouracil and propranolol. Carbimazole and propylthiouracil will inhibit thyroid hormone synthesis whereas propranolol reduces the effect of adrenergic symptoms. To ensure compliance, it is important to discuss the benefits of these drugs with the mother and the minimal problems they pose for the fetus. All these drugs cross the placenta and may alter thyroid function. Although none is an established teratogen, carbimazole has been associated with aplasia cutis, a condition in which small defects of the skin, usually the scalp, occur; however, this is rare. Fetal thyroid function will be reduced by carbimazole and propylthiouracil. The long-term administration of propranolol through the pregnancy may present an increased risk of intrauterine growth restriction which has been shown to occur with chronic adrenoceptor antagonist therapy during pregnancy. Other fetal problems relate to the transfer of thyroid-stimulating antibodies from the mother to the fetus. This can provoke fetal hyperthyroidism. This rarely causes significant problems especially if the mother is taking an antithyroid drug which will suppress fetal thyroid activity, but neonatal thyrotoxicosis can occur in approximately 10% of babies of mothers with Grave's disease. This condition usually lasts only weeks, at most, 2–3 months after delivery, although the situation may be masked at

Thyroid function test results from a patient with hyperthyroidism

	T_4 nmol/L	T_3 nmol/L	Thyroid-stimulating hormone (mU/L)	Free T_4 (pmol/L)
Normal range	55–144	0.9–2.8	0.35–5.0	9–26
Carbimazole started	380	6.6	<0.05	73
13 days later	381	7.2	<0.05	63
24 days later	265	4.2	<0.05	35
38 days later	176	3.4	0.15	17.6

Fig. 6.23 *Thyroid function test results from a patient with hyperthyroidism. Note elevated levels of free thyroxine and normal TSH which normalize after treatment with carbimazole. It is noteworthy that even following treatment with carbimazole total T_3 and T_4 remain elevated above non-pregnant normal levels.*

birth by the maternal administration of antithyroid drugs. There is also a recognized association between hyperthyroidism and increased risk of premature delivery and reduced mean birthweight. It is usual during pregnancy to monitor fetal growth by ultrasound and combine this with assessment of fetal wellbeing if there is any suspicion of disturbance of growth or of serious fetal problems through the transfer of antithyroid antibodies.

On no account should radioactive iodine be used during pregnancy to treat thyrotoxicosis as the fetal thyroid will receive a high concentration of this which, in turn, will precipitate irreversible fetal hypothyroidism. When patients do not respond to drug therapy or there is a serious intolerance along with significant disease, partial thyroidectomy may be required. It is usual to pretreat patients with iodine therapy for 7–10 days to decrease the vascularity of the gland and prevent a thyroid storm. The use of propranolol may also help reduce the symptoms in this situation (**Fig. 6.23**).

HYPOTHYROIDISM

It is unusual for hypothyroidism to cause significant problems during pregnancy. Patients with significant hypothyroidism have reduced fertility. Most patients who conceive are on thyroxine supplements. Thyroid function tests should be monitored intermittently, at least once in each trimester, and the dose of thyroxine adjusted to maintain the patient both clinically and chemically euthyroid. Should dose adjustment occur during pregnancy, this should be reassessed after delivery. The assessment of thyroid status depends not only on the patient's symptoms, but also on the analysis of the thyroid function tests. Thyroid-stimulating hormone will be elevated in hypothyroidism when there is inadequate replacement of thyroxine and free T_4 will be low. Owing to the physiological changes of thyroid-binding globulin during pregnancy, total T_3 and T_4 are not usually helpful in the assessment of this condition (**Fig. 6.24**).

Hypothyroidism in pregnancy			
	T$_4$ nmol/L	Thyroid-stimulating hormone (mU/L)	Free T$_4$ (pmol/L)
Normal range	55–144	0.35–5.0	9–26
Start of treatment	126	11.6	7.2
2 weeks later: thyroxine dose increased	130	32.5	7.6
4 weeks later	178	11.6	9.5
7 weeks later	175	5.2	12
10 weeks later	220	1.4	16

Fig. 6.24 *Hypothyroidism in pregnancy. Note increased TSH and low free T$_4$ with restoration to normal values following an increase in the dose of thyroxine. Total T$_4$ is in the normal non-pregnant range while the patient is hypothyroid.*

CONNECTIVE TISSUE DISEASE

The main connective tissue diseases seen during pregnancy are rheumatoid arthritis and systemic lupus erythmatosus (SLE).

RHEUMATOID ARTHRITIS

Rheumatoid arthritis rarely causes significant problems during pregnancy and the disease often improves during the course of the pregnancy. This may be due to an increased concentration of anti-inflammatory steroid hormones. Thus, for many patients, the need for therapy may be lessened during pregnancy. Simple analgesics such as paracetamol can be used freely during pregnancy. Nonsteroidal anti-inflammatory drugs can also be used. However, the chronic use of these agents may result in oligohydramnios due to suppressed fetal urine production and occasionally, when used in the third trimester, premature closure of the ductus arteriosis which may, in turn, place the fetus at risk of pulmonary hypertension. Thus, if such drugs are used in late pregnancy, the fetus should be regularly monitored for checks on liquor volume. Corticosteroid therapy is satisfactory during pregnancy, however, chronic administration will result in the need for steroid supplements during labour, usually 100mg hydrocortisone intravenously 12-hourly. Fetal adrenal suppression may also occur and the neonate may require steroid supplements after delivery. Cytotoxic agents should obviously be avoided during pregnancy.

SLE

In contrast to rheumatoid arthritis, SLE is associated with particular problems during pregnancy. This autoimmune condition produces specific cytotoxic antibodies, provoking problems such as haemolytic anaemia or thrombocytopaenia, and immune complex problems associated with inflammatory lesions affecting the kidneys, the skin and the central nervous system. The major immune complex implicated is DNA-anti-DNA. Arthritis is a common manifestation of SLE and is not usually deforming in contrast to the arthritis found in rheumatoid arthritis. Evidence of chronic glomerulonephritis is present in 50% or more of patients with SLE. The disease activity can be assessed by the presence of antinative DNA antibodies and depressed levels of the complement components, C3 and C4.

The fetal problems of SLE
- Spontaneous miscarriage.
- Intrauterine death (due to problems such as growth restriction and placental infarction).
- Prematurity (iatrogenic or spontaneous).
- Intrauterine growth restriction (may be associated with pre-eclampsia).
- Congenital heart block and cardiac failure (associated with anti-Ro antibodies).
- Neonatal lupus.

The risks to the mother
- Flare-up of the disease, particularly in early pregnancy and postpartum.
- Pre-eclampsia.
- Deterioration in renal function.
- Arterial and venous thrombotic problems (including DVTs and cerebral thrombosis) often associated with lupus anticoagulant and anticardiolipin antibodies.

In view of the maternal and fetal risks associated with SLE, prepregnancy counselling is important in the management of such patients. This will allow the patient to determine on an informed basis whether or not to become pregnant. If she is in early pregnancy, she may consider whether or not to proceed with the pregnancy. The patient should be advised that it is optimal for her to conceive when the disease is quiescent and when drug therapy is minimal. Drug therapy may have to be modified during pregnancy. Chloroquine was considered to have had adverse effects on the fetal retina but no significant problems are seen and it can be used in pregnancy. Azothiaprine should be avoided if possible, but if required for disease control, then it should not be withheld. As for rheumatoid arthritis, steroids can be safely used during pregnancy with no evidence of teratogenicity in the human, although their administration may cause adrenal suppression in the neonate; this is usually transient and is easily treated. The over-riding interest in SLE is quiescent disease and, thus, steroid administration to the mother should not be withheld. Before and during pregnancy, the mother should be reassured about the effects of steroids on the pregnancy.

It is also worth assessing not only disease activity but also for the presence of anticardiolipin antibodies and lupus anticoagulant in prepregnancy as well as the presence or absence of the anti-Ro antibody. However, should these results be negative, it is often worthwhile repeating them during pregnancy because sometimes anticardiolipin antibodies are only evident during the course of a pregnancy. The presence of anti-Ro antibodies places the fetus at increased risk of congenital heart block because these antibodies cross the placenta and attack the conducting system of the developing fetal heart. This problem is irreversible and babies born with congenital heart block will have this as a persistent problem through their life. *In utero* this can precipitate cardiac failure leading to fetal death, and in labour there is a reduced ability to deal with stress, thus, such fetuses are best delivered by caesarean section.

Lupus anticoagulant and anticardiolipin antibody syndrome
Lupus anticoagulant and anticardiolipin antibodies occur in between 5 and 20% of patients with SLE. However, it should be noted that these antibodies can commonly occur in

patients without underlying SLE, with only approximately 50% of patients with anticardiolipin antibodies and lupus anticoagulant having SLE causing their problem.

Lupus anticoagulant is an IgG or IgM antibody against phospholipids which interferes with the activation of prothrombin by the prothrombin-converting complex of factor Va and factor Xa, calcium and lipid. A variety of laboratory tests are used to determine the presence of lupus anticoagulant, in particular, the activated partial thromboplastin time, the dilute prothrombin time and the Russell's viper venom time. There is a prolongation of these coagulation tests in the laboratory. The name lupus anticoagulant reflects the association with SLE and the prolongation of the coagulation tests *in vitro*. Despite this, *in vivo* problems relate to thrombosis which can occur at the level of the placental bed, so triggering problems such as growth restriction, placental infarction and fetal death, and arterial and venous thromboembolic events as already noted.

Anticardiolipin antibodies are antibodies specifically directed against phospholipids in cell membranes. They often coexist with lupus anticoagulant but they are not the same. High levels of anticardiolipin antibodies are powerful predictors of fetal compromise and are associated with a high risk of fetal death for women with SLE. These antibodies have also been associated with recurrent miscarriage, growth restriction and increased risk of pre-eclampsia as well as arterial and venous thrombotic events as already noted. Patients with lupus anticoagulant and anticardiolipin antibodies are usually treated with low dose aspirin 75mg once a day in an attempt to prevent these thrombotic complications. For patients with a history of thrombotic problems, aspirin can usually be combined with prophylactic heparin. Such combined treatment with low-dose heparin and aspirin appears to be particularly suitable for patients with recurrent miscarriage. The addition of steroids to aspirin or heparin is not usually warranted and would only be used in patients with active SLE, for which steroids would be required in any event. Patients with a history of unexplained fetal loss, growth restriction, severe pre-eclampsia or recurrent miscarriage should be screened for anticardiolipin antibodies and lupus anticoagulant.

The treatment of SLE during pregnancy

In view of the numerous fetal risks associated with SLE, it is usual to prescribe prophylactic low-dose aspirin at a dose of 75mg from the end of the first trimester or earlier should there be a history of miscarriage or previous problems. Low-dose aspirin is not associated with adverse maternal or fetal affects and thus can be used safely throughout pregnancy.

When anticardiolipin antibodies or lupus anticoagulant is found then consideration should be given to thromboprophylaxis. When a patient has such antibodies and a past history of thrombosis, it is usual to prescribe low-dose or low molecular weight heparin through the pregnancy. In any event, postpartum thromboprophylaxis should be used because there may be a substantial risk of venous thromboembolic disease in the puerperium. Postpartum thromboprophylaxis should usually be continued for 6 weeks and low-dose or low molecular weight heparin can be used in this situation.

Careful maternal and fetal monitoring is required throughout the pregnancy. This starts with an accurate determination of gestational age; assessment in the middle of the second trimester of uterine artery blood flow may identify fetuses at an increased risk of adverse perinatal outcome. Patients with normal flow in both the maternal uterine arteries usually have a normal fetal outcome, whereas 'notching' in one uterine artery is associated with increased risk of low birth weight and in both arteries with perinatal loss (see **Fig. 7.6**). Fetal growth should be monitored from approximately 24–26 weeks' gestation by serial ultrasound scans conducted with a minimum of 2 weeks between assessments. Umbilical artery flow velocity waveforms assessed using Doppler ultrasound are also of value to identify fetuses at high risk from growth restriction. A regular assessment of fetal wellbeing should be carried out from late in the second trimester should there be suspicion of any fetal compromise or growth restriction, using biophysical profiles or cardiotocographs combined with the assessment of liquor volume. The intensity of monitoring for fetal wellbeing will depend on the presence of complications such as growth restriction. Maternal monitoring is aimed at detecting any flare-up of the lupus, any deterioration in renal function and the development of superimposed pre-eclampsia. It is often difficult to determine whether the onset of problems such as oedema, hypertension and proteinuria are due to superimposed pre-eclampsia or a flare-up of lupus nephritis. The occurrence of these manifestations in the absence of other evidence of a flare-up in SLE, and in the absence of serological abnormalities, suggests superimposed pre-eclampsia. Elevated DNA antibodies and suppressed complement levels favour the diagnosis of flare in SLE. Should a flare-up of SLE occur, it is usual to treat the patient initially with steroids. If the patient is already on steroids, the dose should be increased.

The timing and mode of delivery will depend on the development of any complications; in the absence of complications, vaginal delivery is not contraindicated. When significant fetal compromise is present, it is usual to perform a caesarean section. Steroid supplements will be needed to cover both the labour and the caesarean section. The treatment of SLE during pregnancy requires a multidisciplinary approach involving physicians, obstetricians and neonatologists.

PROLACTINOMA

Pregnancy is normally associated with a substantial increase in circulating prolactin concentrations of approximately tenfold. It is likely that this reflects a hyperplasia of the pituitary lactotrophs due to the high oestrogen levels associated with pregnancy. There is also an increase in volume of the pituitary gland during pregnancy. Thus, in patients with prolactinomas, there is the risk that the oestrogenic stimulation will provoke tumour expansion and possible deterioration in visual fields. However, in practice, it is unusual for patients with microadenomas to have a clinically significant expansion in their tumour during pregnancy. Patients with hyperprolactinaemia due to prolactinoma will clearly have a problem with fertility; menstruation and ovulation are likely to return to normal after treatment with bromocriptine or cabergoline. When these patients become pregnant, bromocriptine should be discontinued. The patient should be made aware of the risk of tumour expansion and the need to report severe headache or a change in vision during the pregnancy. There may be some merit in monitoring prolactin levels during the pregnancy but this can be difficult to interpret due to the ten- to twentyfold increase in prolactin levels during the course of normal pregnancy. There is also a place for the regular assessment of visual fields but this is unlikely to show any abnormality in the asymptomatic patient. Should symptoms occur, it is important that the multidisciplinary team approach is taken including the endocrinologist, ophthalmologist, obstetrician, and in the case of a microprolactinoma expanding, it is usual to treat the patient with bromocriptine during the pregnancy which is not associated with any apparent risk of miscarriage or teratogenesis.

Macroprolactinomas, that is, prolactinomas greater than 1cm in diameter have a higher risk of tumour expansion during pregnancy but this is minimized if they are treated before pregnancy to reduce their size. A reduction in size should be confirmed objectively by pituitary imaging before pregnancy. Very few patients having had their macroprolactinoma dealt with either surgically or by radiation therapy before pregnancy develop symptomatic tumour expansion. Bromocriptine may be of value in the pretreatment phase to shrink the tumour. In these women, a regular assessment of visual fields may be valuable to look for any recurrent tumour expansion. Should symptoms occur, the first line treatment is to restart bromocriptine. Breast-feeding is not contraindicated in patients with prolactinomas.

RESPIRATORY DISEASE

PHYSIOLOGICAL CHANGES IN THE RESPIRATORY SYSTEM

Oxygen consumption increases during pregnancy by up to 30% because of the demands of the feto-placental unit and increased maternal requirements. This is accompanied by increased carbon dioxide production. Despite this, arterial oxygen tensions are maintained within essentially normal limits, whereas carbon dioxide tension (P_{CO_2}) is approximately 25% below the normal level. These changes are brought about by an increase in tidal volume of approximately 40% over baseline with little change in respiratory rate. These physiological changes appear to be due to increased progesterone sensitizing the respiratory centre. The functional residual capacity will also be reduced during pregnancy in view of the above changes. Women often complain of dyspnoea in early pregnancy if they are aware of these changes.

ASTHMA

Asthma commonly affects young women and is frequently encountered during pregnancy. Pregnancy appears to have a somewhat variable affect on asthma. In some women, the asthma worsens and in others it stays the same, there are others for whom it improves. There are many variables underlying this. It would be unusual for a patient with well-controlled asthma and minimal symptoms to develop significant problems due to the gravid uterus in the third trimester. However, pregnancy is normally associated with an increase in tidal volume which may be interpreted as breathlessness. In addition, many women may adjust their therapy or even halt it as they are worried about the effects of drugs during pregnancy.

Uncontrolled severe asthma can be associated with significant maternal hypoxia which could, in turn, have adverse consequences for the fetus. In modern practice, people with severe uncontrolled asthma are uncommon.

None of the drugs commonly used to treat asthma, including β-sympathomimetics, inhaled and oral steroids, and theophyllines, is associated with teratogenesis or serious risk to the fetus. For virtually all patients, the risks of uncontrolled asthma far outweigh the risks associated with any drug therapy. When theophyllines are used, it should be noted that there is an increased clearance of the drug during pregnancy, making it more difficult to control. Drug levels have to be monitored. It may be more useful to use alternative therapy for such patients. For patients using high-dose steroid therapy in the third trimester, there is a small risk of a degree of suppression of the fetal hypothalamo–pituitary–adrenal axis and the patient should be warned of this in the event the neonate may require steroid supplements.

When the asthmatic patient is seen before pregnancy, the important features are that her asthma is well controlled and to reassure her that the drugs that she is taking will not in any way influence the outcome of the pregnancy and, indeed, that the risk of uncontrolled asthma would be a greater risk to the pregnancy. It should be emphasized that good control of her asthma is critically important to her pregnancy. There is a slight increase in preterm labour and intrauterine growth restriction in patients with asthma. The management of chronic asthma is outlined in **Figure 6.25**. In summary, the patient should avoid triggers, for example, exposure to pollens, etc., as much as possible. The most appropriate inhaler device should be selected, and therapy adjusted up or down steps as required. If stable, the aim would be to reduce inhaled steroids by 25–50% every 1–3 months.

The treatment of asthma during pregnancy is similar to that of the normal individual. In the antenatal period therapy may require to be adjusted to maintain good control similar to patients for whom control is difficult or those that are severely affected. It may be of value to measure routinely diurnal peak flow measurements; a dip, particularly in the evening

Management of chronic asthma in pregnancy

Step 1   Occasional use of short-acting β-sympathomimetic bronchodilators, e.g.
salbutamol or terbutaline.
Reassure the patient about drug safety and encourage compliance.
If required more than once a day, go to Step 2.

Step 2   Inhaled short-acting β-sympathomimetics as required
plus
Regular, inhaled anti-inflammatory agents, e.g. beclomethasone or
budesonide 100–400mg twice daily.
Reassure the patient about drug safety and encourage compliance.

Step 3   Inhaled short-acting β-sympathomimetics as required.
High-dose inhaled steroids, e.g. 800–2000mg of beclomethasone or
budesonide daily
or
Steroid inhalers as Step 2, plus salmeterol (long-acting bronchodilator
50μg twice daily).
Reassure the patient about drug safety and encourage compliance.

Step 4   Inhaled short-acting β-sympathomimetics as required.
High-dose steroid inhalers as Step 3
plus
Sequential trials of additional therapy, e.g. ipratropium, cromoglycate or
high-dose inhaled bronchodilators.
Reassure the patient about drug safety and encourage compliance.

Step 5   Inhaled short-acting β-sympathomimetics as required.
High-dose steroid inhalers as Step 3
plus
One or more long-acting bronchodilators
plus
Regular prednisolone in a single daily dose (steroid supplements will be
required in labour or with caesarean section).

Fig. 6.25 *Management of chronic asthma in pregnancy.*

measurement, may precede the worsening of symptoms. If the patient is taking theophylline, levels need to be monitored. There are no special precautions for fetal wellbeing.

During labour some caution should be exercised with prostaglandin agents used for induction, particularly prostaglandin F_{2a}. General anaesthesia should be avoided for operative delivery if possible. For women with severe disease, it may be useful to obtain the advice of an anaesthetist in the third trimester. There is no contraindication to inhaled β-sympathomimetics during labour.

Postpartum the mother should continue her therapy; breast-feeding is not contraindicated. Physiotherapy may be required particularly if an operative delivery has occurred and pulmonary function is impaired due to a surgical wound or a degree of atelectasis after a general anaesthetic.

Therapy, as already noted, is similar to that of the normal situation. For mildly affected individuals with symptoms once a day, the use of an inhaled β-sympathomimetic such as salbutamol or terbutaline is satisfactory. If more frequent symptoms occur, the regular use of a steroid inhaler should be employed with intermittent inhaled β-agonists as required. When symptoms are not controlled with this therapy, high-dose inhaled steroids may be required and the addition of a long-acting β-sympathomimetic such as salmeterol may be of value. For the most severely affected patients, systemic corticosteroids are required. When systemic corticosteroids have been taken regularly, it is usual to cover delivery with intravenous hydrocortisone 150mg intravenously every 6 hours during labour. Ergometrine should also be avoided during labour.

Acute severe asthma can be extremely dangerous and may require admission to the intensive care unit during pregnancy. As patients can deteriorate very quickly, admission should occur as soon as patients' symptoms start to worsen.

Any evidence of infection should be properly treated with antibiotics. The usual antibiotics can be prescribed for chest infection during pregnancy with the exception of tetracyclines which should be avoided because of their effect on fetal bones and teeth. It should be noted that there is a substantial increase in the clearance of the penicillins and the dose of ampicillin or amoxycillin should be doubled during pregnancy for systemic infections. If the patient is taking long-term systemic corticosteroids, she may develop glucose intolerance and a glucose tolerance test may be required as she may be at risk of gestational diabetes. Furthermore, there may be a possibility of osteopaenia with prolonged systemic steroid therapy. The fetal adrenal gland will also be suppressed after delivery.

TUBERCULOSIS

The incidence of tuberculosis is on the increase and it can be associated with HIV infection. It is essential that tuberculosis during pregnancy is treated by a respiratory physician or infectious diseases physician. When tuberculosis is diagnosed after the first trimester, treatment should follow the established guidelines with combination chemotherapy or pyrazinamide, rifampicin and isoniazid for 2 months followed by a further 4 months of rifampicin and isoniazid. Pyridoxine should be given along with isoniazid to reduce the risk of peripheral neuritis. There is some concern over the use of this regimen in the first trimester. Although ethambutol and isoniazid are considered safe, there are concerns about both rifampicin and streptomycin, the latter having been shown to be ototoxic. There is limited knowledge about the use of pyrazinamide during pregnancy. Thus, in patients who present in the first trimester, it may be best to avoid rifampicin, streptomycin and pyrazinamide if possible, treating the patient with isoniazid and ethambutol alone, moving on the triple therapy after the first trimester. When a patient is seriously ill with tuberculosis in the first trimester, then it would appear prudent to use either pyrazinamide or rifampicin as required.

Extrapulmonary tuberculosis is usually not infectious in patients not coughing sputum or when the sputum has been shown not to contain tubercle bacilli, but when pulmonary sputum is positive, clearly, they are infectious. Treatment will usually result in them becoming noninfectious within 2 weeks or so.

The neonate is usually only at risk of infection if the mother has active tuberculosis at the time of delivery. When the neonate is considered at risk it should be given a BCG injection with a specific strain of BCG which is isoniazid resistant in order to allow prophylactic isoniazid also to be given to the neonate.

RENAL DISEASE

CHANGES IN RENAL FUNCTION
During pregnancy there is a dramatic increase in the glomerular filtration rate. From very early on during pregnancy this is associated with a reduction in the serum concentrations of creatinine and urea. As normal, it is better to use creatinine clearance as a measure of renal function as opposed to serum creatinine because a greater than 50% reduction in renal function must occur before serum creatinine will leave the normal reference range. The kidneys increase in size and the collecting systems dilate. These changes are more marked on the right where the dilatation seen in the ureter may mimic obstructive uropathy. The stasis of urine associated with the dilated collecting system places the patient at risk of urinary tract infection and pyelonephritis. Patients with asymptomatic bacteriuria normally can easily develop significant urinary tract infection during pregnancy.

CHRONIC RENAL DISEASE
The effect of chronic renal disease on pregnancy
In general terms, the problems for the mother and the risk to the fetus are dependent on the degree of renal compromise. Women with mild renal impairment (a serum creatinine of less than 125μmol/L) tend to have a good outcome, whereas those with moderate (a creatinine of 125–275μmol/L) to severe (a creatinine of greater than 275μmol/L) problems have a high incidence of pregnancy problems. The mother will be at risk of pre-eclampsia because of the underlying renal disease, which itself is often associated with hypertension. Pre-eclampsia can be difficult to identify in such women who often have pre-existing proteinuria and hypertension. Thus, blood pressure and renal function must be monitored carefully and hypertension treated appropriately to maintain good control. There is also an association with intrauterine growth restriction. Thus, fetal growth and wellbeing must be monitored regularly. Preterm labour or iatrogenic preterm delivery in the maternal interest is common. Renal function must be monitored carefully because significant decline in renal function will often trigger preterm delivery. When proteinuria appears or worsens but blood pressure remains normal or easily controlled, and overall renal function stable or minimally affected, then the pregnancy can continue with suitable maternal and fetal monitoring.

The effect of pregnancy on chronic renal disease
In connective tissue disorders such as scleroderma, SLE and polyarteritis nodosa, renal function may deteriorate rapidly, particularly with scleroderma and polyarteritis nodosa; in these conditions pregnancy may be best avoided. Patients with moderate to severe renal dysfunction must be warned about the risk of deterioration in their renal function. Reversible causes of reduction in renal function should also be considered, such as urinary tract infection or dehydration.

Women on dialysis and women with transplanted kidneys
Women on long-term haemodialysis or chronic ambulatory peritoneal dialysis have impaired fertility and conception is not common. When it does occur, there is a high miscarriage rate and often the prospects of pregnancy are so poor and the risk to the mother so great that therapeutic termination may be offered and carried out. When pregnancy does occur there is a very high risk of pre-eclampsia, growth restriction, severe hypertension and volume overload.

After renal transplantation, normal endocrine function is often restored relatively rapidly and it is not uncommon for women to become pregnant relatively soon after renal transplantation. Despite the transplant, there is a high incidence of miscarriage and a high risk of pregnancy problems such as intrauterine growth restriction or pre-eclampsia. Although most women will have a successful pregnancy outcome, the pregnancy itself may be complicated. If they do wish to become pregnant, they should ideally wait approximately 2 years after the transplantation to allow graft function to stabilize. The pregnancy does not appear to alter the long-term prognosis for the mother over her renal problems.

Management

In the management of patients with chronic renal disease it is important to have seen them before pregnancy to discuss the implications of pregnancy with them. The implications depend on the severity of the renal compromise, the underlying disease and the presence of hypertension. Particular problems exist for patients on dialysis or with transplants. They must be warned of the very high risk of pregnancy-related problems such as preterm labour, intrauterine growth restriction and pre-eclampsia, as well as the possibility of deteriorating renal function, particularly if renal disease is associated with underlying connective tissue problems. Counsellors should also take into account the overall prognosis for the patient's condition. Many patients with severe renal compromise and underlying disorders may themselves have a limited prognosis for their health and indeed their life and this must be taken into account. They must also be aware of the possibility that, should severe problems occur, termination of pregnancy may be required. Thus, they should enter pregnancy fully armed with the information about the management and possible complications.

If pregnancy does occur, careful monitoring of the maternal and fetal condition must be carried out regularly throughout the pregnancy. This is best done by collaboration between the renal physicians and an obstetrician with a special interest in medical disorders or renal problems during pregnancy. A regular assessment of renal function by creatinine clearance and quantitative proteinuria along with serum biochemistry must be carried out. Anaemia associated with renal compromise will require treatment with haematinics and may on occasion require a blood transfusion or the use of recombinant erythropoetin. Fetal growth should be monitored from the second half of pregnancy and umbilical artery Doppler waveform analysis will be of value in assessing the presence of severe placental problems. Regular biophysical monitoring by cardiotocography or biophysical profiles must be carried out, particularly when intrauterine growth restriction occurs. The clinician must be ever vigilant to the possibilities of pre-eclampsia which can be difficult to diagnose because the patient's biochemistry may be very disturbed and proteinuria and hypertension may already be present. Optimum control of blood pressure must occur. The patient and the clinicians must be aware of and alert to the possibility of preterm labour. After delivery, renal function may deteriorate and it is important to maintain the assessment of renal function and control of blood pressure following delivery. Drugs used to control blood pressure include adrenoceptor antagonists such as labetalol, calcium-channel blockers, such as nifedipine, and methyldopa. Consideration should be given to prescription of low-dose aspirin 75mg daily from the end of the first trimester to prevent problems such as intrauterine growth restriction and pre-eclampsia, particularly in patients with an underlying connective tissue problem such as SLE. However, the decision to use aspirin in patients with moderate to severe renal problems should involve the nephrologist in view of the problems that can arise through chronic inhibition of prostaglandin synthesis in the kidneys.

Chronic hypertension

Chronic hypertension antedating pregnancy is usually due to essential hypertension but renal disorders, connective tissue disease and other less common hypertensive conditions should be considered and excluded if not already done. Before pregnancy it is important to discuss the increased risk of pre-eclampsia and growth restriction associated with chronic hypertension and the need to reconsider antihypertensive medication in order to avoid drugs that may have detrimental effects for the fetus, such as angiotensin converting enzyme inhibitors. In addition, such therapy may be able to be discontinued during pregnancy because of the physiological fall in blood pressure that occurs through the course of a normal pregnancy, even when an underlying problem such as essential hypertension is present. In the antenatal period drug therapy should be reconsidered at the time of booking and often it would be best to change to a drug such as methyldopa in contrast to a β-blocker which may be associated with an increased risk of growth restriction. Urea, electrolytes and uric acid should be checked along with an assessment for proteinuria. If there is any possibility of renal involvement, a creatinine clearance and quantification of proteinuria should be carried out on a 24-hour urine collection. If there is any suspicion of underlying connective tissue disease, screening should be performed for antinuclear antibodies and antiphospholipid antibodies. Regular maternal and fetal surveillance should occur with a careful evaluation of fetal growth and regular assessment of fetal wellbeing if there is a disturbance of fetal growth. These women will be at risk of superimposed pre-eclampsia and this can sometimes be difficult to diagnose in terms of the blood pressure but an increase in plasma urate and the development of proteinuria is usually indicative of pre-eclampsia developing.

Although antihypertensive medication may be stopped in the early part of pregnancy, blood pressure climbs in the second half of pregnancy and it may reach levels that require treatment. Generally, however, if the diastolic blood pressure is maintained below 100mmHg, restarting therapy is not required. If therapy is restarted, then the drugs commonly prescribed for the treatment of hypertension during pregnancy can be used: adrenoceptor antagonists, such as labetalol, methyldopa and calcium-channel blockers such as nifedipine.

HEART DISEASE

CHANGES IN THE CARDIOVASCULAR SYSTEM

There is an increase in plasma volume with a lesser rise in red cell volume, leading to a physiological anaemia of pregnancy as discussed. The total blood volume may increase by up to 50% during pregnancy with an increase starting in the early part of the first trimester. Cardiac output also increases by up to 50%, again, starting from early on during pregnancy. The increase in cardiac output is mainly brought about by an increase in stroke volume with very little increase in resting heart rate. These changes are accompanied by a fall in peripheral resistance, explaining the normal reduction in blood pressure that occurs. Normally, blood pressure falls to reach a nadir at 20 weeks, then gradually climbs again to levels comparable with the normal situation by the mid- to late part of the third trimester. In the third trimester, the gravid uterus may inhibit venous return, particularly in supine positions, compromising cardiac output.

On examination, the woman may be noted to have warm extremities with dilated veins and on auscultation it is not uncommon for a third heart sound or a systolic flow murmur to be heard due to the hyperdynamic circulation of pregnancy.

THE PRESENTATION OF HEART DISEASE

In modern practice in the UK, rheumatic heart disease is rapidly declining and there is an increase in patients with congenital heart disease being seen. Most patients will know at the time of presentation of their history of heart disease and this should be readily evident on history-taking. It is unusual to identify a previously undiagnosed major cardiac problem. A

New York Heart Association Classification

Grades	
1	Patients with cardiac disease but no cardiac decompensation. There is no limitation during ordinary physical exercise.
2	No symptoms of cardiac decompensation at rest but slight limitation by dyspnoea with activities such as walking.
3	Marked limitation of physical activity, although no cardiac symptoms at rest.
4	Breathlessness at rest.

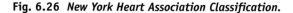

Fig. 6.26 *New York Heart Association Classification.*

history of dyspnoea, particularly on exertion, and at rest, and syncope should be sought. On examination, care should also be taken to identify any scars from previous cardiac surgery and any thrills or murmurs or evidence of heart failure.

Heart disease is usually graded on the basis the New York Heart Association Classification (**Fig. 6.26**).

Regardless of aetiology, patients who are asymptomatic before pregnancy and have only Grade I or II symptoms on the New York Heart Association Classification are unlikely to have major problems during a pregnancy.

VALVULAR HEART DISEASE

Many patients with valvular heart disease will have had a valve replacement before pregnancy. This is usually a mechanical valve as bioprosthetic valves deteriorate more rapidly and are not usually used in young women. The main consideration with valvular heart disease when mechanical valves are in place is that of anticoagulation. As discussed, warfarin places the patient at increased risk of warfarin embryopathy and fetal bleeding, particularly at the time of delivery. However, transferring to heparin is not always easy and may be associated with an increased risk of valve thrombosis. In order to avoid the risk of warfarin embryopathy, transfer to heparin would have to occur by 6 weeks and often this is impractical. In this situation the patient should be aware of the risk of warfarin embryopathy which is approximately 4%, and may be significantly lower than this with good warfarin control. Thus, it is better for the patient to undergo prepregancy counselling before facing these problems during pregnancy. The risk of fetal bleeding with warfarin also has to be appreciated. This is particularly high at the time of delivery and usually patients will be admitted in the late third trimester and switched to therapeutic doses of heparin in anticipation of delivery which may be organized electively. Some women prefer to avoid any risk to the baby and wish to stay on heparin throughout pregnancy, particularly if control is required. The patient must also be aware that she would be at risk of heparin complications such as heparin-induced osteoporosis.

Occasionally, mitral stenosis is encountered during pregnancy. The main risk is of pulmonary oedema developing which may be triggered by problems such as chest infection and situations in which tachycardia occurs. This is because there will be less time to allow adequate left ventricular filling and a subsequent backing up of blood in the left atrium and lungs leading to pulmonary oedema. A reduction in the heart rate by use of β-blockers will increase the left ventricle filling time with subsequent increases in volume. If there is significant deterioration, then surgical treatment may be required by techniques such as baloon valvotomy or closed mitral valvotomy. Situations in which the patient has to be placed on a cardiopulmonary bypass, such as during the valve replacement, place the fetus at considerable risk and ideally should not be performed during pregnancy. The treatment of pulmonary oedema when it arises is similar to normal and diuretics should be administered. If atrial fibrillation occurs, then digoxin can be given and consideration should be given to anticoagulation to prevent development of an atrial thrombus.

CONGENITAL HEART DISEASE

Patients with acyanotic congenital heart disease generally do well during pregnancy. Often the congenital heart disease will have been corrected or they may suffer from a problem such as congenital aortic stenosis. Significant problems tend to occur when there is pulmonary hypertension which may be primary or due to the development of Eisenmenger syndrome. These patients need specialized care and often fetal growth may be affected with an increased risk of a baby that is small for dates. Delivery will usually require to be carried out by caesarean section to avoid the stress of labour in an already seriously compromised patient. These women require careful care by a combined obstetric and cardiology service.

CARDIOMYOPATHY

The most common cardiomyopathy seen is hypertrophic cardiomyopathy. These patients often cope reasonably well with pregnancy and are usually treated with β blockers to allow adequate time for ventricular filling. Thus they will be at risk of growth restriction in the fetus due to long-term administration of β-blockers. Similarly, epidural anaesthesia is usually avoided as it reduces the afterload, in turn, reducing left ventricular filling.

Finally, antibiotic prophylaxis is no longer considered absolutely essential during labour for women with heart disease. However, it is usual practice to treat women undergoing caesarean section with prophylactic antibiotics.

EPILEPSY

Up to 1% of women suffer from epilepsy, thus, this condition is relatively commonplace in obstetric practice. They have particular problems that must be addressed in the period before they become pregnant, including contraception as well as particular problems during the antenatal intrapartum and postpartum periods.

Epilepsy can present for the first time during pregnancy, although this is uncommon. It presents for the first time in between 40 and 50 out of 100,000 women in their reproductive years. Pregnancy has no effect on the incidence of epilepsy first presenting during pregnancy. The important point is to differentiate it from eclampsia which would usually be associated with hypertension or proteinuria. Any patient having such a seizure should have a full neurological assessment and objective investigations to exclude intracerebral tumours, arteriovenous malformations and cerebral venous thrombosis. The assessment will therefore include investigations such as a computerized tomography scan of the head and an electroencephalogram.

THE EFFECT OF EPILEPSY AND ANTICONVULSANTS

Epilepsy and anticonvulsants have several effects on pregnancy. There is an increased incidence of pregnancy complications including hyperemesis, anaemia, vaginal bleeding and having a fetus that is small for dates. The anaemia may be related to folic acid antagonism by anticonvulsant drugs but the other complications mentioned are poorly explained. There is an increased risk of fetal abnormalities which may be related to genetic factors but more particularly to anticonvulsants and this may be due to folic acid antagonism. In addition, some anticonvulsants antagonize vitamin K and will expose the neonate to an increased risk of haemorrhagic disease of the newborn. This may be dealt with by prescribing vitamin K supplements to the mother in late pregnancy and also providing the neonate with vitamin K at the time of delivery. There is no contraindication to women breast-feeding while taking anticonvulsants except for phenobarbitone which is likely to result in the baby being sedated with subsequent difficulties feeding. Mothers often wish to know whether or not their child will be at risk of suffering from epilepsy: the risk to the child is increased from mothers who have had idiopathic seizures before the age of 18 years or if seizures occur during pregnancy. Finally, children born of mothers with epilepsy also suffer from neurodevelopment problems and learning difficulties. This may be related to exposure of the developing brain to anticonvulsants (**Fig. 6.27**).

The risk that mothers tend to worry about most is that of fetal abnormality. The common fetal abnormalities encountered with patients suffering from epilepsy and taking anticonvulsants are cleft lip and palate, cardiac defects and neural tube defects. Minor abnormalities include club foot and hypospadias. Furthermore, dysmorphic features can be seen such as hypoplasia of distal phalanges and nails, hypertelorism, low set ears, long philtrum, irregular teeth and a wide mouth (**Fig. 6.28**).

Effects of epilepsy and anticonvulsants on pregnancy

Pregnancy complications increased
    Hyperemesis
    Anaemia
    Vaginal bleeding
    Small for dates fetus

Vitamin K and folic acid antagonism

Fetal abnormality

Haemorrhagic disease of the newborn

Increased risk of epilepsy in offspring with maternal age of onset at <18 years or seizures in pregnancy

Neurodevelopmental problems and learning difficulties

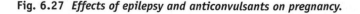

Fig. 6.27 *Effects of epilepsy and anticonvulsants on pregnancy.*

Fig. 6.28 *Fetal abnormality.*

Fetal abnormality	
Major	Neural tube defect Cardiac defect Cleft lip and palate
Minor	Club foot Hypospadias
Dysmorphic feature	Hypertelorism Long philtrum Low set ears Wide mouth Irregular teeth Hypoplasia of distal phalanges and nails

Epilepsy itself may be related to a fetal anomaly in a proportion of patients as opposed to the anticonvulsant drugs, but the majority of problems appear to be linked to the anticonvulsants. No drug is free of risk but the risk increases dramatically when multiple drugs are used, ranging from a risk of significant abnormalities of 3% for women on monotherapy rising to 23% for women on four drugs. Thus, whenever possible, monotherapy should be given.

THE EFFECT OF PREGNANCY ON EPILEPSY AND ON ANTICONVULSANTS

Pregnancy also has an effect on epilepsy and on anticonvulsants. There may be a change in seizure frequency with up to one quarter of women showing an increase in seizure frequency, up to one quarter showing a decline and up to one half staying unchanged. The change in frequency is unpredictable and is not influenced by the type of seizure, drug, the patient's age or the previous pattern in an earlier pregnancy. These changes may be related to problems such as hormonal and metabolic changes of pregnancy, sleep deprivation, stress, hyperventilation and exhaustion, particularly in labour and, in addition, noncompliance. Noncompliance is relatively common as women are aware of the potential problems of anticonvulsant drugs on their baby. However, they often stop their therapy at a stage during pregnancy when they are passed the time of risk for the developing embryo and thus expose themselves to the risk of seizures without having the benefit of prevention of fetal problems. The most worrying abnormality is perhaps neural tube defect. The neural tube closes at 7 weeks' gestation. Stopping therapy after that stage cannot prevent such problems.

Most anticonvulsant drugs show a fall in total levels during pregnancy due to changes in plasma protein binding and drug clearance, yet most patients see no increase in seizure frequency. This is because free drug levels change much less than the total drug level and it is the free drug level that correlates with seizure frequency. This has implications for monitoring therapy during pregnancy. For example, for a decline in total phenytoin levels of approximately 56%, the free drug level will only by altered by just over 30%. Whereas with sodium valproate, the total drug levels may fall by 39% but the free drug levels increase by 25%. Thus, while drug levels may confirm compliance, their assessment does not provide a reliable guide on which to base dose adjustments. Such adjustment, because of the complexity of the levels, requires the input from an obstetrician or a physician with a special interest in this area. In general terms, however, the dose should be increased if there is an increase in seizure frequency, provided compliance is confirmed. If there are side effects, the dose should be lowered.

THE MANAGEMENT OF EPILEPSY

Women with epilepsy should be encouraged to have a planned pregnancy in order to obtain the maximum benefits from periconception care. They should use reliable contraception. The effectiveness of hormonal contraception is reduced in women taking anticonvulsants that are enzyme inducing such as carbemazepine, phenytoin and phenobarbitone. If a combined 'oestrogen-containing' oral contraceptive pill is used, then it should contain at least 50µg of oestradiol/day. Alternatively, nonhormonal methods should be used (**Fig. 6.29**).

Women contemplating pregnancy should be advised about the increased risk of major malformations, minor abnormalities and dysmorphic features, but it should be emphasized to them that the majority of babies born to mothers with epilepsy are normal. In addition, it should be emphasized that the abnormalities may be linked not only to drugs but also to a genetic predisposition. The management of pregnancy should be discussed and, in particular, prenatal screening using serum testing and detailed ultrasound scanning to detect major fetal abnormalities. The patient should be informed that grand mal convulsions during pregnancy carry serious risks for both mother and fetus and that anticonvulsants

---

Hormonal contraception for women taking enzyme-inducing anticonvulsants

Combined oral contraceptive pill: 50µg ethinyl oestradiol pill should be used.

May require even higher dose of oestradiol if breakthrough bleeding occurs.

Reduce pill-free interval to 4 days and use four packs of combined oral contraceptive pills consecutively to enhance contraceptive cover. This may also prevent seizures if they are hormonally triggered at the time of menstruation.

Progesterone-only pill: should only be used if there is no other acceptable method, and doubling of the daily dose may be effective.

Depo-progestogen: reduce dosing interval from 12 weeks to 10 weeks for Depo-Provera®.

Fig. 6.29 *Hormonal contraception for women taking enzyme-inducing anticonvulsants.*

should be continued to avoid such problems. In view of the association between anticonvulsant drugs and neural tube defects and the role of folic acid in preventing such defects, a folic acid supplement should be started before pregnancy. The recommended dose should be 5mg/day while attempting to conceive and for at least the first 12 weeks of the pregnancy. Furthermore, before embarking on a pregnancy, the anticonvulsant therapy should be reviewed. This should include assessment of the continued need for the agents and assessment of the type of agents and number of agents employed. In addition, the need for vitamin K should be discussed. This should be prescribed in a dose of 20mg orally from 36 weeks' gestation to the mother or earlier if a preterm delivery is anticipated and 1mg vitamin K given intramuscularly to the baby at birth. If an adjustment of anticonvulsant drugs is carried out or if anticonvulsant drugs are withdrawn, the clinician must be aware of the possible implications to the patient's life because recurrent seizures in a patient who has been seizure-free for some time may lead to the withdrawal of her driving licence and may have implications for her job.

Antenatal management
Ideally, patients with epilepsy should be managed in a consultant unit with a team with a special interest in such problems but after initial assessment and planning, shared care is appropriate. Seizure control and drugs should be carefully noted and also folic acid prescribed. Further discussion of fetal abnormality and screening for it should be carried out. At 18–20 weeks' gestation detailed anomaly scanning should be performed and this will usually be preceded at 15–16 weeks' gestation by α-fetoprotein testing. Blood levels can be monitored to check compliance. Drugs should not be altered without expert advice simply on the basis of drug levels. Vitamin K should be started at 36 weeks' gestation.

Management during labour
Women with epilepsy should be managed in a consultant unit and obviously should avoid birthing techniques such as a birthing pool. Anticonvulsant agents should be continued throughout labour and ideally doses should not be missed because there is likely to be an increase in stress, hyperventilation and sleep deprivation during the course of labour which may trigger seizures. Postpartum women should be encouraged to breast-feed unless they are on phenobarbitone. If drugs have been increased in dose during pregnancy, they should be reduced to the prepregnancy level after delivery. This reduction should be gradual. Reassurance and care should be given about infant care and the mother should avoid particular risks such as taking baths and ensuring that fires and cookers are guarded. Contraception should be discussed. The baby should be carefully examined for fetal abnormalities.

SKIN DISORDERS

There are normal changes that occur within the skin during pregnancy. There is an increase in spider naevi, and palmar erythema and striae gravidarum are commonplace, a mild degree of gum hypertrophy and gingivitis can occur. Increased pigmentation can occur such as chloasma on the face and a prominent linea nigra on the abdomen and the woman should avoid excess sun exposure. Hair growth can increase, although alopaecia can occur.

PRURITIS GRAVIDARUM
This itching condition is secondary to pregnancy-induced intrahepatic cholestasis. It is also associated with an increased incidence of prematurity and stillbirth, although its course is

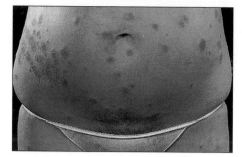

Fig. 6.30 *Pemphigoid gestationis in pregnancy. (From Symonds, E. Malcolm and Macpherson, Marion B. A. 'Diagnosis in Color: Obstetrics and Gynecology' (Mosby-Wolfe, 1997), with permission.)*

benign for the mother. A diagnosis can be made by a modest increase in bilirubin, although the standard liver function test may be normal, jaundice may occur. Other causes of jaundice should be excluded if frank jaundice occurs. The condition will regress with delivery. The best treatment for the itch is cholestyramine for patients with increased bilirubin levels. Antihistamines can be tried but are not usually of value and ultraviolet B radiation can also reduce symptoms. The fetus should be monitored for growth and wellbeing.

PRURIGO OF PREGNANCY

This is an itchy papular eruption which occurs in approximately 1 in 300 pregnancies. It is not associated with any adverse risks to the mother. It usually begins in the early part of the third trimester and manifests as discrete itchy papules over the extensor surfaces of the limbs and the abdomen. It is not vesicular in nature. Oral antihistamines and topical steroid creams are of value in controlling it.

PEMPHIGOID GESTATIONIS

Pemphigoid gestationis – previously named herpes gestationis – is a more worrying condition during pregnancy. This is a rare condition which may be associated with autoimmune disease. It usually starts in the second trimester with itching preceding a widespread polymorphic eruption with vescicles and bullae formation. Pruritis is a major symptom and a definitive diagnosis can be made with skin biopsy. Treatment includes oral antihistamine to relieve the itch, topical steroids and, if severe, oral steroids will be required (**Fig. 6.30**).

chapter 7

The Complications of Pregnancy

INTRAUTERINE GROWTH RESTRICTION AND FETAL MONITORING

Although the World Health Organization definition of low birth weight is 2.5kg, it is also important to consider maturity. Gestation must be taken into account with regard to birth weight. For example, an infant weighing 2.5kg born at term would be small for dates, whereas an infant of 2.5kg at 33 weeks' gestation would be appropriately grown. Thus, it is important to be aware of the use of birth weight centiles in the assessment of fetal growth. This is critically important in assessing pregnancies in which the fetal growth rate is considered to be impaired: intrauterine growth restriction (IUGR). In the assessment of the fetus *in utero*, it can often be difficult, even with the use of birth weight centiles, to determine whether a baby is congenitally small, that is, small because it is normal and destined to be small, or small because of placental dysfunction leading to poor fetal growth or another pathological cause of poor growth.

Fetal growth can be influenced by many factors including chromosomal constitution and genetic factors such as race and sex, exposure to toxins such as alcohol and tobacco, the development of intrauterine infection, maternal nutrition and the extent of trophoblastic invasion into the mother to allow the development of an adequate utero–placental circulation to supply the fetus with nutrients and oxygen. Ultrasound is used to examine fetal growth *in utero* by performing serial scans. Critical to the assessment of fetal growth is an accurate knowledge of the stage of gestation. This illustrates the importance of establishing an accurate gestational age early during the pregnancy. The time of conception it is not usually known, except in women having fertility treatment. It is usual to accept the menstrual dates if the mother is certain of the date of the last menstrual period, the cycle is regular (ideally 28 days in duration), there has been no vaginal bleeding and no recent use of hormonal contraception (the pill withdrawal bleed is an inaccurate event by which to judge subsequent ovulation). When the ultrasound dates are within a week of the certain menstrual dates, the menstrual dates are accepted. When there is a discrepancy or one of the factors is an irregular cycle or the last period was a pill withdrawal bleed, then the ultrasound date is used. When doubt still exists, a second ultrasound scan can be performed later (**Fig. 7.1**).

THE DETECTION OF INTRAUTERINE GROWTH RESTRICTION

A great deal of an obstetrician's time and energy is spent on attempts to identify a fetus which is small for dates. Subsequently, attempts are made to determine whether a small-for-dates fetus is pathologically small due to factors such as placental insufficiency, or whether it is congenitally small. Thereafter, appropriate monitoring of the pregnancy is required.

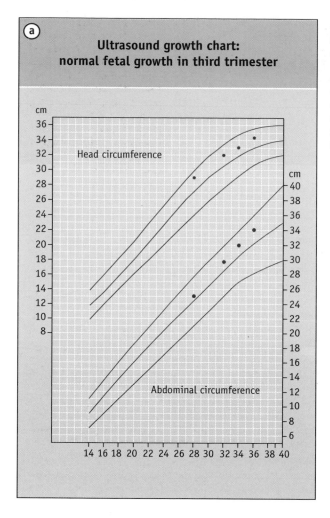

Fig. 7.1 *(a) Ultrasound growth chart illustrating normal fetal growth in the third trimester on measurement of abdominal circumference and head circumference (lines on the circumference charts indicate mean +/- 2 standard deviations).*

Traditionally, abdominal palpation has been used to assess uterine size and indirectly fetal growth. Although it may pick up the extremes, such as a baby which is very small for dates or very large for dates, it cannot be considered reliable or accurate.

In an attempt to improve the situation, many obstetricians now measure the symphysis–fundal height in an attempt to give a more objective assessment of fetal growth. This is done by placing a measuring tape on the upper border of the symphysis pubis and measuring the height of the uterine fundus in centimetres. This, particularly if the measurements are carried out by the same individual in a serial manner, is usually regarded as being better than abdominal palpation alone.

Perhaps the most objective assessment is that of ultrasound and various parameters are employed. The best parameters to identify poor fetal growth are usually considered to be the abdominal circumference or area. This is particularly useful because it includes the fetal liver which will be rich in glycogen stores in a well-nourished fetus and consequently will be smaller if the fetus were undernourished. In addition, combinations of measurements or ratios are also used, such as the ratio of the head area to the trunk area or the crown–rump

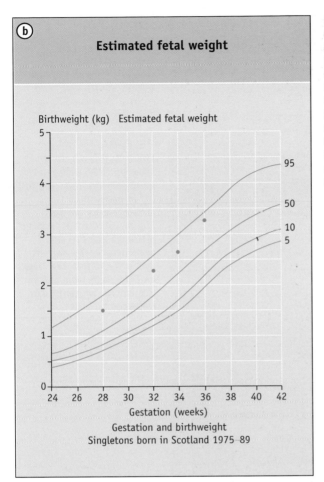

Fig. 7.1 *(b) The abdominal circumference measurement is converted to an estimate of fetal weight which lies between the 50th and 95th centiles in this case. (c) Ultrasound image of abdominal circumference being measured. (d) Ultrasound image of head circumference being measured.*

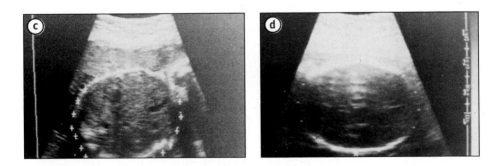

length coupled with the trunk area. In placental insufficiency, the growth within the trunk area will fall off before the head because there is head-sparing by the fetus to allow brain development. Thus, the most common measurements employed are usually of the head, such as head circumference, and abdominal circumference (**Fig. 7.2**).

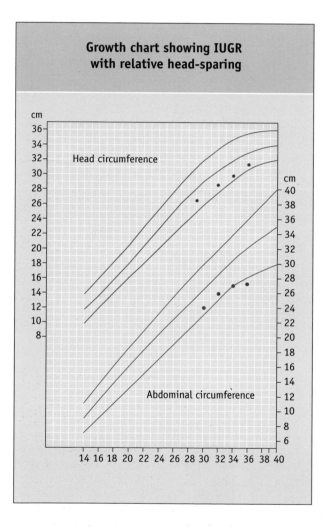

Fig. 7.2 *Growth chart showing IUGR with relative head-sparing. Note the fall off in abdominal circumference growth. Liquor volume was reduced although the CTG was satisfactory. The patient was delivered at 36+ weeks and the baby weighed 2.1 kg. The placenta was infarcted.*

Fig. 7.2 *cont.*

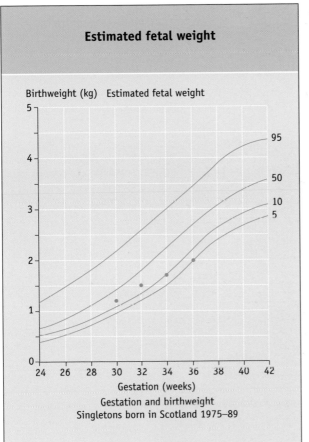

Ultrasound alone does not provide a sufficient accuracy to identify a fetus that is truly growth restricted with a significant degree of placental insufficiency. As a result of this, several other techniques have been developed. Doppler ultrasound is used to assess blood flow in the umbilical artery (**Fig. 7.3**). It can measure blood flow velocity waveforms which can be indicative of a high resistance in the fetal part of the placenta which is associated with abnormalities in the placental vasculature seen in IUGR. The high resistance in the fetal placenta will result in a reduction or loss of flow during diastole of the fetal cardiac cycle and this can be seen using Doppler ultrasound. A fetus with loss of end diastolic flow is usually considered to be at extremely high risk (**Figs 7.4** and **7.5**).

In an attempt to screen for underlying placental insufficiency, many tests have been evaluated. The one that currently appears most effective is to perform Doppler flow velocity waveform analysis of the utero–placental circulation, that is, the maternal blood vessels supplying the placenta, at 18–22 weeks' gestation. In a normal situation, a notch will be seen in the Doppler waveform (**Fig. 7.6**). By 22 weeks' gestation, the notch will usually have disappeared. This disappearance is thought to be caused by the second wave of

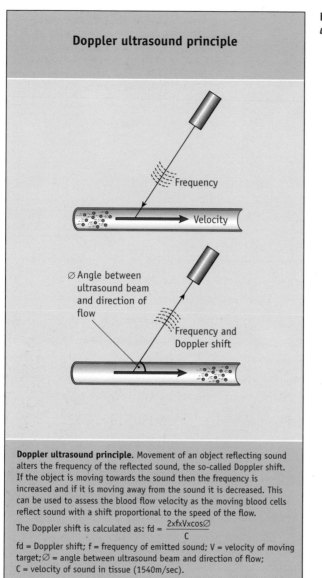

Doppler ultrasound principle

Frequency

Velocity

∅ Angle between
ultrasound beam
and direction of
flow

Frequency and
Doppler shift

Fig. 7.3 *Doppler
ultrasound principle.*

Doppler ultrasound principle. Movement of an object reflecting sound
alters the frequency of the reflected sound, the so-called Doppler shift.
If the object is moving towards the sound then the frequency is
increased and if it is moving away from the sound it is decreased. This
can be used to assess the blood flow velocity as the moving blood cells
reflect sound with a shift proportional to the speed of the flow.

The Doppler shift is calculated as: $fd = \dfrac{2 \times f \times V \times \cos \varnothing}{C}$

fd = Doppler shift; f = frequency of emitted sound; V = velocity of moving
target; ∅ = angle between ultrasound beam and direction of flow;
C = velocity of sound in tissue (1540m/sec).

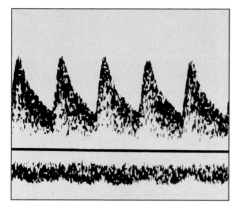

Fig. 7.4 *Normal umbilical artery flow velocity waveform (upper part) showing systolic peaks and continued flow in diastole. The lower part shows umbilical venous flow which can be seen to fluctuate with fetal breathing movements.*

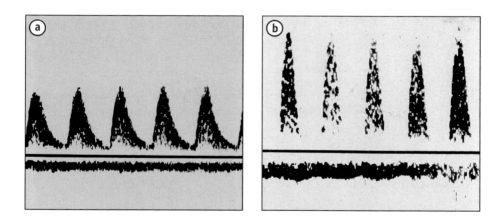

Fig. 7.5 *Doppler flow velocity waveforms showing reduced (a) and absent (b) end diastolic flow in a fetus with severe growth restriction.*

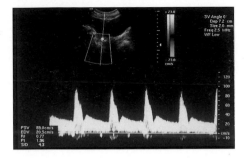

Fig. 7.6 *Uterine artery Doppler ultrasound examination showing notching.*

Factors associated with the small for gestational age fetus

Pre-existing maternal problems	Chronic hypertension Connective tissue disease, such as systemic lupus erythematosus Social deprivation Environmental problems Smoking High altitude Drug abuse Poor nutrition Low body weight (<50kg at booking)
Medical or obstetric conditions arising in pregnancy	Pre-eclampsia Antepartum haemorrhage
Fetal factors	Chromosomal abnormalities, e.g. triploidy Structural abnormalities Congenital infections, e.g. rubella
Placental problems	Impaired trophoblast invasion

Fig. 7.7 *Factors associated with the small for gestational age fetus.*

trophoblastic invasion into the maternal circulation, which allows the final development of a high-flow, low-pressure system supplying the placenta. Persistence of the notch suggests that the second wave of trophoblastic invasion has not occurred satisfactorily and such pregnancies are considered to be at high risk of growth restriction or pre-eclampsia.

THE INVASION OF THE MATERNAL CIRCULATION BY TROPHOBLASTS

The maternal blood supplies the placenta via the uterine, arcuate and spiral arteries which normally supply the endometrium. After implantation, an increase in blood flow to the placental implantation site is required and these spiral arteries undergo profound changes. Trophoblasts from the invading placenta invade these vessels, destroying the muscular and elastic layers and replacing them with fibrinoid material and lining the vessels with trophoblasts. This process occurs in two waves, the first at the primary implantation time in early pregnancy lasting for several weeks. This reaches the decidual layer of the spiral arteries. The second wave starts at 14–16 weeks' gestation and is completed in 4 weeks. This wave of invasion allows the spiral arteries to be invaded by trophoblasts to a much greater depth, resulting in a high-flow, low-pressure circulation in contrast to the high-pressure, low-flow circulation of the non-pregnant situation. The blood from the spiral arteries bathes the trophoblastic villi of the placenta and oxygen and nutrients are transferred across to the fetal circulation. This change allows a dramatic increase in blood flow from approximately 50ml/min in the first trimester to 500ml/min at term. This process is inadequate in pre-eclampsia and IUGR (**Fig. 7.8**) resulting in placental insufficiency. When the process fails there is a reduced perfusion of the intervillus space (**Fig. 7.9**). In pre-eclampsia this is associated with maternal hypertension and a disturbance of metabolism, whereas in IUGR, in the absence of pre-eclampsia, there appears to be minimal maternal derangement.

It has been usual in the past to divide IUGR into two types, symmetrical in which both the head and the abdomen are reduced in growth, and asymmetrical in which there is sparing of the head. The former is more characteristic of underlying congenital problems such as viral infections or genetic or chromosomal problems, whereas the latter is associated with placental insufficiency (**Fig. 7.7**).

THE MANAGEMENT OF INTRAUTERINE GROWTH RESTRICTION

Identification

The currently available methods for screening in an unselected population are not considered accurate for widespread clinical use. However, screening should be carried out for patients at an increased risk such as those with a past history of severe or recurrent IUGR, or pre-eclampsia, and patients with established medical conditions associated with growth restriction such as chronic hypertension or systemic lupus erythematosus. The usual screening technique is to perform an assessment of the utero–placental blood flow at 18 and 22 weeks' gestation to look for notching. Fetal growth is assessed starting in the late second trimester or early third trimester with measurements carried out every 14 days, with abdominal circumference being the usual ultrasound-based method of screening. If a problem is identified, there is little that can be done as intervention. Low-dose aspirin has been used in an attempt to prevent the problem by inhibiting platelet function, which may be responsible for some of the vascular abnormalities seen in conditions such as IUGR or pre-eclampsia, but there is no good evidence that this is successful. Some obstetricians still use this for high-risk patients such as those with notching or a bad past history, but its efficacy remains uncertain. Recent evidence suggests that supplementing anti-oxidant vitamins (vitamins C and E) may be of value where persistent notching is found. The important factor is to detect the problem and monitor the pregnancy carefully when it arises. It should also be noted that women with an unexplained elevated α-fetoprotein result on testing at 15 weeks' gestation have a higher incidence of IUGR (and other complications such as abruption).

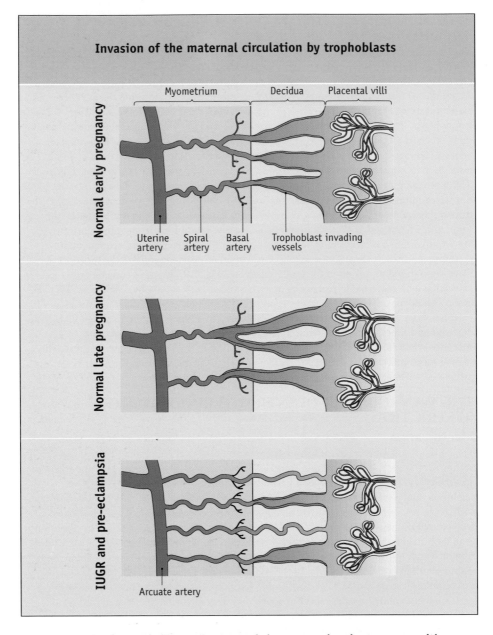

Fig 7.8 *Invasion by trophoblasts. Upper panel shows normal early pregnancy with invasion to level of the decidua. Middle panel shows invasion to level of myometrium following second wave of trophoblast invasion. Lower panel: inadequate implantation of IUGR and pre-eclampsia. Broken lines indicate trophoblast invading blood vessels.*

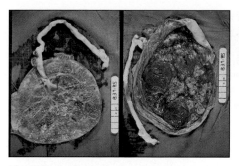

Fig. 7.9 *A placenta showing severe infarction on the fetal surface from a pregnancy with pre-eclampsia and IUGR delivered at 28 weeks' gestation. Left: fetal surface, right: maternal surface.*

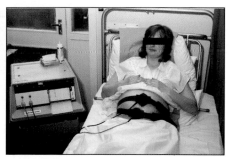

Fig. 7.10 *Patient undergoing antenatal cardiotocography.*

The further management of suspected IUGR

Once suspected IUGR has been identified through clinical assessment or ultrasound, it is important to evaluate the pregnancy for any underlying cause of growth restriction and monitor the fetal condition. Critical to this assessment is the gestation at which the IUGR becomes apparent.

In early-onset IUGR (before 32–34 weeks' gestation), the fetus may be symmetrically small. Many of these fetuses represent the lower end of the normal spectrum of fetal size, but when the symmetrical growth restriction appears more severe, consideration should be given to underlying problems such as chromosomal abnormalities or congenital infections. The fetus should therefore be scanned for underlying structural anomalies or ultrasound markers indicating chromosomal problems such as Down syndrome in which duodenal atresia or congenital heart problems can occur and for which nuchal thickening is evident on ultrasound. When there is a strong risk of chromosomal abnormality, then karyotyping of the fetus by fetal blood sampling should be considered.

The most common situation is late-onset IUGR (beyond 34 weeks' gestation), this is usually due to placental insufficiency and an asymmetric pattern of growth will be seen. Umbilical artery flow velocity waveforms assessed by Doppler ultrasound are also valuable. In this situation loss of end diastolic flow suggests that the fetus is at high risk.

ANTENATAL MONITORING OF THE FETUS

It is critically important in the management of IUGR to determine whether or not the fetal condition is satisfactory or whether there is any evidence of fetal compromise. Should there be evidence of fetal compromise, then if the fetus is potentially viable, delivery usually by caesarean section is required. If the fetal condition is satisfactory and monitoring tests are indicative of fetal wellbeing, then the pregnancy can continue with further monitoring until gestation is judged to be sufficient to allow a delivery without the risks of prematurity. When there is a concomitant maternal problem such as pre-eclampsia, delivery may be required in the interests of the mother regardless of the fetal condition. The mainstay of fetal monitoring is antenatal fetal cardiotocography (**Fig. 7.10**).

The cardiotocograph (CTG) consists of two transducers. The first of these is the cardiograph transducer which is a Doppler ultrasound device to measure fetal heart rate. This is held in place with a strap around the mother's abdomen, the fetal heart having been localized. A further device, the tocodynamometer, is also strapped to the mother's abdomen and picks up contractions: during a contraction the uterus moves forward compressing the tocodynamometer. The information from these two devices is shown graphically on the cardiotocograph. The upper channel shows the heart rate and the lower shows any contractions. In the antenatal period the uterus is not entirely quiescent and irregular contractions occur but are not usually painful. These are termed Braxton–Hicks contractions and represent part of the normal uterine physiology with their frequency increasing towards term. The normal fetal heart rate lies between 110 and 160 beats/minute with a reduction towards the lower end of this range occurring towards term. There are short-term fluctuations in the fetal heart rate due to changes in the activity of the autonomic nervous system. This is termed beat-to-beat variability and is usually greater than 5 and 10 beats/minute. In addition, accelerations and decelerations can occur.

Accelerations can be defined as an increase in fetal heart rate over the baseline by a minimum of 15 beats/minute for a minimum of 15 seconds. Accelerations on an antenatal cardiotocograph are usually seen in conjunction with fetal movements or with a uterine contraction. In the normal course of events, a minimum of two accelerations will be seen in a 20-minute period in an antenatal cardiotocograph. Often they are present at a much higher rate than this. On occasion, there may be periods when the accelerations are not seen due to periods of fetal sleep. However, a period of 40 minutes is sufficient to allow for this, hence the absence of accelerations on an antenatal cardiotocograph over a 40-minute period is a worrying feature because accelerations are rarely present in a compromised fetus.

Decelerations can also occur. Variable decelerations can be indicative of a reduced amniotic fluid volume with cord compression during fetal movements or contraction. This is a worrying situation. Variable decelerations are irregular in their character. When the umbilical cord is compressed, the venous flow returning to the fetus is impaired, first resulting in reduced venous return to the heart and a transient minor increase in heart rate is occasionally seen. With arterial compression there is a reflex slowing of the heart which returns to normal as the arterial pressure eases off. There may again be a minor acceleration at the end of the deceleration as venous return will be impaired for slightly longer than the arterial compression. Late decelerations on an antenatal tracing are usually indicative of hypoxia.

Thus, when assessing an antenatal cardiotocograph, it is important to be aware of the underlying basal rate, the basal variability, the presence of acceleration and any decelerations (**Fig. 7.11** and **7.12**).

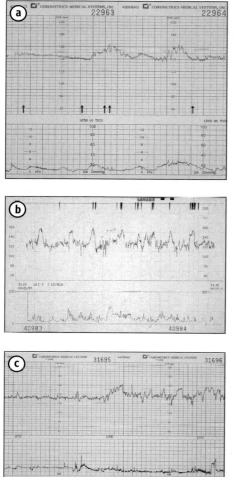

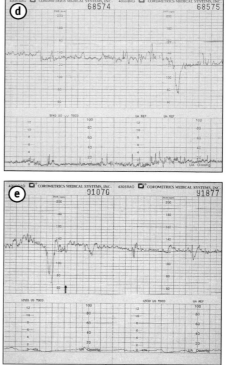

Fig. 7.11 *Normal antenatal CTGs (a, b) showing accelerations and marks on the trace indicating the timing of fetal movements; (c) shows a normal pattern without fetal movement marks. Antenatal CTGs (d, e) show variable decelerations in fetuses compromised by IUGR and oligohydramnios.*

The use of cardiotocography on its own is also termed the nonstress test as various techniques have been employed in an attempt to stimulate the fetus and look at the resulting fetal behaviour. These have included the oxytocin stress test in which an oxytocin infusion is set up until mild uterine activity occurs and the response of the fetal heart to this can be assessed. Vibroacoustic stimulation has also been used in which a device is held against the mother's abdomen which produces noise and vibration and the fetal response can be studied. A physiologically based test is the nipple stimulation test which uses stimulation to the nipples to produce oxytocin which in turn can trigger uterine contractility. However, none of these tests is widely used in practice in the UK and the mainstay is cardiotocography without any stress being applied.

FETAL MOVEMENT COUNTING

The use of fetal movement counts can be of value in assessing fetal wellbeing. The most commonly used technique used in the UK is the Cardiff Kick Chart in which mothers record

Fetal heart rate patterns and possible diagnoses

Antenatal heart rate pattern	Abnormalities and possible causes
Fetal tachycardia	Maternal pyrexia Chorionamnionitis Fetal anaemia
Variable decelerations	Cord compression during fetal movement usually associated with oligohydramnios
Late deceleration	Fetal hypoxia
Reduced beat-to-beat variability	Mild due to fetal sleep or opiate exposure Marked or associated with other abnormalities such as late decelerations indicative of hypoxia
Persistent, marked bradycardia	Uncommon, can be associated with congenital heart block

Fig. 7.12 *Fetal heart rate patterns and possible diagnoses.*

the time taken each day to feel 10 fetal movements. A reduction in fetal movements, and particularly the absence of fetal movements, can be indicative of an underlying problem with the fetus. If this does occur, the mother will require to be reassured and usually a cardiotocograph and/or ultrasound assessment of the fetus will be performed to allay her fears. It should noted that some women are unable to perceive fetal movements and an ultrasound scan is employed so that fetal movements can be seen of which the mother is unaware.

FETAL BIOPHYSICAL PROFILE

This is an ultrasound-based method of determining fetal wellbeing (**Fig. 7.13**). The profile has five variables, the first of these is the nonstress cardiotocograph, the other variables are 'fetal breathing' movements, gross fetal body movements, fetal tone and amniotic fluid volume. In practice it is unusual to perform all five of the variables and modifications include an assessment of the three movement parameters and amniotic fluid volume or a combination of the nonstress cardiotocograph and amniotic fluid volume. When the ultrasound-based test is employed because of variations in fetal activity, observation may have to continue for up to 40 minutes before the test can be considered abnormal. The parameters that are used in the biophysical profile represent a series of markers of fetal behaviour which give an idea of the fetal condition at that time, whereas a reduction of amniotic fluid volume is considered to be due to a reduction in perfusion of the fetal kidney and thereby reduced fetal urine production. This, therefore, is a marker of chronic stress on the fetus with a resultant redistribution in organ perfusion favouring the brain and away from the abdominal viscera and fetal kidneys. Thus, the combination of a nonstress cardiotocography and amniotic fluid volume give an assessment of both acute and chronic fetal condition.

The biophysical profile

		Score
Nonstress test	Reactive is two or more fetal heart rate accelerations in a 20-min period	2
	Nonreactive is none or one fetal heart rate acceleration	0
Fetal breathing movements	One episode of prolonged breathing (>60 s) within 30-min	2
	Fetal breathing movement absent	0
Gross fetal body movements, i.e. movements of the trunk	Fetal movements present with a minimum of three movements within a 30-min period	2
	Fetal movements absent or reduced	0
Fetal tone, i.e. limb flexion and extension	Normal: one episode of limb flexion and extension	2
	Abnormal: extremities extended with no return to flexion	0
Amniotic fluid volume	Normal: largest pocket of fluid is >1cm in vertical diameter in a cord-free pool*	2
	Decreased liquor volume	0
		Total score = 0–10

*Many obstetricians prefer to use a greater limit than 1cm in assessing liquor volume and many use a cut off of 2 or 3cm.
Alternatively, the amniotic fluid index, derived from measuring fluid volume in four quadrants of the uterus, can be used.

Fig. 7.13 *The biophysical profile.*

A normal score lies between 8 and 10 and an abnormal score is in the range of 0–4. A score of 6 is equivocal and would usually lead to the tests being repeated. Although a biophysical profile may take 30 minutes to complete, in practice, for a normal fetus it is common for all the parameters to have been reached within 5–10 minutes, in which case the tests can be terminated and classified as normal. It is also noteworthy that the parameters from which the score is derived are important and more weight should be applied to certain parameters. For example, a fetus with a normal liquor volume and a normal reactive cardiotocograph but for whom fetal breathing movements have not been seen is not usually a cause for great concern, although it would be unusual for this situation to occur because normally, movements will be seen and will be associated with a normal reactive cardiotocograph.

A SUMMARY OF THE MANAGEMENT OF A FETUS THAT IS SMALL FOR DATES

- Identification and confirmation that the fetus is small for gestational age by serial ultrasound scans.
- Assessment of Doppler ultrasound umbilical flow velocity waveform.
- Regular fetal monitoring by biophysical profile or cardiotocography coupled with liquor volume measurement.
- If umbilical flow velocity waveform and fetal monitoring tests are normal, continue with pregnancy with regular monitoring.
- If the umbilical artery flow velocity waveform is abnormal showing loss of end diastolic flow but monitoring tests are normal, continue with the pregnancy with careful frequent monitoring because an abnormal umbilical artery blood flow is associated with a potentially poor outcome for the fetus. Should the fetus have reached an adequate gestational age, deliver.
- Should cardiotocography or biophysical profile show clear abnormalities compatible with hypoxia, proceed to immediate delivery by caesarean section.

BACKGROUND INFORMATION ON THE PHYSIOLOGY OF PLACENTAL FUNCTION AND FETAL DEVELOPMENT

The placenta is important in supplying oxygen and nutrients to the fetus and also acts as an endocrine organ. Oxygen diffuses from the maternal blood with a gradient favouring the oxygen transfer from the maternal to the fetal circulation. Fetal haemoglobin has a higher affinity for oxygen than maternal, favouring the uptake of oxygen. Fetal red blood cells are more resistant to acid and alkaline environments and this forms the basis of the Kleihauer test (**Figs 5.10** and **7.26**) to determine whether fetal cells are present in the maternal circulation. Carbon dioxide which is readily soluble in fetal blood diffuses across the placenta.

Glucose crosses the placenta by facilitated diffusion which is a saturable process, protecting the fetus to a certain extent from the extremities of hyperglycaemia in women with diabetes. The placenta will consume a considerable portion of the glucose being transferred from the mother. Glucose stores are held in the liver as glycogen. Insulin does not cross the placenta and fetal insulin functions as a growth hormone in the fetus as opposed to being primarily a regulator of blood glucose. It will, however, respond to high blood glucose levels and this is thought to be the mechanism underlying macrosomia in the babies of diabetic mothers. If sufficient oxygen supplies are not present, the metabolism of glucose by anaerobic metabolism and acidosis will occur.

The fatty acids that the fetus needs for development, particularly in the formation of cell membranes, are transported in lipoproteins. In normal pregnancy there is a physiological hyperlipidaemia, presumably to supply the fetus with triglyceride and cholesterol. This is exaggerted in pre-eclampsia in which high levels of certain lipoproteins can promote vascular damage. In contrast, the hyperlipidaemia of pregnancy is less marked in pregnancies complicated by IUGR and this presumably contributes to the fetal undernutrition seen in this condition. Essential fatty acids are also important for fetal development.

The fetus synthesizes protein from free amino acids which are actively transported across the placenta. One hormone produced by the placenta is human placental lactogen which is similar to growth hormone. It is produced from the syncytiotrophoblast and levels rise throughout pregnancy. It appears to antagonize insulin. In the past it was used as a marker of placental function. Human chorionic gonadotrophin is also produced by the trophoblast and is very similar to luteinizing hormone. It reaches a peak in the first trimester and then declines and is the basis for the pregnancy test performed in urine or blood. The placenta is a major source of progesterone production which is dependent on

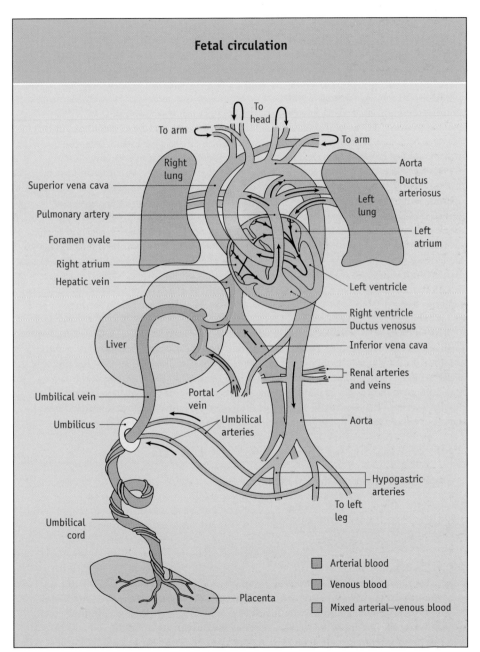

Fig. 7.14 *Fetal circulation.*

cholesterol being supplied to the placenta. Oestrogens, particularly oestriol, are produced in the placenta and oestriol was in the past used as a biochemical test of placental function. It is produced from dehydroepiandrosterone, synthesized by the fetal adrenal gland; levels of this hormone increase through pregnancy.

DEVELOPMENT OF THE FETUS

The fetal circulation is shown in **Figure 7.14**.

Oxygenated blood returning from the placenta in the umbilical vein enters the right atrium with approximately 40% crossing through the foramen ovale to the left atrium and then to the left ventricle, where it is ejected into the aorta and will perfuse the brain and other organs with oxygenated blood. The remainder of the blood entering the right atrium will flow into the right ventricle where it is ejected into the pulmonary vessels but instead of going to the lungs it flows mainly through the ductus arteriosus and joins the blood in the aorta, bypassing the lungs. There is a small flow of blood to and from the lungs but this does not become significant until after birth when the ductus arteriosus closes and there is a major shunting of blood into the pulmonary circulation for oxygen transfer.

The fetus makes breathing-like movements and these appear to be important for lung development. The movements result in an influx of amniotic fluid in and out of the lungs. Chronic reduction in amniotic fluid such as in the patient with prolonged rupture of membranes from an early point in pregnancy will be associated with poor pulmonary development and pulmonary hypoplasia. The lungs appear to be the last organ to become sufficiently mature to cope with preterm birth. Infant respiratory distress syndrome due to immaturity of the fetal lungs after birth is a major cause of morbidity and mortality. Lung maturation may not be complete until 36–37 weeks' gestation, when sufficient surfactant is produced to allow adequate expansion of the alveoli at birth. The production of surfactant can be enhanced by the administration of high doses of corticosteroids to the mother and this is employed in preterm labour.

The fetal kidney is a major source of amniotic fluid production in the second half of pregnancy. Renal agenesis or an obstruction to urine outflow is associated with reduced amniotic fluid volume: oligohydramnios. The fetus also swallows amniotic fluid and it is absorbed in the gut before being excreted again as urine into the amniotic sac. In a fetus that cannot swallow, such as with oesophageal atresia, excess fluid volume, polyhydramnios, may occur. Early during pregnancy the amniotic fluid is mostly formed by the secretion of fluid from the amnion and across the fetal skin before keratinization.

THE FETUS THAT IS LARGE FOR DATES

In a fetus that is large for dates it is important to:

- Check that the dates are accurate.
- Exclude twins if this has not already been done.
- Assess for the presence of polyhydramnios.
- Consider the possibility of fetal macrosomia due to gestational or pre-existing diabetes.
- Exclude any underlying fetal abnormalities.

Polyhydramnios can be defined by an increase in amniotic fluid on ultrasound with a single pool of greater than 8cm in depth or an amniotic fluid index above the 95th centile (the amniotic fluid index is the sum of the liquor depth in each of the four quadrants of the uterus as assessed on ultrasound scan). The four measurements of cord-free pools of amniotic fluid are summated. A value of greater than 24cm would be compatible with polyhydramnios. The causes of polyhydramnios are shown in **Figure 7.15**.

Fig. 7.15 *Causes of polyhydramnios.*

Causes of polyhydramnios
Maternal diabetes
Multiple pregnancy, particularly monovular twins
Fetal anomaly, including neural tube defect, oesophageal atresia, duodenal atresia
Fetal hydrops such as occurs with severe fetal anaemia

Polyhydramnios can precipitate preterm labour. The presenting part may be ill fitting in the pelvis and cord prolapse can occur as a result. The increased uterine volume also puts the pregnancy at risk of malpresentation, and after delivery, postpartum haemorrhage can occur due to the previous overextension of the uterus.

Treatment

Exclude or identify any underlying conditions. Care must be taken in labour at the time of the rupture of the membranes to ensure that the presenting part is well fitted into the pelvis and that there is no cord prolapse. In severe cases, such as those associated with twin–twin transfusion, amniotic fluid is sometimes removed by amniocentesis and attempts have also been made to reduce fetal urine production by administering indomethacin to the mother. If the mother is very uncomfortable, she may require admission to hospital.

HYPERTENSION DURING PREGNANCY

Hypertension during pregnancy may be due to pre-existing hypertension. This is usually identifiable by an elevated diastolic blood pressure ($\geq$90mmHg at booking in the first trimester or before the pregnancy). Pre-existing hypertension may be essential hypertension in which the cause is unknown, but often a familial predisposition exists, or due to an underlying medical condition such as renal disease. Occasionally, a new cause of hypertension can develop during pregnancy due to the coincidental occurrence of a new medical condition. However, the most common problem is women who have a normal blood pressure before pregnancy and during early pregnancy, but subsequently develop high blood pressure in the second half of pregnancy. This problem will remit within a few weeks or months of delivery. When such an increase in blood pressure is combined with proteinuria, this is called pre-eclampsia. Changes in biochemistry, typically an increased concentration of uric acid, sometimes an upset in liver function and also a disturbance in the coagulation system, particularly a reduction of platelet count, will also be present. When gestational hypertension occurs without proteinuria, this is termed pregnancy-induced hypertension, which can be mild–moderate (diastolic blood pressure of 90–110mmHg) or severe (diastolic blood pressure >110mmHg).

Eclampsia is the occurrence of convulsions during pregnancy not due to a primary neurological problem in a patient with features of pre-eclampsia. It is caused by cerebral oedema and vasospasm. It is a rare (1 in 2500 maternities), but nonetheless important, obstetric emergency in the West. It may be the first manifestation of pre-eclampsia and can occur without any obvious pre-eclampsia. The woman may be totally asymptomatic or have headache, visual disturbance or epigastric pain prior to the seizure. Over 40% of cases occur after delivery and approximately 25% of cases occur during labour.

Pre-eclampsia/pregnancy-induced hypertension is a hypertensive disorder peculiar to pregnancy. Pregnancy-induced hypertension occurs in 10–15% of pregnancies and pre-eclampsia in 2–3%. The classic features are hypertension, oedema and proteinuria. It usually occurs in the second half of pregnancy. Once established, it progresses at a variable and unpredictable pace until delivery. The cause of this disorder remains unknown. The primary pathology appears to be defective implantation which appears to trigger maternal endothelial dysfunction and damage (**Fig. 7.16**). Thus, it is not simply a disorder associated with high blood pressure and proteinuria, the main clinical manifestations, but rather it is a

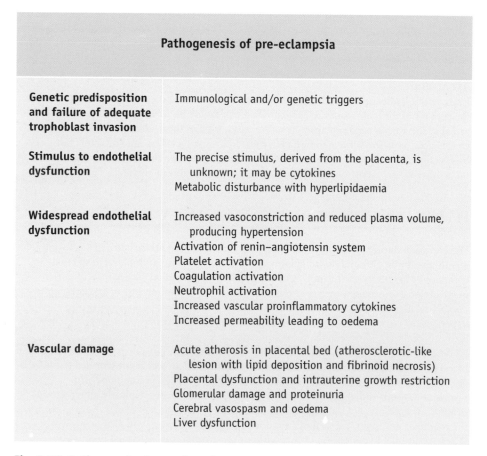

Pathogenesis of pre-eclampsia	
Genetic predisposition and failure of adequate trophoblast invasion	Immunological and/or genetic triggers
Stimulus to endothelial dysfunction	The precise stimulus, derived from the placenta, is unknown; it may be cytokines Metabolic disturbance with hyperlipidaemia
Widespread endothelial dysfunction	Increased vasoconstriction and reduced plasma volume, producing hypertension Activation of renin–angiotensin system Platelet activation Coagulation activation Neutrophil activation Increased vascular proinflammatory cytokines Increased permeability leading to oedema
Vascular damage	Acute atherosis in placental bed (atherosclerotic-like lesion with lipid deposition and fibrinoid necrosis) Placental dysfunction and intrauterine growth restriction Glomerular damage and proteinuria Cerebral vasospasm and oedema Liver dysfunction

Fig. 7.16 *Pathogenesis of pre-eclampsia.*

Fig. 7.17 *Risk factors for pre-eclampsia.*

Risk factors for pre-eclampsia

Chronic hypertension
Renal disease
Connective tissue disease
Primigravida
Diabetes
Previous severe pre-eclampsia or
    intrauterine growth restriction
Migraine
Central obesity
Age <20 years and >35 years
Family history on maternal side (genetic
    component)

serious multisystem disorder that can affect every organ and system in the body by this endothelial damage and dysfunction. Many risk factors have now been identified (**Fig. 7.17**). Pre-eclampsia is traditionally regarded as a disease of primigravidae (although primipaternity would be a more accurate description) with a higher level of risk in the first pregnancy. A previously uncomplicated pregnancy with the same partner can be regarded as a protective factor against the development of pre-eclampsia. The risk of pre-eclampsia will be substantially increased if there is an underlying medical condition such as renal disease or essential hypertension. For patients with unusual or recurrent forms, it is important to assess them for any underlying renal or cardiovascular disease. It is one of the major causes of maternal death in the West with the most common modes of death being cerebral haemorrhage, pulmonary oedema, adult respiratory distress syndrome and liver failure. The fetus can also be affected by placental damage resulting in insufficiency which may impair fetal growth or precipitate the need for preterm delivery. In view of its multisystem nature, it has many unusual presentations.

CLINICAL AND LABORATORY FEATURES

Hypertension is normally diagnosed when the diastolic blood pressure is greater than 90mmHg, provided that the booking blood pressure has been less than this, or when there has been a rise of 20–25mmHg over the diastolic blood pressure at booking, in early pregnancy or a combination of both. When the diastolic blood pressure exceeds 110mmHg, this is severe hypertension and carries a significant risk to the mother including that of cerebral haemorrhage.

Proteinuria is more easily diagnosed and it is normally regarded as significant when there is more than 0.3g of protein in 24 hours collected urine, or on Dipstick testing, '++' or more. When a '+' is persistent, this, in the absence of other causes of proteinuria such as urinary tract infection, would be regarded as significant. It is noteworthy that proteinuria occurring in the absence of significant hypertension can still be attributable to pre-eclampsia and, indeed, would denote a severe form of the disease.

171

Although oedema is included in the classic definition of pre-eclampsia, its use as a diagnostic feature is poor as normal pregnancy is associated with oedema in more than two-thirds of patients. Furthermore, severe pre-eclampsia and eclampsia can occur without oedema. Thus, although oedema is a common feature of pre-eclampsia, it is not of value as a diagnostic sign.

Of more importance are the biochemical and haematological changes. An increase in uric acid is one of the most useful features of the disease. An increase in uric acid can occur in advance of proteinuria, will increase as the disease progresses and is, therefore, a marker of disease severity. Although, significant increases occur, these may not lie outside the normal non-pregnant range and attention should be paid to the range for uric acid during pregnancy. At 32 weeks' gestation, the upper limit of normal is 0.34mmol/L; at 36 weeks, 0.39mmol/L, as there is a change with gestation. The platelet count is another useful marker of disease progression: it falls as the disease advances. However, it is not a useful diagnostic sign as, although the platelet count may be reduced, it usually stays within the normal non-pregnant range. However, serial platelet counts can be helpful. There will be alterations in renal function, in particular, increasing urea, although, again, this may stay within the normal range. Liver function abnormalities can occur, particularly, in severe forms of the disorder and it is important to assess these in any patient with significant disease. Severe haematological changes including haemolytic anaemia, in which the red blood cells are broken down, can occur, as can coagulation disturbances such as disseminated intravascular coagulation (DIC). Again, these complications should be sought in more severely affected patients (**Fig. 7.18**).

THE LIVER AND COAGULATION SYSTEM IN PRE-ECLAMPSIA

The liver is often affected in pre-eclampsia but usually this is to a minor degree. This will manifest as a modest elevation in the transaminases, such as AST. However, as noted, pre-eclampsia is a protean condition with many atypical presentations, including the situation in which there is a substantial liver involvement with a gross elevation of transaminases and bilirubin, often with minimal presence of other symptoms. HELLP syndrome is one variant of this condition: Haemolysis, Elevated Liver enzymes and Low Platelets. There is usually no gross DIC, even though haemolysis is occurring and hypertension is often mild. Jaundice may be present. When there is major liver involvement, this is often associated with DIC.

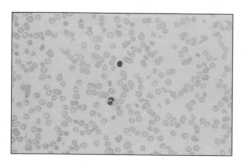

Fig. 7.18 *Blood film showing microangiopathic haemolytic anaemia with fragmentation of red cells.*

The main pathological lesions with hepatic involvement in pre-eclampsia are areas of infarction and necrosis. Necrosis of the small blood vessels in the hepatic portal system (the blood flow from the gut to the liver) and also in small branches of the hepatic arteries can been seen. Hepatic involvement will be seen in more than 50% of women dying from pre-eclampsia. The hepatic lesion is probably related to the activation of the coagulation system and intravascular damage. The situation can progress to liver failure. In addition, there may be swelling of the liver, resulting in stretching of Glissons's capsule. This will provoke significant pain and often vomiting. Haematoma can also occur in the liver where bleeding occurs at sites of infarction. This is usually subcapsular and may progress to liver rupture with massive intra-abdominal and intrahepatic bleeding. Such bleeding is likely to be associated with, or lead to, DIC. Thus, in patients presenting with possible pre-eclampsia, with symptoms such as right upper quadrant pain, epigastric tenderness and vomiting, it is likely that liver involvement is present and this is extremely worrying feature that usually leads to immediate delivery. Liver rupture carries a high level of maternal mortality.

THE MANAGEMENT OF PRE-ECLAMPSIA

Much of the antenatal care is focused on making a diagnosis of pre-eclampsia. Care should be taken when assessing blood pressure and detecting the presence of proteinuria. Once diagnosed, the severity of the disease and the rate of progression must be regularly assessed (**Figs 7.19**). This will require a regular assessment of blood pressure, proteinuria and also laboratory investigations, including a full blood and platelet count, along with a biochemical assessment of urea, electrolytes and plasma urate. Liver function tests should be checked, particularly, in severe or atypical forms of the disease. Patients with severe disease will require a coagulation screen. The fetus should be assessed for growth and wellbeing, usually by regular assessment of fetal growth by ultrasound scans. These should be repeated at least at 14-day intervals. In addition, ultrasound should be used to document the amniotic fluid because a chronic reduction in amniotic fluid is associated with fetal compromise. Fetal wellbeing can also be assessed using cardiotocography which can warn of any fetal distress. Doppler ultrasound assessment of the umbilical artery blood flow can be helpful in identifying patients at high risk of compromise.

The initial assessment can usually be carried out in a Day Assessment Unit, which will allow an appropriate assessment of the patient's problem and will guide subsequent care. This assessment should guide whether or not to admit the patient, as well as, the frequency of maternal and fetal monitoring and the need for delivery. The aim of treatment is to protect the mother and the fetus from the consequences of high blood pressure to allow the pregnancy to be prolonged to avoid the problems of prematurity. This will require a constant evaluation, weighing up the risk to the mother and fetus of continuing the pregnancy against those of delivery. It is important when delivery occurs before 36 weeks' gestation, that consideration is given to treatment with high-dose steroids which, when administered to the mother, can promote increased fetal lung maturity and minimize the problems after delivery. When hypertension is not severe, proteinuria absent and there is no fetal compromise, then outpatient monitoring can occur (**Fig. 7.20**).

THE TREATMENT OF HYPERTENSION

Pre-eclampsia can be regarded as the most common curable form of hypertension because delivery will result in the resolution of the disease process. The philosophy of antihypertensive therapy is to protect the mother from the effects of hypertension, such as cerebral vascular haemorrhage and eclampsia. This will allow the pregnancy to advance and reduce the risk of premature delivery. When diastolic blood pressure exceeds

Assessment of pre-eclampsia

Check for symptoms	Headache Visual disturbance Epigastric pain
Monitor blood pressure	Usually 4-hourly
Haematology	Full blood count Monitor platelet count Coagulation screen in severe cases
Biochemistry	Urea and electrolytes, including uric acid Liver function tests Monitor proteinuria and urine output
Assess fetal growth and wellbeing	Ultrasound to check growth parameters Cardiotocograph or biophysical profile Umbilical artery Doppler ultrasound

Fig. 7.19 *Assessment of pre-eclampsia.*

110mmHg, there is no doubt that treatment of the hypertension is required. When diastolic blood pressure is between 90 and 110mmHg, then there is controversy over the management as blood pressure levels in this range are not usually associated with a major hazard to the mother. Thus, some obstetricians will treat if diastolic blood pressure is in excess of 90mmHg, whereas others will delay antihypertensive therapy until blood pressure exceeds 110mmHg. A variety of drugs are available for treatment of the hypertension, including methyldopa, labetalol, atenolol, nifedipine and hydralazine. There is no evidence that any one drug is superior to the other. Perhaps, most experience and information is available for methyldopa. Although safe for mother and fetus, it is associated with minor, although troublesome, side effects, including tiredness, loss of energy, dizziness, depression, flushes, headaches and vomiting, and palpitations. It is normally started as a dose of 250mg, two or three times each day, increasing to 500mg four times each day as required. Alternative medication is labetalol 200mg three times each day to a maximum of 300mg

Laboratory investigations into severe pre-eclampsia at 27-weeks' gestation

Date	14.11.96	15.11.96	15.11.96	15.11.96	16.11.96	22.11.96	Normal range
Time	1630 h	0915 h	1500 h	2100 h	0900 h	0900 h	
Urea (mmol/L)	8.2	10.7	12.6	12.6	12.1	2.0	2.5–8
Creatinine (µmol/L)	76	85	96	90	83	70	40–130
Urate (µmol/L)	548	571	581	580	570	330	160–480
Bilirubin (µmol/L)	17	25	31	–	–	20	3–22
Aspartate aminotransfe--rase (U/L)	74	90	88	–	–	34	12–48
Albumin g/L	27	27	24	23	24	30	40–52
Platelets × 10⁹/L	120	–	96	–	–	259	150–400
Haemoglobin (g/dl)	12.8	–	10.6	–	–	11.3	10.5–15

Fig. 7.20 *Laboratory investigations in a patient with severe pre-eclampsia at 27 weeks' gestation admitted with blood pressure of 170/120mmHg and "+++" of proteinuria and a severely growth restricted fetus which suffered an intrauterine death shortly after admission. Note the elevated urea and urate and mild liver dysfunction with slightly elevated bilirubin and AST. The albumen is also low reflecting severe proteinuria.*

(a)

Drug treatment of hypertension in pregnancy

Step 1	Methyldopa 250mg b.i.d. or t.i.d. or Labetalol 200mg t.i.d.
Step 2	Increase methyldopa to 500–750mg q.i.d. or Increase labetalol to 300mg q.i.d.
Step 3	Add second line agent: nifedipine 30–60mg daily (long acting preparation)
Step 4	If blood pressure remains uncontrolled, consider delivery in maternal interest or Increase dose of nifedipine And/or Add methyldopa or labetalol (whichever not previously used)

Fig. 7.21 *(a) Drug treatment of hypertension in pregnancy.*

four times each day. If this fails, nifedipine is added as a second line agent (**Fig. 7.21(a)**). If premature delivery is required in the maternal or fetal interest, then high-dose steroids should be given to mature the fetal lungs.

SYMPTOMATIC PRE-ECLAMPSIA

When blood pressure is uncontrolled or the patient becomes symptomatic, delivery is indicated. Worrying symptoms include abdominal pain, which is usually indicative of liver involvement, headache and visual disturbances. Such signs and symptoms may be a prelude to the most severe form of the disorder, namely, eclampsia, when seizures occur. It is important to elicit any such symptoms and to consider them carefully in the assessment of the disease process and the management plan. When such symptoms are present, it is usual to control the blood pressure, institute therapy to avoid seizures (magnesium sulphate) and arrange delivery. When this is several weeks from term, it would be usual to perform caesarean section.

Delivery

Delivery will result in disease regression. Thus, for patients who have significant disease and in whom prematurity is not a problem, that is, the pregnancy is advanced to 34–36 weeks and beyond, then there is really little place for conservative management. Decisions about

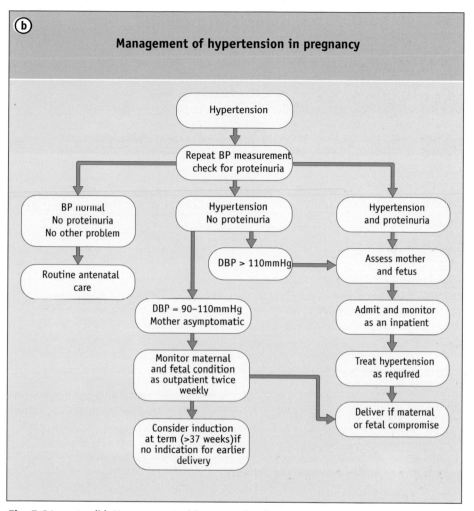

Fig. 7.21 *cont.* *(b) Management of hypertension in pregnancy.*

delivery may be difficult, particularly when the fetus is very preterm, as in addition to the *in utero* risks from the disorder, the risks resulting from premature delivery have to be taken into account. Nonetheless, if there is any suspicion about impaired fetal wellbeing *in utero*, delivery should take place if the fetus is considered viable. This would usually be by caesarean section if delivery is preterm or if there is significant risk of fetal distress or urgency. When the mother has severe disease and, in particular, if there is uncontrolled blood pressure or symptoms, such as epigastric pain or severe headache, then urgent delivery is essential to protect the mother from the risks of severe hypertension and the widespread systemic disturbance that can occur with this condition. When intrauterine death occurs, it is usual to induce labour to avoid major surgery for the mother.

TREATMENT OF ECLAMPSIA

- Obtain venous access.
- Stop convulsions (intravenous magnesium sulphate 4g over 20 min or diazepam 10mg bolus repeated if required).
- Prevent further convulsions (magnesium sulphate 1g/h by intravenous infusion).
- Control blood pressure (intravenous labetalol as the first line).
- Catheterize: monitor urine output, check for proteinuria.
- Assess cardiovascular, respiratory and neurological systems.
- Check full blood count, coagulation screen, urea and electrolytes, urate, liver function tests.
- Assess fetal wellbeing (ultrasound, cardiotocography).
- Check chest radiograph and pulse oximetry or blood gases if there is a suspicion of pulmonary oedema.
- Deliver.
- Consider the need for computerized tomography or magnetic resonance imaging of the brain (cerebral haemorrhage can occur in severe disease).
- Consider other causes of convulsions.
- Continue to monitor the mother (biochemistry, coagulation, urine output).

Fluid management

It is not uncommon in severe disease, particularly after delivery, to have a transient oliguria which may last for 24 hours or more. In the management of patients with severe disease, in whom urinary output is reduced, it is important to be aware of the risk of fluid overload, as this can precipitate pulmonary oedema. This occurs, not simply due to the increased volume of fluid that may be administered to the patient during the course of labour or in an attempt to increase urine output, but more importantly, because of damage to the blood vessels throughout the body that can also occur in the lung, whereby fluid is more able to leak from the blood vessels into the soft tissues. In the lung, this manifests itself as pulmonary oedema. This condition can cause serious problems for the mother and, thus, careful monitoring of her fluid balance must be conducted. In patients with severe problems, a central venous pressure line is often inserted to monitor the fluid status. Generally, no more than 500 ml of fluid should be given intravenously over each 6 hour period. However, even with this, it is still possible to develop conditions such as pulmonary oedema due to 'leaky' blood vessels.

Postpartum care

After delivery, it may be some time before the disease process resolves. During this period the mother will still be exposed to the risks and hazards of high blood pressure as well as the systemic upset of pre-eclampsia. Thus, in the severe forms of this disorder, it is imperative that, not only is antenatal and intrapartum care optimal, but that postpartum care is also regarded carefully as antihypertensive problems may persist. It is important in the postpartum period to document adequate disease control and resolution as many complications can occur in the few days after delivery and it may take several weeks for blood pressure to regress to normal levels. In severe cases, it is usual to follow-up patients and exclude any underlying medical condition such as connective tissue disease or renal disease.

ANTEPARTUM HAEMORRHAGE

PLACENTAL ABRUPTION

Placental abruption is the premature separation of the normally implanted placenta from the uterine wall resulting in haemorrhage before the delivery of the fetus. It occurs in approximately 1 in 80 deliveries and the more severe forms are associated with a high degree of perinatal mortality and morbidity. The risk to the fetus depends on the severity of the abruption, the gestation, the birth weight and the amount of concealed haemorrhage. Abruption is initiated by bleeding into the decidua basalis of the placenta and with the hydrostatic pressure associated with this bleeding and the development of decidual haematoma, this leads to the separation of the adjacent placenta. As the uterus is still distended with the pregnancy, it is unable to contract around the uterine vessels at the placental site and thus bleeding continues. As the haematoma expands, it can dissect between the fetal membranes leading to vaginal bleeding. The bleeding, however, may be in whole or in part concealed if the haematoma does not reach the margin of the placenta and cervix so that the blood loss is revealed. It can therefore be seen that the amount of revealed blood loss can be a poor guide to the degree of haemorrhage as an enlarged haematoma may be concealed within the uterus. The haematoma may also result in bleeding into the amniotic cavity with subsequent blood-stained liquor being noted when the membranes rupture. Furthermore, the bleeding may infiltrate the myometrium resulting in so-called Couvelaire uterus. This infiltration of blood into the myometrium is associated with sustained uterine contraction, making the uterus feel very 'solid' on examination provoking labour and reducing utero–placental blood flow with serious compromise to the fetus (**Figs 7.22–24**).

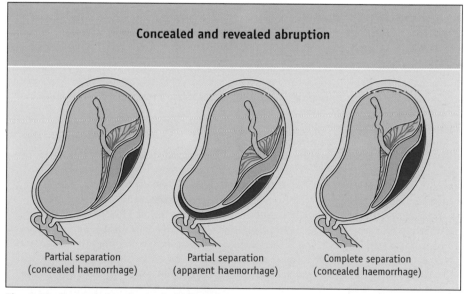

Fig. 7.22 *Concealed and revealed abruption.*

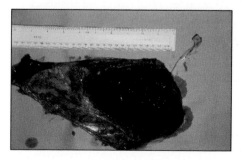

Fig. 7.23 *A large placental abruption showing extensive clot attached to the fetal side of the placenta following delivery by emergency section for severe fetal distress.*

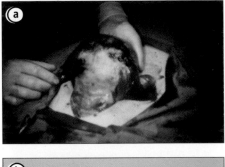

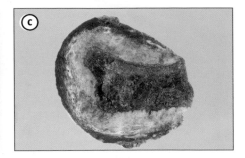

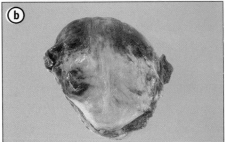

Fig. 7.24 *(a) Couvelaire uterus following abruption. This resulted in severe intractable postpartum haemorrhage leading to hysterectomy to control bleeding. (b) Pathological hysterectomy specimen showing the Couvelaire features. (c) Specimen from (b) opened showing clot within the uterus.*

The aetiology of abruption is essentially unknown. It may reflect abnormal placentation as necrosis of the decidua basalis and placental infarcts are often seen in association with abruption. Risk factors associated with abruption include severe external trauma, uterine abnormality, maternal age, parity, deficiency in folic acid, low socioeconomic status, sudden uterine decompression, smoking and an unexplained elevation of maternal serum α-fetoprotein in the second trimester, which may itself be an indication of a placental abnormality. Women who give up smoking during pregnancy will reduce the incidence of abruption by approximately 25% and of stillbirth and neonatal death associated with abruption by approximately 50% compared with women who continue to smoke. There is also a high risk of recurrence of abruption in subsequent pregnancies.

Placental abruption is frequently associated with hypertension. However, the causal relationship between hypertension and abruption is somewhat controversial as hypertension can result from the sudden release of vasoactive substances generated from the disturbance created by the abruption itself into the maternal circulation. In addition, although there are associations between pre-eclampsia, chronic hypertension and abruption, this could be in keeping with the theory of defective placentation being responsible for abruption because significant abnormalities in placentation occur in pre-eclampsia and intrauterine growth restriction, and patients with chronic hypertension are at increased risk of pre-eclampsia. In any event, when hypertension and abruption coexist the perinatal mortality is increased. The classical presentation of severe abruption (**Fig. 7.25**) is vaginal bleeding, uterine tenderness and irritability with contractions or uterine hypertonus, often resulting in premature labour. Fetal distress or intrauterine fetal death may be present.

The diagnosis of placental abruption may not be obvious, particularly if the abruption is largely concealed and it may be misdiagnosed as a premature labour of an unknown cause. Thus, abruption should be considered in any patient presenting with unexplained vaginal bleeding or possible preterm labour, particularly if fetal distress is present. As the bleeding may be concealed, it is possible that hypovolemic shock may be present, due to blood loss

Fig. 7.25 *Features of abruption.*

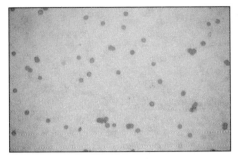

Features of abruption

Vaginal bleeding

Abdominal pain

Uterine contractility or premature labour

Uterine tenderness

Fetal compromise

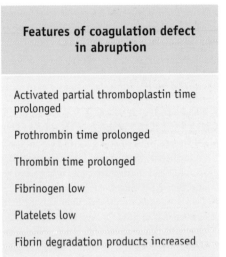

Features of coagulation defect in abruption

Activated partial thromboplastin time prolonged

Prothrombin time prolonged

Thrombin time prolonged

Fibrinogen low

Platelets low

Fibrin degradation products increased

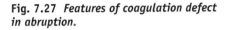

Fig. 7.26 *Positive Kleihauer test showing persistent fetal cells which are resistant to acidification in contrast to adult red cells.*

Fig. 7.27 *Features of coagulation defect in abruption.*

which is contained within the uterus with only minimal or even absent vaginal bleeding. As well as severe maternal haemorrhage, feto–maternal bleeding can also occur and can result in severe fetal anaemia or even death. If the patient is Rhesus negative, she should obviously receive anti-D immunoglobulin in the event of abruption regardless of the size. A Kleihauer test (**Fig. 7.26**) will be required to diagnose the presence of feto–maternal bleeding and also to estimate the volume of haemorrhage to provide sufficient anti-D.

Abruption is a common cause of coagulation failure in pregnancy and the degree of coagulation disturbance tends to correlate with the size of abruption and blood loss. The features of coagulation defects are shown in **Figure 7.27**.

The management of abruption is to correct the hypovolaemia, deliver the fetus and observe for and correct any coagulation defect that arises. This requires management in a labour ward with intensive monitoring of both mother and fetus. Guidelines for obstetric haemorrhage management are set out below. Ultrasound is useful in confirming viability and presentation with clinical diagnosis often difficult due to uterine hypertonicity. It is also of value in excluding an alternative diagnosis of placenta praevia. As abruption often precipitates rapid labour, vaginal delivery may be possible. The assessment in a severe case should be in theatre set for section with an anaesthetist present. The examination aims to assess the stage of labour and exclude the alternative or coexisting diagnosis of placenta praevia. If the woman is in labour, the membranes should be ruptured as this will advance labour and an electrode can be applied to the fetal scalp to assess fetal distress. Clearly, if intrauterine death has already occurred vaginal delivery would be ideal. If fetal distress is present, then caesarean section should be performed in the fetal interest. In the absence of fetal distress, labour which is usually rapid should be allowed to progress with continuous monitoring. Abruption also places the patient at risk of severe postpartum haemorrhage. In milder degrees of abruption, in which small episodes of vaginal bleeding occur with some transient uterine activity and no evidence of fetal compromise, conservative management is indicated particularly if the patient is far from term. The mother should initially be admitted for a full maternal and fetal assessment. This will include full blood count and coagulation screen, cardiotocograph or biophysical profile to confirm fetal wellbeing and ultrasound scan to assess fetal growth, liquor volume and also to exclude placenta praevia. If no adverse features are present and the condition settles, the patient can be discharged but must be carefully and regularly followed as an outpatient because the risk of recurrent abruption and preterm labour and associated problems remains.

COMMON ASPECTS OF THE MANAGEMENT OF MAJOR OBSTETRIC HAEMORRHAGE

- Obstetric, anaesthetic and midwifery staff should be summoned urgently. Senior anaesthetists and obstetricians are usually required. Haematology and blood transfusion should be alerted. Porters should be immediately available to transport samples of blood and blood products.
- Two 14-gauge peripheral lines should be set up and if possible central venous monitoring carried out to guide therapy, ensuring adequate volume replacement while avoiding fluid overload. An arterial line, if available is also extremely useful for monitoring the patient's condition. A urinary catheter should be inserted with hourly assessment of urinary output.
- Continuous monitoring of blood pressure, pulse and electrocardiography should be performed. Blood gas and acid base status should be assessed regularly.
- While setting up the infusion, a sample of venous blood usually approximately 20ml is required for blood grouping and cross-match and assessment of coagulation status. Six units of blood should be cross-matched initially. Plasma expansion can be provided with human albumin solution or artificial plasma expanders such as polygeline (Haemaccel®) will be needed. Dextran should not be used as it can interfere with cross-matching, and is associated with risks of allergic and anaphylactic reactions. In particular, administration antenatally can result in an anaphylactoid reaction within the uterus resulting in severe uterine hypertonus which has been associated with fetal distress and a high level of perinatal mortality and serious morbidity. In very severe haemorrhage uncross-matched blood may be life saving and two units of blood group O, Rhesus negative can be kept available at all times for such overwhelming emergencies. The blood can be administered rapidly using a pressure cuff and blood warming equipment should be used. In major haemorrhage a blood filter should not be used routinely as it may slow blood administration.
- Haemoglobin concentration and coagulation status should be monitored regularly. The coagulation tests required are platelet count, prothrombin time and activated partial thromboplastin time to assess the extrinsic and intrinsic coagulation pathways, respectively. The thrombin time should be performed to measure thrombin clottable fibrinogen and also measure the fibrinogen itself. Fibrin degradation products should be measured to determine whether increased fibrinolysis is occurring. Blood products such

as fresh frozen plasma or platelets may be required if there is a degree of coagulation failure which can occur with massive blood loss itself.

- Recourse to procedures such as uterine artery, internal iliac artery ligation or caesarean hysterectomy should not be left until the patient is moribund and an experienced obstetrician is essential in such cases.
- Depending on staffing and resources in the labour ward and the patient's condition, the patient may be better transferred to the intensive care unit.

PLACENTA PRAEVIA

Placenta praevia is when the placental site is abnormally low and encroaches into the lower uterine segment, including the situation in which it covers the cervix. Bleeding occurs as the lower uterine segment forms or the cervix dilates.

Placenta praevia is divided into types of severity. Type 1 encroaches into the lower uterine segment, type 2 reaches the edge of the cervical os but does not cover it, type 3 covers the cervical os but the placental site is asymmetric with most of the placenta being on one side of the cervical os and type 4 is centrally located over the cervical os (**Fig. 7.28**). In clinical practice, however, types 1 and 2 are regarded as minor degrees of placenta praevia and types 3 and 4 as major placenta praevia. In the major forms, bleeding is inevitable as the cervix dilates. In contrast, types 1 and 2 may present with minor, painless degrees of bleeding as the lower uterine segment forms over the latter few weeks of pregnancy but may in the course of the formation of the lower uterine segment in the weeks leading up to term, 'move' out of the vicinity of the cervix as the lower uterine segment below the level of the placental implantation site expands. Although the placenta will be readily visualized with ultrasound it may be difficult accurately to delineate the relationship of the placenta to the lower uterine segment and cervix, and in addition it may be difficult to exclude a succenturiate placental lobe (an extra lobe of the placenta attached to the main body by a thin vascular connection). Placenta praevia occurs in approximately 0.5% of pregnancies. It is associated with multiparity, high maternal age and previous caesarean section. As with the placenta implanted within a caesarean section scar, it may be more difficult for this to 'move clear' of the cervix as the lower segment forms due to the previous scarring. Large placentae such as those associated with multiple pregnancy are clearly at increased risk of being praevia simply because of their size. Furthermore, placenta accreta is also more common with placenta praevia.

Classically, placenta praevia presents with minor degrees of painless vaginal bleeding starting spontaneously. They tend to occur at the time of formation of the lower uterine segment in the first half of the third trimester. Such warning haemorrhages may herald the diagnosis but up to one third of patients have no history of such haemorrhages and on some occasions diagnosis will only become apparent during labour. Other clinical clues to placenta praevia are malpresentations, unstable lie or a high presenting part as the lower portion of the uterus is occupied by the placenta. This should raise suspicion of placenta praevia. On examination (**Fig. 7.29**) of the patient presenting with painless vaginal bleeding associated with placenta praevia, the uterus will be found to be soft and nontender. Vaginal and speculum examination must be avoided in all cases of indeterminate vaginal bleeding until placenta praevia has been excluded because in the case of placenta praevia, digital examination can initiate major placental separation with life-threatening haemorrhage.

Management

The management of placenta praevia depends on gestation and presentation, severity of the bleeding and degree of praevia. When the bleeding is severe, delivery by caesarean section is required immediately in the maternal interest regardless of fetal maturity or condition.

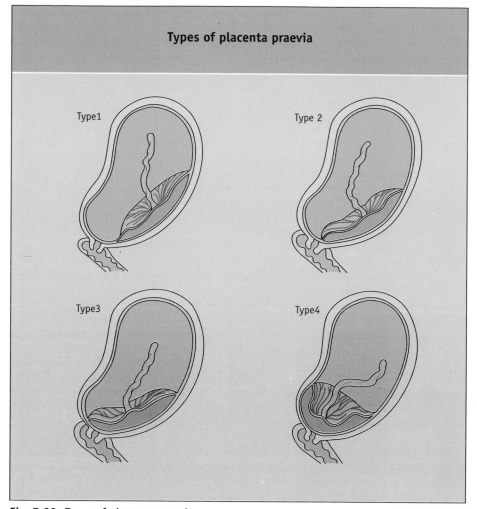

Fig. 7.28 *Types of placenta praevia.*

If major placenta praevia presents at 36 weeks' gestation or more, then delivery is indicated by caesarean section. When bleeding occurs before 36 weeks' gestation, (i.e. the fetus is significantly preterm) and the bleeding has been of a minor nature and stops spontaneously then conservative management is warranted. The patient should remain in hospital with blood immediately available at all times in case of severe haemorrhage. When the fetus is considered mature, delivery by caesarean section is performed usually at approximately 37 weeks' gestation, before the onset of spontaneous labour which would inevitably provoke bleeding.

Minor degrees of placenta praevia can be managed conservatively with the possibility of subsequent vaginal delivery. In this situation, ultrasound is used to monitor the placental site at 14-day intervals. If the placenta is found to move clear of the cervix as gestation advances as the lower uterine segment forms, and clinically there is no other contraindication, then vaginal delivery may be anticipated. In borderline and minor degrees of placenta praevia,

Clinical features of placenta praevia
Minor degrees of vaginal bleeding in the first half of the third trimester
Painless
Associated with malpresentation, unstable lie or high presenting part
Uterus is soft and not tender
Avoid vaginal and speculum examination until placenta praevia is excluded

Fig. 7.29 *Clinical features of placenta praevia.*

examination and theatre set for section may be required to delineate whether the placenta will be disturbed by or interfere with the process of labour and delivery. A decision can then be made whether to proceed directly to caesarean section or whether to allow vaginal delivery. The latter can only be accomplished in the most minor degrees of placenta praevia and should bleeding occur, early recourse to caesarean section will be required. With good obstetric ultrasound, the need for such examination in theatre is very limited.

Caesarean section for patients with placenta praevia can be extremely hazardous particularly if the placenta is anterior. A lower uterine segment incision will inevitably encounter heavy bleeding as the incision will impinge directly on to the placental bed. Significant damage to the fetal placenta may also result in fetal bleeding. Thus, an experienced surgeon is required. The fetus is delivered by separating the placenta from the uterus, rupturing the membranes and delivering the fetus round the side of the placenta through the lower uterine segment wound. However, on occasion the placenta itself may have to be divided and the fetus delivered through it. This can be associated with a high risk of fetal bleeding. As in any major obstetric haemorrhage, blood needs to be cross-matched and available, particularly when a section is being performed. Furthermore, serious bleeding may lead to disseminated intravascular coagulation (DIC).

DISSEMINATED INTRAVASCULAR COAGULATION

DIC occurs when there is a gross activation of the coagulation system leading to the generation of fibrinogen (the protein used to seal blood vessels and stop bleeding). However, at the same time, there is activation of the fibrinolytic system, the system used to break down fibrin, which protects from excessive coagulation. When both systems are activated, the fibrinogen which is generated is rapidly broken down by the active fibrinolytic system. Thus, there is insufficient fibrinogen to allow blood vessels to be sealed and bleeding to stop. As the coagulation system continues to be activated in an attempt to prevent bleeding, there is gross consumption of the coagulation factors, many of which are produced by the liver. Effectively, the body runs out of coagulation factors. There will usually be clinical evidence of bleeding and an underlying clinical problem such as severe pre-eclampsia or abruption. The woman may have spontaneous bleeding from mucus membranes such as within the mouth or from the sites of needle sticks. They may also have severe bleeding from surgical wounds. It can be diagnosed by prolongations of the main coagulation tests, namely, the activated partial thromboplastin time, which tests the intrinsic pathway of coagulation containing factors such as factor XII, XI, VIII and IX, and the prothrombin time which tests the so-called extrinsic pathway of coagulation which focuses mainly on factor VII. In addition, it is usual to measure the concentration of fibrinogen which will be low in DIC. As the fibrinogen is rapidly broken down, there is an excess amount of fibrin degradation products (**Fig. 7.30**). In DIC, platelets are also consumed and the platelet count, which is normally measured along with a coagulation screen, will fall. In addition, there may be fragmentation of red blood cells. This is thought to be due to the formation of fibrin mesh within the small blood vessels throughout the body which breaks up the red cells as they pass through the microcirculation. This is termed microangiopathic haemolytic anaemia and would be seen as a marked reduction in haemoglobin, and on examination of the blood film, red cell fragments would be seen.

There are many triggers for DIC. In obstetric practice, the common ones are abruption of the placenta, excessive blood loss in the course of delivery (major postpartum haemorrhage) and pre-eclampsia in its more severe forms.

An amniotic fluid embolus is a rare cause of sudden cardiorespiratory collapse which usually occurs in labour. It is due to the entry of amniotic fluid, which triggers DIC, into the maternal circulation. It is often fatal. Treatment is by support of the cardiovascular and coagulation systems.

The treatment of DIC is, firstly, to deal with the cause. If it is abruption or pre-eclampsia, then the patient requires urgent delivery, and, secondly, to restore the coagulation system and haemoglobin levels by administration of blood products such as fresh frozen plasma and red cell concentrate.

The prognosis for a patient with severe DIC varies according to the precipitant, the presence of any comorbid condition, the magnitude of blood loss, the severity of the DIC and

A typical coagulation screen result from a patient with DIC following an abruption	
Platelets	39×10^9/L
Haemoglobin	5.4 g/dl
Activated partial thromboplastin time	75 s (normal = 38 s)
Prothrombin time	29 s (normal = 14 s)
Fibrinogen	0.3 g/L
Fibrin degradation products	8–16 mg/L

Fig. 7.30 *A typical coagulation screen result from a patient with DIC following an abruption.*

the extent of other organ involvement. Other organ involvement can occur due to the nature of the intravascular coagulation and the blood loss; it is established that problems such as renal failure or hepatic damage can occur. Once problems, such as adult respiratory distress syndrome occur, with associated multiorgan failure, the mortality is greater than 50%.

INTRAUTERINE DEATH

Intrauterine death can be associated with underlying problems such as IUGR, cord accidents, abruption of the placenta or maternal problems such as pre-eclampsia or underlying chronic medical conditions such as systemic lupus erythematosus. In a large number of cases no cause is found. If intrauterine death is suspected, such as a woman presenting with no fetal movements, particularly in an at-risk pregnancy, it is important to confirm rapidly the diagnosis and establish the possible cause. Ultrasound will show no fetal heart pulsation or movement. Spalding's sign which is the overlapping of skull bones in the absence of labour may be seen. This was used in the past when radiography was employed to help to identify intrauterine death. It is important to screen for an underlying problem. These are shown in **Figure 7.31**.

Investigations performed with an intrauterine death

Full blood count and coagulation screen (disseminated intravascular coagulation can be associated with prolonged retention of a dead fetus or with abruption which may be a cause of fetal death).

Kleihauer test to check for major fetal–maternal haemorrhage.

HbA1C and random glucose to exclude maternal diabetes which is a recognized cause of intrauterine death.

Viral screen for underlying infection including rubella, cytomegalovirus, herpes and toxoplasma. When there is evidence of fetal hydrops, it would also be useful to screen for parvovirus infection.

Look for the presence of underlying connective tissue problems such as antinuclear factor, and particularly screen for lupus anticoagulant and anticardiolipin antibodies.

If fetal blood or tissue is available, it is often useful to karyotype the fetus.

A radiograph of the fetus should be performed to help with the identification of abnormalities.

A postmortem should be requested, with the parents' consent, on all intrauterine deaths.

Pathological examination of the placenta.

Fig. 7.31 *Investigations performed with an intrauterine death.*

The management of intrauterine death should be prompt. The patient should be counselled about the event and given time to take the events on board before proceeding to induction of labour. This is usually done with prostaglandins pretreatment with mifepristone may be used. Mothers often wish to see the baby when it is born and may wish a photograph or a handprint of the baby. This can be important to help with their grieving process. After delivery, lactation should be suppressed with bromocriptine or cobergaline. The stillbirth requires to be registered and the parents will have to be given a stillbirth certificate which has to be taken to the Registrar of Births and Deaths within 42 days of the delivery. There are many support groups available that can help the patient with this problem and appropriate follow-up should be discussed to go over the events of the past pregnancy and discuss implications for the future.

MULTIPLE PREGNANCY

Twin pregnancy occurs in approximately 1 in 80 conceptions, being higher in Black populations. Twin gestation can either be dizygotic (nonidentical twins) or monozygotic (identical twins). Dizygotic twins occur when two separate ova are fertilized. In contrast, monozygotic twins occur after the division of a fertilized ovum at various times after conception. Such monozygotic twinning occurs in approximately 1 in 250 pregnancies. A familial factor may be present being passed from mother to daughter, thus, a family history of twins on the paternal side does not present an increased risk of twins in pregnancy. The likelihood of multiple pregnancy is increased in assisted conception techniques, particularly with ovulation induction. With *in vitro* fertilization, in which two or three embryos may be replaced, there is clearly an increased chance of multiple pregnancy occurring.

Although a woman with a history of infertility may view twin pregnancy as a good outcome, it must be noted that there are significant problems with twin pregnancies. There is an increased risk of miscarriage. Furthermore, it is clear from ultrasound studies in early pregnancy that often one of the twins may perish *in utero* and either be resorbed if death

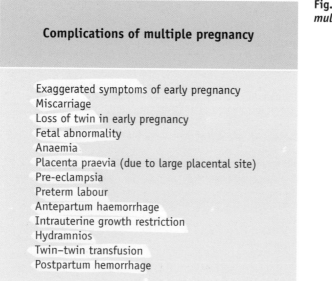

Complications of multiple pregnancy

Exaggerated symptoms of early pregnancy
Miscarriage
Loss of twin in early pregnancy
Fetal abnormality
Anaemia
Placenta praevia (due to large placental site)
Pre-eclampsia
Preterm labour
Antepartum haemorrhage
Intrauterine growth restriction
Hydramnios
Twin–twin transfusion
Postpartum hemorrhage

Fig. 7.32 *Complications of multiple pregnancy.*

Length of gestation in multiple pregnancies

Singleton	40 weeks
Twins	37 weeks
Triplets	33 weeks
Quadruplets	29 weeks

Fig. 7.33 *Length of gestation in multiple pregnancies.*

Categories of monozygotic twins

Category	Time of separation	Placenta and membranes
Diamniotic, dichorionic	Division within 3 days of fertilization	2 placentae 2 chorions 2 amnii
Diamniotic, monochorionic	Division 4–8 days after fertilization	1 placenta 1 chorion 2 amnii
Monoamniotic, monochorionic	Division 9–12 days after fertilization	1 placenta 1 chorion 1 amnion

Fig. 7.34 *Categories of monozygotic twins.*

occurs at an early stage or be retained in the uterus and be noted at delivery as a so-called fetal papyraceous (an amorphous shrivelled and compressed fetal body). Congenital abnormalities are also more common and such women should be screened with detailed ultrasound in the second trimester. There is increased risk of pregnancy complications (**Fig. 7.32**) including anaemia, disorders of fetal growth, pre-eclampsia and preterm labour. Twin pregnancies as a group tend to deliver approximately 3 weeks in advance of singleton pregnancies, with triplets, a further 3–4 weeks earlier and with quadruplets a further 4 weeks earlier. Thus, with increasing number of fetuses the length of gestation shortens (**Fig. 7.33**).

Division after 12 days may be incomplete and results in conjoined (Siamese) twins. Such joining may be at the chest or abdomen. These categories reflect the fact that the chorion begins to develop between days 4 and 8 after fertilization whereas the amnion does not. Between day 9 and day 12, both the amnion and chorion develop (**Figs 7.34 and 7.35**).

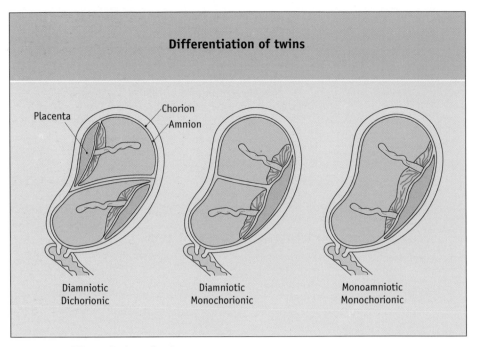

Differentiation of twins

Placenta Chorion Amnion

Diamniotic
Dichorionic

Diamniotic
Monochorionic

Monoamniotic
Monochorionic

Fig. 7.35 *Differentiation of twins.*

A particular problem that can occur is twin–twin transfusion syndrome. In this situation, the placental circulations are linked in such a way that one twin loses blood from its circulation while the other gains it. The 'donor' twin will usually have impaired growth, anaemia and hypovolaemia, whereas the 'recipient' twin may have problems from hypervolaemia, hypertension, polycythaemia and heart failure. The recipient twin may also have increased amniotic fluid due to its hypervolaemia, increasing renal perfusion and urine production, whereas the donor twin may have oligohydramnios because of reduced renal perfusion.

THE MANAGEMENT OF MULTIPLE GESTATION

The diagnosis of multiple pregnancy is usually made at an early stage in modern obstetrics because of routine ultrasound scanning for dating. However, when a woman is considered large for dates, it is obvious that multiple pregnancy should be excluded if that has not already occurred. In view of the problems raised by twin pregnancies, particular consideration should be given to the problems that may develop. These problems are often best managed at a specialist clinic where fetal growth and wellbeing can be monitored carefully.

The mother should receive prophylactic haematinics, that is, folic acid and iron supplements, as anaemia is common. She should be advised of the excess risk of preterm labour and told to report to hospital or seek advice if there is any evidence of preterm labour such as uterine contractility, show or spontaneous rupture of the membranes.

The mother must be monitored carefully for the development of pre-eclampsia with blood pressure and urinary protein being checked for at every visit. It is usual to see patients with multiple pregnancy more often, and as well as monitoring the maternal condition, it is important to monitor fetal growth and wellbeing. As already noted, this will include an assessment of fetal abnormality by way of detailed anomaly scanning at 18 weeks' gestation and if α-fetoprotein testing is performed then special consideration has to be given to its interpretation because twin pregnancy results in a different normal range for α-fetoprotein. It is important to try to determine whether there is any discrepancy in fetal growth and, in particular, examine for situations such as twin–twin transfusion and growth disturbance. Thus, growth should be measured at regular intervals from the end of the second trimester to term and, in addition, amniotic fluid volume should also be assessed. If growth is discordant, and this is usually considered if the difference in estimated weight is greater than 20%, then more frequent assessment may be required. As fetal movements perceived by the mother cannot accurately define the wellbeing of both fetuses, an objective assessment of fetal wellbeing is required. This can be carried out by ultrasound or by cardiotocography using a specific monitor able to pick up two fetal hearts independently. If the fetal heart is to be auscultated, again it is impossible to distinguish which fetal heart is being listened to. Thus, if this is to be assessed clinically then two independent observers are required to listen to the fetal heart simultaneously, count the pulse rate and if the pulse rate is different from that of the other observer and is not that of the mother, then fetal viability can be confirmed. In view of the difficulties with cardiotocography in reliably picking up both hearts simultaneously, biophysical profiles are often employed in the assessment of fetal wellbeing.

It is generally considered that if a twin pregnancy has any complication, delivery should be by caesarean section. For example, if the first twin is breech then delivery would usually be by caesarean section or if there is a complication such as disturbance in fetal growth or significant pre-eclampsia. When the leading twin has a cephalic presentation and there are no other complications, in particular, both twins have estimated weights of greater than 1.5kg, labour may be allowed to progress in the anticipation of vaginal delivery. During labour, the fetal heart rate for both fetuses must be monitored separately, often the leading twin can have a fetal scalp electrode applied and the other twin can be monitored by way of Doppler ultrasound transducer for cardiotocography. It is usual to have an anaesthetist in attendance and the paediatricians alerted, particularly if the delivery is likely to be preterm. As operative delivery is often required, it is useful to have had epidural anaesthesia established for the course of labour. When there are more than two fetuses, it is usual to perform a caesarean section rather than allow labour to develop because of the high possibility of complications.

Once the vaginal delivery of the first twin occurs, then an assessment can be made of the lie, presentation and position of the second twin. There is no point in trying to assess this before delivery as once the first twin is born, there is a substantial amount of space within the uterus and the second twin can change position. Once the first twin is delivered, it is usual to clamp and cut the cord and often it is useful to place a ligature round it to identify it as that of the first twin. Abdominal examination can then determine the lie and presentation of the fetus and if the presentation cannot be confirmed, then vaginal examination or transabdominal ultrasound will reveal whether it is a head or a breech. When the lie is other than longitudinal, then external version, in which the fetus is gently rotated round by gentle pressure on the abdomen, is usually required to make the lie longitudinal. Occasionally, internal podalic version may be required in which the fetus is grasped by the legs which are brought down to the vagina to allow breech delivery to ensue. Clearly, in the course of the delivery of a second twin, it is important to assess for problems such as cord prolapse. Thus, once the lie and presentation have been confirmed, if the amniotic sac is intact, it is usual to rupture the sac and allow the head or breech to descend into the pelvis. Thereafter, the delivery is carried out in a routine way for any vaginal cephalic or breech presentation. It is not uncommon that forceps may be required in the second stage. In addition, occasionally uterine contractions diminish and it is usual to have an oxytocin infusion ready to establish and maintain uterine contractility if it is required. This also is of value postpartum, as the uterus which has been overdistended during the pregnancy may not contract normally and there is a higher risk of uterine atony and postpartum haemorrhage. Thus, the management of the third stage should be active. Should significant problems such as fetal distress occur in the course of a labour, it is usual to proceed to caesarean section with a lower threshold for such operative intervention. A rare complication is that of locked twins, in which fetal parts interlock preventing completion of the vaginal delivery of the first twin. It usually occurs if twin one is breech and twin two cephalic with the heads locking in the pelvis. If vaginal manipulation fails to release them, then caesarean section is required.

NERVE ENTRAPMENT PROBLEMS IN PREGNANCY

The most common nerve entrapment problem in pregnancy is carpal tunnel syndrome. It is caused by the compression of the median nerve with tingling and parasthesia over its distribution in the hand over the area of the thumb and the lateral two and a half fingers. It is likely to be due to fluid retention with compression of the nerve within the tunnel. It can be minimized by wearing splints at night. A physiotherapist's advice should be sought. The lateral cutaneous nerve of the thigh can also undergo a similar entrapment giving pain and discomfort within its area of distribution. Occasionally, a Bell's palsy can occur during pregnancy.

chapter 8

Normal Labour and Delivery

DEFINITION AND STAGES

Labour is defined as the expulsion of the uterine contents after the 24th week of pregnancy. Before 24 weeks, the correct term is spontaneous abortion or miscarriage; between 24 and 37 weeks, the process is called preterm labour. Labour is divided into three stages. The first stage is from the onset of labour to full dilatation of the cervix, the second stage is from full dilatation of the cervix to the delivery of the baby and the third stage is from the delivery of the baby to the delivery of the placenta (**Fig. 8.1**).

THE DIAGNOSIS OF LABOUR

It can be very difficult to make a correct diagnosis of labour during the early stages, and the diagnosis is often delayed until labour is more advanced and obvious. However, it is important to make an accurate diagnosis of labour as early as possible because this will influence the subsequent management, particularly if the labour does not progress normally. The onset of labour is defined as regular, painful uterine contractions accompanied by effacement and progressive dilatation of the cervix. This is often accompanied by a 'show': a discharge of the blood-stained mucus plug, or 'operculum', from the cervical canal as it shortens and begins to dilate. Rupture of the membranes is not in itself diagnostic of labour

The three stages of labour	
First stage	**Dilatation of the cervix:** from onset of labour to full dilatation of the cervix.
Second stage	**Delivery of the baby:** from full dilatation to delivery of the baby.
Third stage	**Delivery of the placenta:** from delivery of the baby to completion of delivery of the placenta.

Fig. 8.1 *The three stages of labour.*

Fig. 8.2 *The diagnosis of labour.*

The diagnosis of labour
Regular, painful contractions Effacement and dilatation of the cervix

in the absence of other features, although in most cases of prelabour rupture of the membranes at term, labour will be established within 24 hours (**Fig. 8.2**).

TERMS USED TO DESCRIBE THE RELATION OF THE FETUS TO THE UTERUS AND PELVIS

The 'lie' of the fetus describes the relationship of the long axis of the fetus to the long axis of the uterus. The most common (normal) lie is longitudinal, the others being transverse and oblique.

'Presentation' refers to the part of the fetus that is leading in relation to the cervix. The most common presentation is cephalic, in which the baby is delivered head first. This can be subclassified into vertex presentation, in which the neck is flexed and the top of the head is leading, brow presentation in which the forehead comes first, or face presentation in which the neck is extended and the fetal face leads. The normal presentation is vertex.

The 'position' describes the relationship between the fetal denominator, the occiput in a vertex presentation (occipito-O), the chin in a face presentation (mento-M) and the sacrum in a breech presentation (sacro-S), and the maternal pelvis. The positions are described as anterior (A), transverse (T) or posterior (P), and are divided into right (R) and left (L), according to which side of the maternal pelvis the denominator lies in. If the denominator is directly (D) anterior or posterior, then it is described accordingly. For example, the position of the head might be described as 'left occipitoanterior' or LOA.

The 'attitude' describes flexion or extension of different parts of the fetus. The usual attitude is one of flexion of the spine, neck and limbs (**Fig. 8.3**).

THE MECHANISMS OF LABOUR

The fetal head usually engages in the pelvis in the occipitotransverse position, but during labour, as all diameters of the fetal head cannot pass through all diameters of the maternal pelvis, the head and trunk of the fetus follow a series of well-described manoeuvres known as the mechanisms of labour (**Fig. 8.4**).

- The descent of the presenting part into the pelvis can occur either before or during labour. This brings the leading part of the fetus into contact with the pelvic floor muscles.
- During descent, flexion of the fetal neck occurs, resulting in a smaller diameter of the fetal head entering the pelvis, as well as ensuring that the leading part that reaches the pelvic floor first is the vertex.

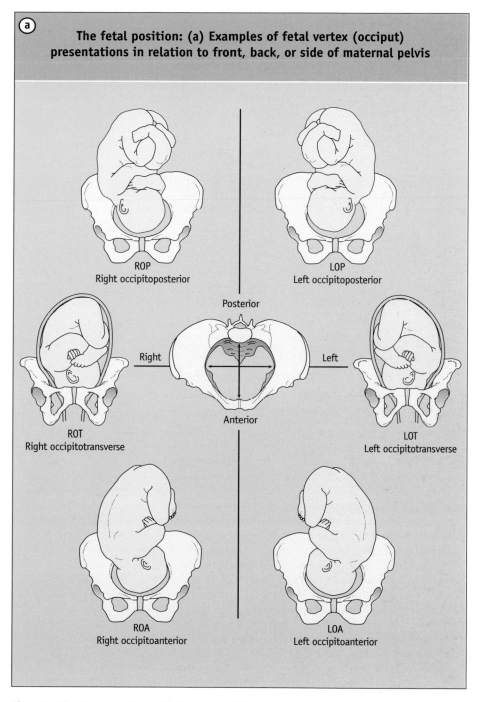

The fetal position: (a) Examples of fetal vertex (occiput) presentations in relation to front, back, or side of maternal pelvis

ROP
Right occipitoposterior

LOP
Left occipitoposterior

Posterior

Right

Left

Anterior

ROT
Right occipitotransverse

LOT
Left occipitotransverse

ROA
Right occipitoanterior

LOA
Left occipitoanterior

Fig. 8.3 *The fetal position. (a) Examples of fetal vertex (occiput) presentations in relation to front, back, or side of maternal pelvis.*

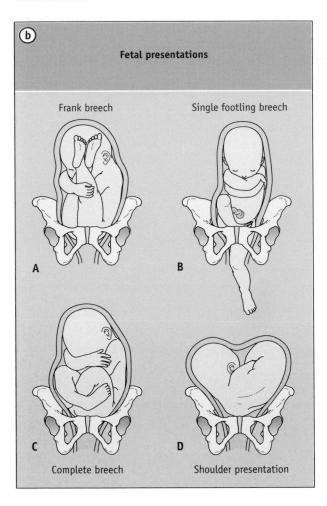

(b)

Fetal presentations

Frank breech

Single footling breech

A

B

Complete breech

Shoulder presentation

C

D

Fig. 8.3 *cont. (b) Fetal presentations. A–C: Breech (sacral) presentation. D: Shoulder presentation.*

- As the pelvic floor is an anteriorly sloping shelf of muscle, the first part of the fetus to reach it will rotate anteriorly (internal rotation). If the fetal neck is well flexed and the vertex is leading, this will result in an occipitoanterior position. However, if there is inadequate flexion of the neck, internal rotation will result in the occiput being posterior.
- During delivery, as the vertex becomes visible at the introitus, the fetal neck undergoes extension while the head follows the upward curve of the pelvis. The time when the vertex no longer recedes from the introitus during contractions, and perineal stretch is maximal, is known as crowning. There is further extension of the neck after delivery of the head to free the face and chin from the introitus.
- Once the head is delivered, restitution takes place as the head assumes the correct orientation in relation to the fetal shoulders.
- The shoulders then reach the pelvic floor and rotate into the anteroposterior position. This is followed by external rotation of the head so that the face looks at the maternal thigh.
- Delivery is completed by lateral flexion, first posteriorly to deliver the anterior shoulder, then anteriorly over the maternal abdomen to deliver the posterior shoulder and trunk (**Fig. 8.4**).

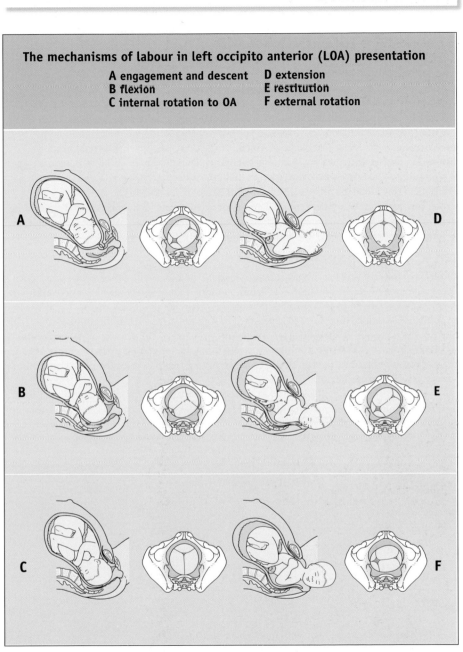

Fig. 8.4 *The mechanisms of labour in left occipitoanterior (LOA) presentation. A: engagement and descent; B: flexion; C: internal rotation to OA; D: extension; E: restitution; F: external rotation.*

THE FIRST STAGE OF LABOUR

The first stage of labour lasts from the onset of labour until full dilatation of the cervix. During this time it is important to ensure that both the mother and the fetus are well, that the mother has adequate analgesia should she wish this and that the labour is progressing normally. On admission to the labour ward, the maternal pulse, temperature and blood pressure are noted. Abdominal palpation is performed to determine the lie and the presentation of the fetus, and the engagement of the presenting part. The fetal heart is listened to and contractions are assessed. Vaginal examination is essential to diagnose labour and to assess progress. The position and consistency of the cervix, and its degree of effacement (or thickness) and dilatation should be noted, as should the station of the presenting part in relation to the ischial spines of the maternal pelvis (**Fig. 8.5**). It should be determined whether the membranes are intact or ruptured, and the colour of liquor should be documented. Vaginal bleeding should be noted.

PROGRESS IN LABOUR

Progress in the first stage of labour is determined by the rate of dilatation of the cervix. An acceptable rate of cervical dilatation is 1cm/hour, although progress may be more rapid than this, especially in parous women. During the first stage of labour, vaginal examinations should be performed at least every 4 hours, to ensure that progress is adequate. Progress in the second stage of labour is gauged by the descent of the presenting part and ultimately delivery. Overall progress in labour is influenced by the 'powers', the uterine contractions, the 'passages', the bony pelvis and soft tissues of the pelvis, and the 'passenger', the fetus.

The partogram is a visual record of progress in labour. Maternal and fetal observations are recorded, and each vaginal examination is charted so that the rate of cervical dilatation is easily seen (**Fig. 8.6**).

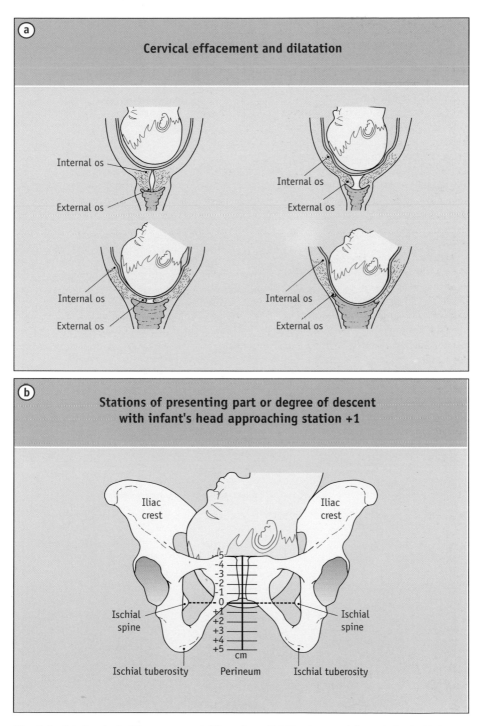

Fig. 8.5 *(a) Cervical effacement and dilatation. (b) The bony pelvis and the ischial spines are landmarks to gauge descent of the head.*

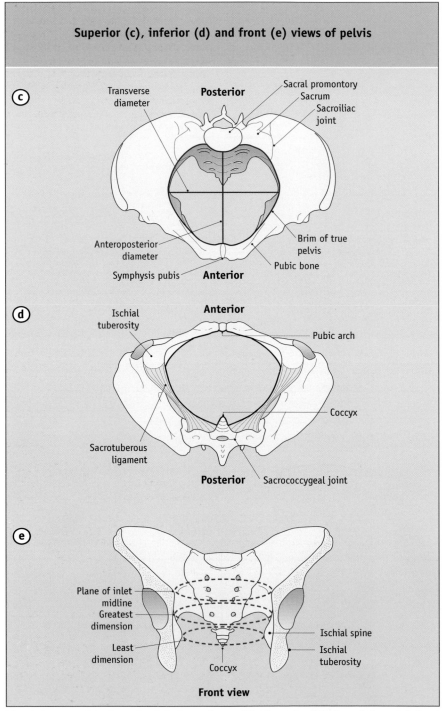

Superior (c), inferior (d) and front (e) views of pelvis

c

Transverse diameter
Posterior
Sacral promontory
Sacrum
Sacroiliac joint
Anteroposterior diameter
Brim of true pelvis
Symphysis pubis
Pubic bone
Anterior

d

Ischial tuberosity
Anterior
Pubic arch
Coccyx
Sacrotuberous ligament
Posterior
Sacrococcygeal joint

e

Plane of inlet
midline
Greatest dimension
Least dimension
Coccyx
Ischial spine
Ischial tuberosity
Front view

Fig. 8.5 cont. *(c) view of pelvis from above, (d) view of pelvis from below, (e) front view of pelvis.*

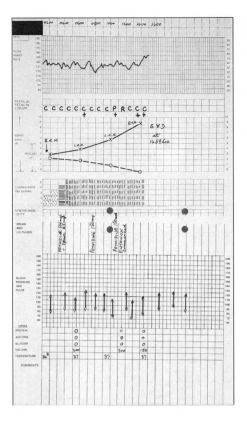

Fig. 8.6 *A partogram. This shows that labour started following a spontaneous ruture of membranes (SRM). Contractions were initially mild occurring twice in each 10-minute period and increased in strength and frequency over 4 h. Progress was relatively slow (0.5 cm/h) in this woman who was primigravid but spontaneous delivery occurred without augmentation of the labour.*

PROLONGED LABOUR

This is much more common in primigravidae than in parous women. It is usually secondary to inefficient uterine activity or a malpresentation or malposition (which in itself may be secondary to inefficient uterine activity). In the primigravid population, prolonged labour may occur in 30–40% of patients, usually because of poor uterine activity. Parous women rarely have inefficient uterine activity; if labour is prolonged in a parous woman, obstruction must be excluded. This may be secondary to true cephalopelvic disproportion, where the fetal head is too large to pass through the pelvis, but it is more likely to be due to a malposition such as an occipitoposterior position, or a malpresentation, such as a brow (**Fig. 8.7**).

THE TREATMENT OF PROLONGED LABOUR

Once a diagnosis of prolonged labour has been made it is important to determine the reason: inefficient uterine activity, malposition, malpresentation or cephalopelvic disproportion (**Fig. 8.8**). The most common cause is inefficient uterine activity, which is corrected by augmenting labour with intravenous oxytocin to increase the strength and frequency of contractions. Oxytocin is also helpful for malposition because efficient uterine action is required to aid the rotation and descent of the head. A diagnosis of cephalopelvic disproportion cannot be made in a primigravida until adequate uterine contractility has been ensured by the use of oxytocin. Intravenous oxytocin should be used with extreme caution in prolonged labour in parous women, and only when obstruction has been

201

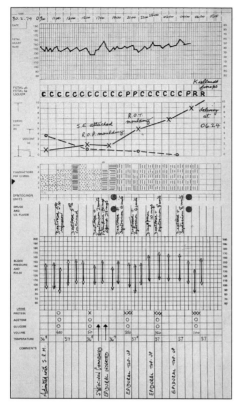

Fig. 8.7 *Partogram showing prolonged labour. This primigravida woman was slow to establish in labour following spontaneous rupture of membranes. After minimal progress to 2cm dilatation uterine activity was augmented with oxytocin. Labour then progressed but was not at an optimal speed due to the fetus being in the ROP/ROT position and delivery was effected by Kjelland's forceps. Epidural analgesia was employed.*

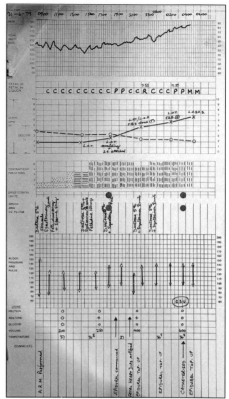

Fig. 8.8 *Partogram showing poor progress in labour. Despite augmentation of labour with oxytocin this primigravida failed to progress and there was excessive moulding of the fetal skull. A diagnosis of cephalopelvic disproportion was made and delivery was effected by caesarean section under epidural analgesia. Fetal blood samples had also been obtained for suspected fetal distress as decelerations had been seen on the CTG, but both samples had a satisfactory pH (7.31 and 7.29).*

excluded as far as possible. If a genuine obstruction exists, increasing the strength of the contractions could result in uterine rupture. The treatment for absolute cephalopelvic disproportion and relative disproportion not responding to intravenous oxytocin is caesarean section.

MALPOSITIONS

The normal position is occipitoanterior. Occipitotransverse and occipitoposterior positions are malpositions (**Fig. 8.3**). They can occur by chance, or may be secondary to poor fetal flexion, inefficient uterine contractions, a flat sacrum, android or anthropoid pelvic shapes or an anterior placenta. Malpositions are associated with long labours, a greater need for oxytocin and epidural analgesia, and higher operative delivery rates. In the majority of cases of malposition diagnosed during labour, spontaneous rotation to occipitoanterior and vaginal delivery will occur. However, up to 25% will require operative vaginal delivery or caesarean section. If labour is progressing well and a malposition is diagnosed, no treatment is indicated unless the labour becomes prolonged or the malposition remains in the second stage. If there is poor progress, adequate analgesia and intravenous oxytocin is the management of choice, even at full dilatation.

ABNORMALITIES OF THE PASSAGES

Abnormalities of the bony pelvis may result in prolonged or obstructed labour. Bony abnormalities of the pelvis can be developmental or acquired. Developmental abnormalities are rare. The incidence of acquired abnormalities has decreased over recent years in many countries, mainly as a result of the prevention of rickets. The most common pelvic abnormalities seen now are the results of trauma. Abnormalities of the soft tissues of the pelvis can also interfere with the progress of labour. The classic example is a large ovarian cyst impacted in the pouch of Douglas preventing the descent of the presenting part. Other examples include uterine or cervical fibroids or a pelvic kidney.

FETAL FACTORS: THE PASSENGER

Malpositions and malpresentations are the most common fetal factors in prolonged labour. Macrosomia, classically seen in the fetus of a diabetic mother, can result in prolonged labour, difficult delivery and shoulder dystocia, in which the head has been delivered but the shoulders become impacted in the pelvis. This obstetric emergency requires the use of specific manoeuvres and controlled strength to negotiate the shoulders under the pubic symphysis and through the pelvis before severe hypoxia affects the baby. Injuries to the clavicles and brachial plexus (resulting in Erb's palsy) are recognized complications of severe shoulder dystocia. Prolonged and obstructed labour can also be caused by fetal abnormalities, such as hydrocephalus, hydrops fetalis, gross ascites or abdominal tumours.

FETAL MONITORING DURING LABOUR

Labour is a time of potential danger for the fetus. The blood flow to the placenta decreases during uterine contractions. This can lead to reduced blood flow to the fetus itself. These events rarely cause a problem if the placenta and fetus are healthy, but if the contractions are too frequent or last too long, or placental function is already compromised, the fetus may become hypoxic and even acidotic. For these reasons, fetal monitoring may be employed during labour in an attempt to detect early signs of hypoxia and acidosis. Methods for fetal monitoring include assessment of the liquor for meconium staining, intermittent auscultation of the fetal heart rate, electronic fetal monitoring and fetal blood sampling. In the low-risk pregnancy during uncomplicated labour, electronic fetal monitoring has not been shown to confer any benefit over intermittent auscultation, but it has been demonstrated to increase the operative intervention rate. Abnormalities of the cardiotocograph (CTG) are not always associated with fetal distress. On the other hand, fetal distress can be seen in the presence of a normal fetal heart trace. Even if the CTG were 100% reliable as an indicator of hypoxia, electronic monitoring in labour would not eliminate cerebral palsy completely, for the brain damage sustained by these infants is thought to be suffered before labour in 90% of cases (**Fig. 8.9**).

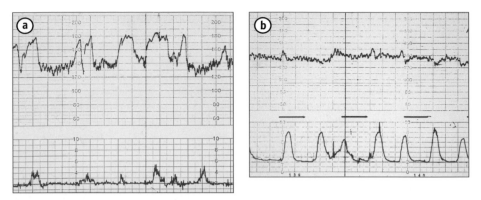

Fig. 8.9 *The cardiotocograph (CTG). At term, the normal CTG has a baseline heart rate of 110 to 160 beats per minute. The fetal heart rate normally varies from beat to beat and this is called the variability. The heart rate normally reacts with movement and uterine contractions. This reaction takes the form of an acceleration of the fetal heart rate. A normal CTG should have 3 accelerations of at least 15 bpm lasting at least 15 s in a 20 min period. This CTG (a) from a patient in early labour shows accelerations in response to contractions. It is not unusual in labour for accelerations to be infrequent or even absent (b). This is not of concern in the absence of other abnormalities in the fetal heart rate.*

MECONIUM STAINING OF THE LIQUOR

Meconium is the term used to describe the fetal bowel motions. The passage of meconium when the membranes are intact results in meconium staining of the liquor. There are two main reasons for meconium staining of the liquor: maturity and fetal compromise. The passage of meconium is not uncommon at and beyond term. This reflects a maturation of the fetal nervous system leading to increased gut motility. When released at the time of membrane rupture, the meconium-stained amniotic fluid is thin and has a brownish-yellow colour (Grade I meconium/old meconium). The clinical significance of this is very different to meconium staining that occurs in association with fetal compromise. Fetal hypoxia stimulates the autonomic nervous system. This increased autonomic activity can result in contraction of the smooth muscle of the bowel, with passage of meconium into the amniotic fluid. The degree of meconium staining is influenced by the liquor volume available to dilute the meconium. Thus, dark green, viscous meconium (Grade III meconium/thick, fresh meconium) indicates recent passage into a decreased liquor volume, which in itself may be indicative of placental dysfunction. In this situation, the index of suspicion of fetal compromise leading to hypoxia and acidosis must be high. The premature fetus rarely passes meconium due to immaturity of the autonomic nervous system.

INTERMITTENT AUSCULTATION

This is performed using a Pinard stethoscope. It is usually performed for 1 minute every 15 minutes during labour, and after every contraction in the second stage. The normal fetal heart rate at term is 120–160 beats/minute. An increase in the heart rate (acceleration) may be heard in response to fetal movement or contractions. If the heart rate is heard to slow down (deceleration), or the baseline rate lies outside the normal range, electronic monitoring should be commenced. An advantage of intermittent auscultation is that it is noninvasive, so it does not interfere with the woman's mobility during labour. However, the disadvantage is that due to the intermittent nature of the auscultation, abnormalities may

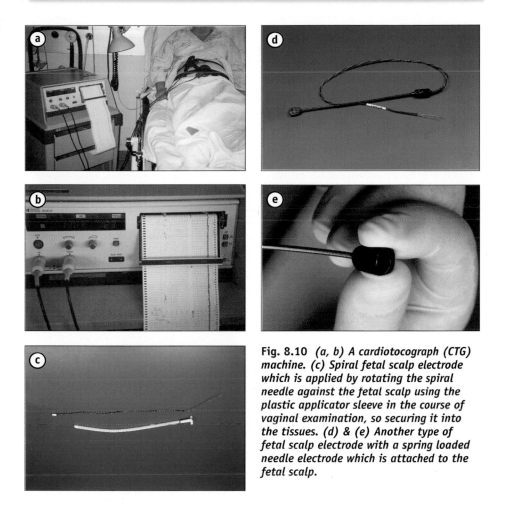

Fig. 8.10 *(a, b) A cardiotocograph (CTG) machine. (c) Spiral fetal scalp electrode which is applied by rotating the spiral needle against the fetal scalp using the plastic applicator sleeve in the course of vaginal examination, so securing it into the tissues. (d) & (e) Another type of fetal scalp electrode with a spring loaded needle electrode which is attached to the fetal scalp.*

be missed if the fetal heart rate was normal at the time of auscultation. This is particularly true of fetal heart rate changes during contractions, as it is difficult to auscultate at this time. For this reason, auscultation is generally performed as soon after a contraction as possible.

ELECTRONIC FETAL MONITORING

The CTG combines a continuous recording of both the fetal heart rate (the cardiograph) and uterine contractility (the tocograph). The cardiograph is recorded by an ultrasound transducer placed on the maternal abdomen (**Fig. 8.10**). The transducer picks up movement of the fetal heart during the cardiac cycle. The tocograph gives a graphical representation of the pattern of uterine contractions, but does not quantify contractility. Direct fetal monitoring involves the attachment of an electrode to the fetus (usually the scalp) to detect the cardiac impulses. This is not the same as an electrocardiogram. Uterine contractility can also be measured directly and quantitatively by the insertion of an intrauterine pressure catheter, usually after the membranes have been ruptured (**Fig. 8.11**).

EARLY DECELERATIONS

These are not thought to be sinister. The onset of the deceleration is with the start of the contraction. The nadir of the deceleration coincides with the peak of the contraction and the heart rate returns to normal by the end of the contraction. The heart rate rarely drops below 100 beats/minute. Early decelerations are usually repetitive and are thought to be due to head compression (**Fig. 8.12**).

VARIABLE DECELERATIONS

These decelerations are variable in both shape (amplitude and duration) and onset in relation to the contractions. The most common cause is cord compression. Variable decelerations are most often seen in the second stage of labour. They usually occur with each contraction and have a rapid onset and recovery. Many variable decelerations are benign. Reassuring signs are rapid onset and recovery, good baseline variability and an acceleration at the onset of the contraction. If these signs are absent or disappear, or if there is progressive worsening of the decelerations, fetal blood sampling should be considered to exclude acidosis (**Figs 8.13** and **8.14**).

LATE DECELERATIONS

The onset of this type of deceleration is after the start of the contraction. The nadir is reached once the peak of the contraction has passed and recovery takes place after the

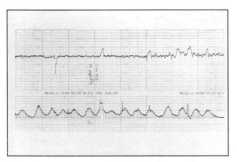

Fig. 8.11 *A normal CTG in labour where the uterine activity is being quantified by an intrauterine pressure catheter. The printout from this is on the lower part of the trace.*

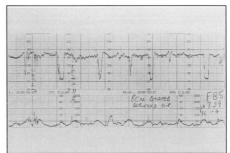

Fig. 8.13 *Variable decelerations of the fetal heart rate. Note that as they were recurrent a fetal blood sample was performed.*

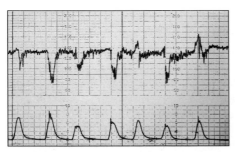

Fig. 8.12 *Early decelerations of the fetal heart rate.*

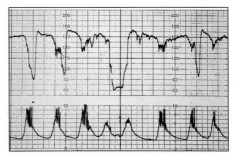

Fig. 8.14 *Variable decelerations with a baseline tachycardia and reduced variability in second stage of labour. Note the contraction pattern is suggestive of the mother pushing with contractions.*

contraction has ended. Late decelerations can be shallow and subtle, and are often associated with reduced or absent baseline variability. They are usually a result of uteroplacental insufficiency and can signify significant hypoxia. Fetal blood sampling should be performed, if it is possible, to assess fetal acidosis (**Figs 8.15–18**).

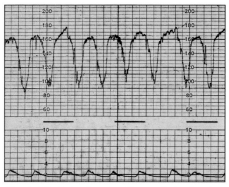

Fig. 8.15 *Late decelerations of the fetal heart rate. Note the baseline tachycardia and some loss of variability.*

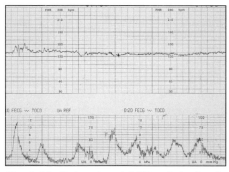

Fig. 8.16 *Reduced variability of the fetal heart rate in labour. The mother had received narcotic analgesics which can reduce variability.*

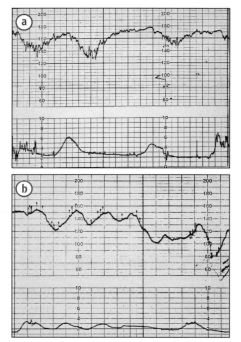

Fig. 8.17 *(a) Late decelerations followed by a grossly abnormal CTG representing an essentially moribund fetus (b) which suffered from birth asphyxia.*

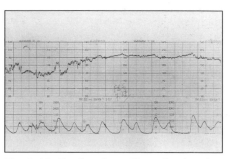

Fig. 8.18 *Fetal tachycardia and reduced variability. Fetal blood sampling showed a normal pH. The fetal tachycardia was due to maternal pyrexia.*

Fetal blood sampling

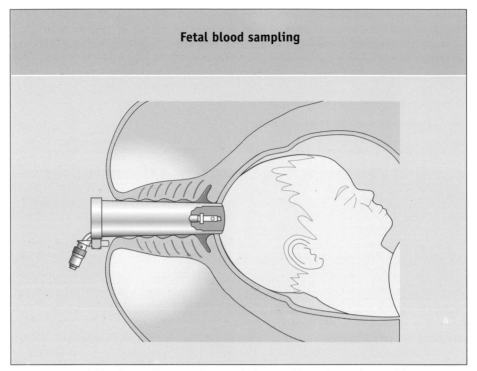

Fig. 8.19 *Fetal blood sampling. Amnioscope is inserted into the vagina, guided into the cervix by the examiner's fingers, and pressed against the presenting part. A small 2mm deep blade is used to puncture the fetal scalp.*

FETAL BLOOD SAMPLING

It must be remembered that electronic fetal monitoring is a screening test for fetal hypoxia and acidosis, and not a diagnostic test. All studies in which electronic fetal monitoring has been employed have shown increased operative intervention on the basis of abnormal electronic fetal monitoring. If monitoring is abnormal, this only indicates that fetal hypoxia may be present. If feasible, diagnostic testing should be performed. This takes the form of fetal blood sampling to measure the oxygen content or pH of the fetal blood. This can be performed once the cervix is dilated enough to pass an amnioscope to access the fetal scalp (or buttock in the case of breech presentation). The fetal skin is cleaned and a small scratch is made to cause bleeding. Fetal blood is collected in a capillary tube and analysed. A pH above 7.25 is normal. A pH between 7.20 and 7.25 indicates a degree of acidosis, and sampling should be repeated in 30 minutes. A pH below 7.20 indicates significant hypoxia and delivery should be expedited (**Fig 8.19**).

ANALGESIA IN LABOUR

Different types of pain are experienced during labour. Pain during uterine contractions is thought to be secondary to ischaemia of the myometrium. Dilatation and stretching of the cervix also causes pain, as does distension of the perineum during delivery itself. Womens' perception of pain during labour varies enormously, as do analgesic requirements.

Antenatal education is important to remove the fear of the unknown. If women know what to expect during labour, and are aware of the different methods of pain relief available to them, they are likely to cope better during labour itself. One of the most important factors, however, is the constant presence of a supportive person during labour. It is now normal for the partner to be present during labour and delivery, and this may well provide the necessary psychological support for the woman. However, the ideal is the continuous presence of an experienced midwife.

INHALATIONAL ANALGESIA

Entonox®, a mixture of 50% nitrous oxide and 50% oxygen, is widely used in the UK for analgesia during labour. It is self-administered via a mask or mouthpiece. Entonox® rarely provides complete pain relief, but is effective in reducing pain, allowing the woman to cope better. If used for prolonged periods, it can be tiring, and in large doses it can cause disorientation and hallucinations. On the whole, it is a safe and effective self-administered method of analgesia, with no adverse effects on the baby.

TRANSCUTANEOUS ELECTRICAL NERVE STIMULATION (TENS)

This is another self-administered method of analgesia. It works by electrically stimulating large myelinated afferent fibres, thereby reducing the pain impulses conducted by smaller myelinated and nonmyelinated nerve fibres. The exact mechanism of action is unclear, but in well-motivated individuals, a reasonable degree of analgesia can be obtained. It is essential that the machine is applied very early in labour, usually before hospital admission.

INTRAMUSCULAR NARCOTIC ANALGESIA

The most commonly used agents are pethidine (50mg to 150mg) and diamorphine (5mg to 10mg). These drugs are widely used and can provide effective pain relief, although there is good evidence to suggest that diamorphine is the more effective of the two. Narcotic administration can be repeated every 3 hours and the concurrent use of an antiemetic such

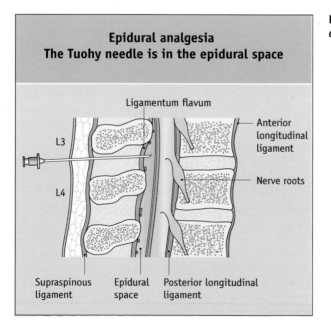

Fig. 8.20 *Epidural analgesia.*

Epidural analgesia
The Tuohy needle is in the epidural space

Ligamentum flavum

L3

L4

Anterior longitudinal ligament

Nerve roots

Supraspinous ligament

Epidural space

Posterior longitudinal ligament

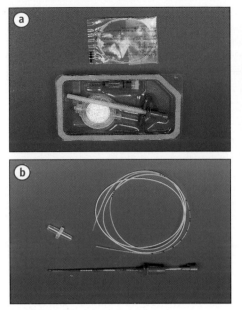

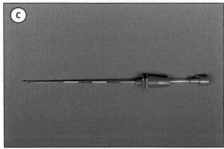

Fig. 8.21 *(a) & (b) Epidural pack, (c) epidural needle.*

as prochlorperazine is recommended as both pethidine and diamorphine cause nausea and vomiting. They also increase gastric stasis, and thus the risk of aspiration, particularly if maternal sedation is excessive. Another significant problem is respiratory depression in the neonate. This is more likely if the drugs have been given within 2 hours of delivery, but the depressive effects can be reversed quickly by administering the opiate antagonist naloxone.

EPIDURAL ANALGESIA

This is the most effective method of analgesia available for labour but it is also the most invasive. An intravenous infusion must be in place because epidural blockade can cause profound hypotension (this usually responds rapidly to intravenous fluids, failing this, the vasoconstrictor ephedrine is effective). A needle is inserted into the epidural space in the lumbar spine and a fine catheter introduced. Local anaesthetic agents (usually bupivacaine) are then injected through the catheter via a filter, resulting in both sensory and motor blockade. This limits mobility and is therefore seen by many as a major disadvantage. The other main disadvantage of epidural blockade is that it appears to lengthen the second stage of labour, and thus it is often implicated in higher operative vaginal delivery rates. However, it may be that women whose labours are difficult and prolonged are more likely to be offered epidural analgesia in the first place (**Figs 8.20** and **8.21**).

THE SECOND STAGE OF LABOUR

The second stage of labour lasts from the diagnosis of full dilatation of the cervix to the delivery of the baby. It is divided into a passive phase, in which descent and possibly rotation of the presenting part take place, and an active phase, during which the mother pushes. Many regard the passive phase as an extension of the first stage of labour, with no increased risk to the baby with time. However, there is evidence to suggest that a prolonged second stage, with the baby's head sitting deep in the pelvis for a long time may result in not only fetal hypoxia, but maternal pelvic nerve injury with bladder and/or bowel dysfunction in later life. As a result of this, the passive second stage is often limited to 1 hour unless an epidural is being

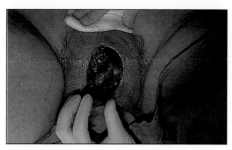

Fig. 8.22 *Crowning of the head.*

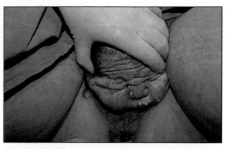

Fig. 8.23 *The head emerges at delivery.*

Figs. 8.22–24 *Normal vaginal delivery. (From Symonds, E. Malcolm and Macpherson, Marion B. A. 'Diagnosis in Color: Obstetrics and Gynecology' (Mosby-Wolfe, 1997), with permission.)*

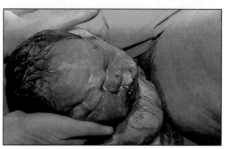

Fig. 8.24 *Delivery of the head and shoulders.*

used for analgesia, in which case 2 hours are often allowed to ensure the maximal descent of the presenting part before pushing. The active second stage usually begins in response to a strong maternal urge to bear down during contractions, or after instruction from the midwife because of the time already spent in the second stage or fetal distress. Most women, especially those who are parous, will deliver within 1 hour of starting to push.

DELIVERY

Pushing continues until the vertex no longer recedes into the vagina between contractions. This indicates that the head has passed through the pelvic floor and that delivery is imminent. This is referred to as crowning. The midwife will control the head to avoid damage to the perineum, by keeping the head flexed until the widest part is delivered, while 'guarding' the perineum with the other hand to prevent lacerations. Once the head crowns, the woman is asked to stop pushing and to pant to allow a slow, controlled delivery of the fetal head. If it is thought that tearing is going to occur, an episiotomy may be performed. The need for an episiotomy can only be assessed by the person doing the delivery. Some women would rather be allowed to tear than have an episiotomy, and their wishes should be respected. Once the head is delivered, nuchal cord should be excluded by inserting a finger under the subpubic arch to the anterior shoulder. If present, the cord should be slipped over the baby's head if possible, or clamped and cut before the rest of the baby is delivered. If the baby is slow to breathe, or if meconium is present, the nasopharynx should be sucked out (**Figs 8.22–24**).

THE INDUCTION OF LABOUR

The induction of labour is the initiation of labour by artificial means. There are many indications such as maternal hypertension or a gestation beyond 41 weeks. In view of the increased risk of fetal death in pregnancies going beyond 42 weeks' gestation, it is usual to offer induction at 41–42 weeks. Should the mother not wish induction, then it is essential to monitor the pregnancy twice a week and, in particular, assess the fetal condition by CTG and liquor volume. The outcome of a spontaneous labour may be slightly better than that of an induced labour and the mother may prefer a spontaneous labour. It is usually considered that induction should only be performed when the risks to either the mother or the fetus of continuing the pregnancy outweigh the risks of delivery. However, in contemporary practice, with appropriate patient selection, cervical ripening as required and the good management of induction, the outcome is not appreciably different from spontaneous labour and many inductions are performed for social reasons or because of maternal request. For some patients, the risks of labour or delivery are such that caesarean section is a safer option, such as for a growth-restricted fetus which would be unable to withstand the stress of labour or a severely ill mother. Many indications for the induction of labour are relative, and delay in intervention is often possible if the induction process is likely to be prolonged and arduous. An assessment of the cervix gives an indication of how easy induction will be (**Fig. 8.25**). A low cervical score (less than 4) suggests that the induction process may be difficult, and if the indication for induction is not pressing, it may be better to delay intervention to allow spontaneous cervical ripening. Cervical ripening can be induced medically as a prelude to induction proper. Primigravidae, in particular, often require cervical ripening which will increase, substantially, the success of induction.

Cervical ripening

When the cervix is unfavourable, there may be time to use pharmacological methods of cervical ripening to improve the cervical score before the induction of labour. This makes the subsequent labour shorter and less painful, reduces maternal and neonatal morbidity, and lowers the caesarean section rate. It is common for primigravidae to require cervical ripening but much less common for parous women. The agent of choice for cervical ripening is vaginally administered prostaglandin E_2 which can be given in various forms such as gel, pessary or a sustained-release device. The prostaglandin causes the softening and effacement of the cervix, and a degree of cervical dilatation. Once adequate ripening has occurred, that is, the cervix is well effaced and is approximately 3cm dilated, amniotomy is usually performed, following which intravenous oxytocin may be required to ensure adequate progress in labour.

The Bishop score to assess cervical ripening The score is made up from the sum of the individual scores				
Score	**0**	**1**	**2**	**3**
Cervical length	3cm	2cm	1cm	Effaced
Cervical dilatation	Closed	1–2cm	3–4cm	>5cm
Cervical consistency	Hard	Intermediate	Soft	Not applicable
Cervical position	Posterior	Intermediate	Anterior	Not applicable
Presenting part related to ischial spines	>3cm above	2–3cm above	<2cm above	Below

Fig. 8.25 *The Bishop score to assess cervical ripening.*

The induction process

If the cervix is ripe or has been ripened with prostaglandins, then induction can be carried out. This can be by amniotomy (**Fig. 8.26**) followed by escalating doses of intravenous oxytocin to stimulate uterine activity or by vaginal prostaglandin E_2 administration. Women generally prefer the latter as it is more like normal labour. Uterine activity does not usually commence for 3–4 hours after prostaglandin E_2 treatment and often a second dose is required. It is essential to monitor the fetus during induction. Occasionally uterine hypertonus can occur with frequent strong contractions which can precipitate fetal distress. If this happens with oxytocin, the infusion can be stopped but if severe and if there is concern for the fetus, then caesarean section may be required (**Fig. 8.27**).

The outcome of the induction of labour

The induction of labour can be associated with higher intervention rates than spontaneous labour. However, it must be borne in mind that the indication for induction may well influence how well the mother or the fetus can tolerate labour. The obstetrician's threshold for intervention may be lowered for a patient who is at risk. Intervention before 41–42 weeks can be associated with higher forceps and caesarean section rates. Beyond 42 weeks, the situation is reversed: women who labour spontaneously have a higher intervention rate compared with women induced just before 42 weeks. The increased caesarean section rate in the spontaneous labouring group is usually secondary to fetal distress in labour, indicating that prolonged pregnancy beyond 42 weeks is associated with the fetus being less able to tolerate the stresses of labour.

BREECH PRESENTATION

Approximately 3% of fetuses present by the breech at term. Breech presentation is associated with prematurity, and it is therefore much more common in preterm labour. It is also more common if a fetal anomaly is present, or if there is something holding the presenting part out of the pelvis, such as placenta praevia, a pelvic tumour or a contracted pelvis. It is thought that the fetus 'kicks' itself round into a cephalic presentation, so persistent extension of the knees or neurological abnormalities have also been implicated. There are three types of breech presentation (**Fig. 8.3(b)**). The first is when the hips are flexed and the knees are extended: extended or frank breech. The second is when both the hips and knees are flexed: flexed or full breech. The third is when the hips and knees are not completely flexed, resulting in the feet presenting (and sometimes the cord) without the breech being in the pelvis: footling breech. Many women with a breech presentation are now delivered by elective caesarean section if external cephalic version (turning the baby to cephalic by

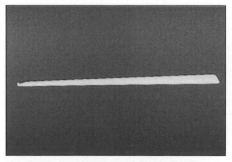

Fig. 8.26 *Amnihook used for rupturing membranes in the course of vaginal examination for induction of labour.*

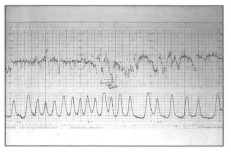

Fig. 8.27 *Hypertonic uterine action resulting in fetal distress. Note the late decelerations. The fetus was promptly delivered by caesarean section and recovered without complication.*

213

abdominal palpation and manipulation) has not been attempted or has failed. This is because of the concern that the largest part of the baby, the head, is delivered last, and may become stuck after the body has been delivered, and the suggestion that intracranial trauma and hypoxic brain damage are more common after vaginal breech deliveries.

VAGINAL BREECH DELIVERY

It is wise to select patients before the onset of labour. In most instances it is feasible to attempt external cephalic version after fetal anomaly and placenta praevia have been excluded, liquor volume has been confirmed as normal and fetal weight has been estimated by ultrasound scanning. Very big babies are more difficult to turn, and oligohydramnios makes it almost impossible. If external cephalic version is not attempted or fails, positive factors in favour of a vaginal breech delivery include an estimated fetal weight between 2.5kg and 3.5kg, a well-flexed neck and extended knees. A flexed breech is not a contraindication to vaginal delivery but the risk of cord prolapse and poor progress in labour associated with a footling breech makes caesarean section a better option (**Fig. 8.3b**). If a breech presentation is diagnosed during labour, many obstetricians will deliver the woman by emergency caesarean section.

FACE PRESENTATION

This occurs with a cephalic presentation when the fetal neck is fully extended, making the presenting part the face. The incidence is approximately 1 in 500 deliveries at term, and the aetiology is usually a normal fetus holding its neck in extension. A brow presentation may convert to a face presentation during descent through the pelvis. Tumours of the fetal neck, such as cystic hygroma may also result in a face presentation. Face presentations can deliver vaginally if the position is mentoanterior, as flexion of the neck allows the delivery of the head. Forceps can be used in a face presentation with a mentoanterior position if necessary. In a mentoposterior position, however, further extension of the neck is required to allow the delivery of the head, and as the neck is already fully extended, this is not possible. The

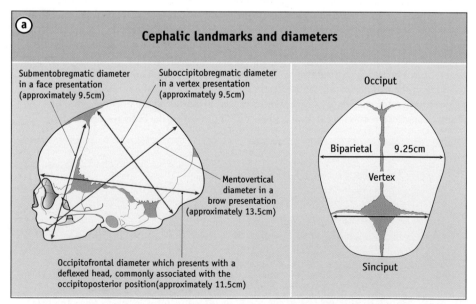

Fig. 8.28 (a) *Brow presentation. This figure illustrates the different diameters of the fetal head which can present to the mother's pelvis and illustrates how a brow presentation cannot deliver vaginally.*

forehead becomes jammed behind the symphysis, and the face and thorax become impacted in the pelvis resulting in obstructed labour. A face presentation with a persistent mentoposterior position is an indication for caesarean section. Diagnosis is by vaginal examination, when the eyes, nose and mouth can be felt. Marked oedema may result in a breech presentation being wrongly diagnosed. The parents should be advised that swelling and bruising of the face will resolve spontaneously.

BROW PRESENTATION

This occurs when the presenting part is the fetal forehead, secondary to partial extension of the fetal neck. The incidence is approximately 1 in 5000 deliveries at term. Diagnosis is by vaginal examination, during which the sutures cannot be felt but the supraorbital ridges and the bridge of the nose are palpable. A brow presentation is unstable in that it will usually convert to a face or a vertex presentation during labour. However, with a normal-sized baby, the presenting diameter of the fetal head with a brow presentation is too large to pass through the pelvis, so if it persists or is diagnosed in advanced labour, delivery should be by caesarean section. Vaginal delivery is only possible if the baby is very small (**Fig. 8.28**).

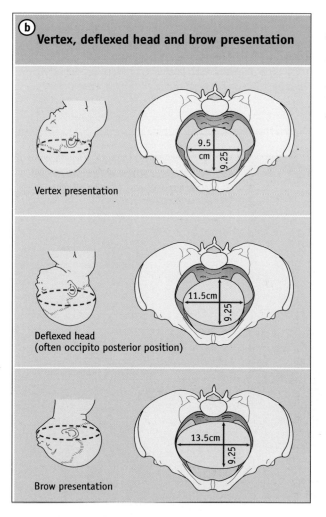

(b)

Vertex, deflexed head and brow presentation

Vertex presentation

9.5 cm / 9.25

Deflexed head
(often occipito posterior position)

11.5cm / 9.25

Brow presentation

13.5cm / 9.25

Fig. 8.28 (b) *Brow presentation. This figure illustrates the different diameters of the fetal head which can present to the mother's pelvis and illustrates how a brow presentation cannot deliver vaginally.*

TRANSVERSE AND OBLIQUE LIES

With a transverse lie (**Fig. 8.3b**), the long axis of the fetus is transverse in the uterus, and the shoulder is usually the presenting part. In an oblique lie, the head or the breech are usually in the iliac fossa. The diagnosis is generally made on abdominal palpation, and may be confirmed by ultrasound. These lies are often secondary to poor uterine tone in the parous woman or polyhydramnios. If the membranes are intact, both lies can usually be corrected by external version at term. The membranes can then be ruptured, after which contractions should maintain the lie. If the membranes are already ruptured or the lie reverts, delivery should be by caesarean section because only a longitudinal lie can deliver vaginally. Both transverse and oblique lies predispose to cord presentation, with the consequent risk of cord prolapse.

VENTOUSE EXTRACTION

This method of delivery involves fitting a cup over the vertex of the fetal head and applying suction. A vacuum is created and the pressure is increased slowly to reach 0.8kg/cm^2. The fetal scalp is sucked into the cup of the ventouse, forming the chignon, and delivery is then effected by traction. If rotation is necessary it usually occurs spontaneously as the head crosses the pelvic floor. Ventouse extraction is associated with less maternal soft tissue injury than is the case with obstetric forceps. In addition, it requires less analgesia. On the other hand, the failure rate is higher with the ventouse than with forceps in the case of malpositions, and forceps deliver more quickly if there is acute fetal distress. The most common side effect of the ventouse is cephalhaematoma. Scalp necrosis, subaponeurotic haematoma and intracranial haemorrhage have also been reported (**Figs 8.29** and **8.30**).

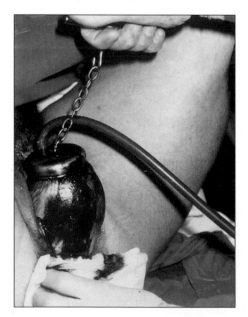

Fig. 8.29 Ventouse delivery. (From Al-Azzawi, F. 'Color Atlas of Childbirth and Obstetric Techniques' (Mosby-Wolfe, 1990), with permsission.)

FORCEPS DELIVERY

There are three types of obstetric forceps: short curved (Wrigley's), for low pelvic cavity deliveries, long curved (various), for nonrotational deliveries from the pelvic midcavity, and long straight (Kjelland's), for rotational deliveries in the case of malpositions. All forceps have a cephalic curve to allow the blades to fit over the fetal head. Curved forceps also have a pelvic curve which makes rotation within the pelvis impossible, thus rotational forceps have no pelvic curve and are therefore termed straight. The prerequisites that must be fulfilled before operative vaginal delivery are that there should be minimal head palpable in the abdomen, the cervix should be fully dilated, with the vertex below the ischial spines, the membranes should be ruptured, the operator must be certain of the position of the fetal head, and adequate maternal analgesia should be provided (**Figs 8.31–34**).

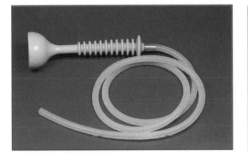

Fig. 8.30 *A ventouse.*

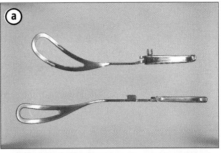

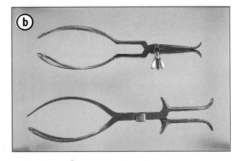

Fig. 8.31 *Different types of obstetric forceps. Haig Ferguson forceps are typical of those used for mid and low cavity forceps delivery (a), note the presence of a cephalic curve to accommodate the fetal head, and a pelvic curve to allow the forceps to fit the birth canal. This contrasts with Kjellands forceps (b) which only have a cephalic curve. The absence of the pelvic curve allows these forceps to be used for rotation of the fetal head.*

217

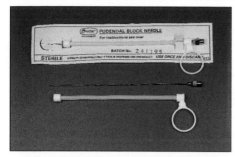

Fig. 8.32 *Pudendal block needle used to provide a local anaesthetic block in the course of a forceps or ventouse delivery. The needle protected by the needle guard is guided within the vagina to the ischial spine. The needle is advanced into the tissues and local anaesthetic injected posterior to the spine to provide a block to the pudendal nerve. The procedure is repeated on the other side.*

Forceps delivery

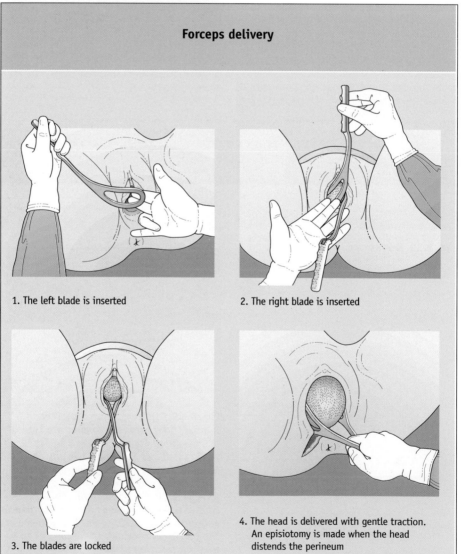

1. The left blade is inserted

2. The right blade is inserted

3. The blades are locked

4. The head is delivered with gentle traction. An episiotomy is made when the head distends the perineum

Fig. 8.33 *Forceps delivery.*

Rotational forceps (Kjelland's forceps)

Rotational forceps are used when a malposition is present. It is essential that the correct position is clearly identified before application of the blades to avoid fetal and maternal trauma. Kjelland's forceps have a sliding lock on the shank to enable correction of asynclitism (when the fetal neck is flexed laterally), which is especially common with occipitotransverse positions. There are small knobs on the handles of the forceps for orientation. These knobs point towards the occiput after application. The left or anterior blade is applied first. With an occipitoposterior position the blades are applied directly. With an occipitotransverse position, the anterior blade can be applied directly, or inserted laterally then 'wandered' over the fetal head into the correct position under the symphysis. The second blade is applied directly and the blades are locked. Rotation by the short route is then performed to the occipitoanterior position. The position of the head must be checked after rotation before traction is applied.

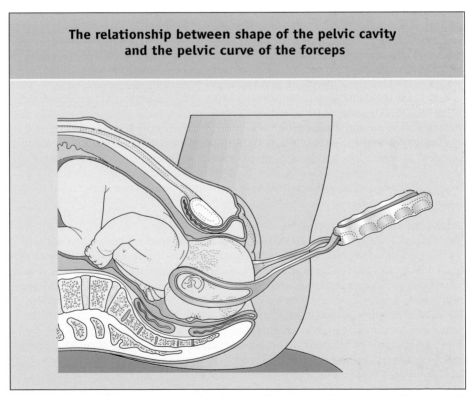

The relationship between shape of the pelvic cavity and the pelvic curve of the forceps

Fig. 8.34 *The relationship between the shape of the pelvic cavity and the pelvic curve of the forceps.*

CAESAREAN SECTION

In this operation the baby is delivered abdominally, after the abdominal cavity and the uterus have been opened. There are many indications for caesarean section. It can be performed electively before the onset of labour, for example, because of a previous section for cephalopelvic disproportion or for breech presentation, or as an emergency, for example, for fetal distress, either before or during labour. Caesarean section is associated with a significantly higher maternal morbidity and mortality than vaginal delivery. There are few absolute indications for caesarean section (such as major placenta praevia). For most patients, the benefits to the mother and baby have to be balanced against the risks of the operation. The procedure leaves a scar on the uterus. This influences the woman's obstetric future and leads to a significantly higher chance of delivery by caesarean section in subsequent pregnancies.

Lower uterine segment caesarean section

This is the most common type of caesarean section, often performed under regional anaesthesia. The anterior abdominal wall is usually opened through a transverse suprapubic incision, and the peritoneal cavity is entered. The lower uterine segment is exposed by opening the uterine peritoneum transversely where it lies loose above the uterovesical fold. The bladder is then reflected down to prevent trauma and the lower segment of the uterus is opened transversely. The fetus is delivered through the incision. The placenta and membranes are then delivered and the uterine cavity is confirmed empty. The uterine incision is closed in two layers. Most women are able to eat and drink later the same day, and are mobile within 24 hours. As a result of the increased thrombotic tendency in pregnancy and the association between deep venous thrombosis and pelvic surgery, consideration should be given to thromboprophylaxis (e.g. with low-dose or low molecular weight heparin). It is also usual for women to receive prophylactic antibiotics to reduce the risk of infective complications.

The incidence of scar rupture in a future pregnancy after a lower segment caesarean section is extremely low. Labour and vaginal delivery are feasible after a lower segment caesarean section as long as the indication for the initial procedure is not recurrent (e.g. breech presentation) and care is taken to monitor the fetal condition and avoid overstimulation of the uterus.

Classical caesarean section

In a classical caesarean section, the body of the uterus is opened vertically in the midline. Compared with a lower segment caesarean section, the classical operation is associated with greater blood loss and healing is poorer. As a result there is an increased risk of scar rupture in subsequent pregnancies, both spontaneously and during labour. As a result of this, labour and vaginal delivery are contraindicated after classical caesarean section. The indications for classical caesarean section include instances in which delivery is performed before the lower segment is formed (such as extreme prematurity), instances in which entry into the lower segment may be hazardous (some cases of placenta praevia, large fibroids), and some cases of transverse lie with ruptured membranes when it may not be possible to reach a limb or deliver a fetal pole through the lower segment.

PRETERM LABOUR

Prematurity accounts for more than 50% of cases of neonatal morbidity and mortality. It is defined as labour before 37 completed weeks of gestation. In general, poor maternal nutrition and low social class are associated with an increased incidence of preterm delivery, as is smoking and a maternal age of younger than 20 years. A past history of preterm labour and delivery is predictive of recurrence, particularly if this has happened more than

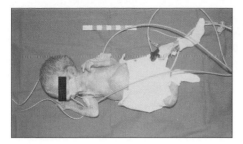

Fig. 8.35 *Preterm neonate in incubator.*

once. In most cases, however, no cause is found. Infection has been implicated in the aetiology of a significant number of cases but it is still not clearly established whether antibiotics are of benefit in the absence of clear indicators of infection. Uterine malformations and congenital fetal abnormalities, especially those linked with polyhydramnios, are also associated with preterm labour. Multiple pregnancy can lead to preterm labour in the same way that polyhydramnios seems to, by overdistension of the uterus. Antepartum haemorrhage, particularly placental abruption, can initiate labour at any gestation (**Fig. 8.35**).

Cervical incompetence

This is a condition in which the cervix dilates spontaneously. The problem usually occurs without warning. The patient often presents in the second trimester with an effaced, dilating cervix in the absence of uterine contractions or vaginal bleeding. Cervical incompetence may be diagnosed because of a previous history of second trimester miscarriage or may follow cervical surgery (such as a cone biopsy). Delivery is usually inevitable but a cervical suture can be inserted as an emergency if there is no bleeding, no infection, no uterine activity and enough cervix in which to place a stitch. The only effective treatment is cervical cerclage which should be done electively at approximately 14 weeks' gestation. This is carried out with a heavy tape which is tightly tied. It is released at approximately 36 weeks, before labour, or when the patient presents in labour if it is still *in situ* (**Fig. 8.36**).

The management of preterm labour

Unless the benefits of delivery outweigh the risks of prematurity, then an attempt should be made to arrest preterm labour if this is possible. In the short term this may allow *in utero* transfer to a unit more equipped to look after a preterm baby, and the administration of high-dose corticosteroids (two 12mg doses of betamethasone or dexamethasone given intramuscularly 12–24 hours apart) to the mother to promote fetal lung maturity. This will significantly reduce the risk of infant respiratory distress syndrome and its complications, and represents the biggest single contribution an obstetrician can make to influence the outcome of preterm labour. The short-term use of a tocolytic therapy such as ritodrine may be of value to allow steroid administration to occur.

In the long term, the prolongation of pregnancy, ideally to term, will avoid the risks of prematurity. However, the drugs available to inhibit preterm labour are not ideal. β-sympathomimetics given intravenously, such as ritodrine, terbutaline and salbutamol, are useful for short-term therapy, but do not decrease the incidence of preterm delivery or reduce neonatal morbidity or mortality. They are also associated with significant maternal side effects: tachycardia, tremor, palpitations and pulmonary oedema. Cyclo-oxygenase inhibitors such as indomethacin, which decrease prostaglandin production, have been shown to inhibit preterm labour and decrease the incidence of preterm delivery, but there is a risk of premature closure of the ductus arteriosus. Other drugs that may have a role

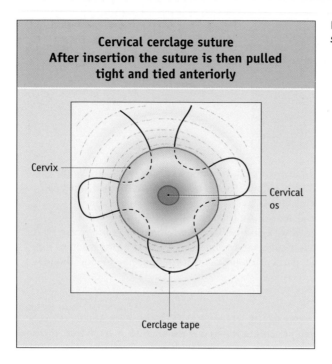

Cervical cerclage suture
After insertion the suture is then pulled
tight and tied anteriorly

Cervix

Cervical
os

Cerclage tape

Fig. 8.36 *Cervical cerclage suture.*

include calcium channel antagonists and oxytocin antagonists. If infection is present, it should be treated. If the presentation is cephalic and labour becomes established, it should be managed as normal, with intervention based on fetal and maternal monitoring. If the presentation is breech, there is good evidence to suggest that caesarean section is safer than vaginal delivery below 35 weeks' gestation.

Preterm, prelabour rupture of the membranes

This is defined as the spontaneous rupture of the membranes before 37 weeks' gestation (**Fig. 8.37**) and before the onset of labour. It is important to confirm the diagnosis, usually by speculum examination to reveal the presence of a pool of liquor in the vagina. Ultrasound may be helpful to assess liquor volume. Digital vaginal examination should be avoided as this will only serve to introduce infection. In many cases, uterine activity will follow shortly after membrane rupture, but if labour does not supervene in the first few days, there may be a prolonged latent period. Labour can be precipitated by the development of infection which is a significant risk in the presence of ruptured membranes. The development of chorioamnionitis is a serious complication and usually warrants delivery. Intrauterine infection should be suspected if the uterus becomes tender or if other indices of infection develop, such as maternal or fetal tachycardia, maternal pyrexia, elevated white cell count, elevated C-reactive protein, vaginal discharge or a positive high vaginal swab. If there is a long-standing oligohydramnios secondary to membrane rupture, fetal flexion contractures can develop. Pulmonary hypoplasia is often a fatal consequence of preterm, prelabour rupture of the membranes between 18 and 22 weeks' gestation.

Prelabour rupture of the membranes

This is defined as the rupture of the membranes at term, before the onset of labour. A confirmation of the diagnosis by speculum examination is important if doubt exists because

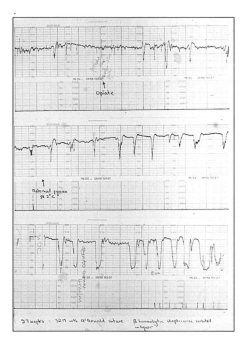

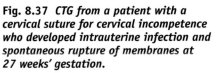

Fig. 8.37 *CTG from a patient with a cervical suture for cervical incompetence who developed intrauterine infection and spontaneous rupture of membranes at 27 weeks' gestation.*

at term intervention is common if labour does not become established. It is also important to exclude any fetal distress by assessing the fetal heart rate because cord prolapse and cord compression may occur. In the majority of cases, labour will become established in the next 24 hours. Thus, it is worth managing these cases conservatively at first if there is no other abnormality. The main risk is infection. Digital examination should be avoided if a conservative approach is to be adopted. For patients who do not establish labour within 24 hours, induction is usually recommended, although recent evidence suggests that expectant management for up to 4 days does not result in a significant increase in the risk of infection.

Cord prolapse

Cord presentation is when the umbilical cord lies beside or in front of the presenting part. It is more common in malpresentations, polyhydramnios, during breech deliveries and with preterm rupture of the membranes. It is an obstetric emergency. The umbilical vessels will constrict once exposed to the extrauterine environment, the cord will stop pulsating and the fetus will perish from asphyxia. Unless the cervix is fully dilated, when an operative vaginal delivery can be conducted, then caesarean section is required. During the transfer to theatre, the woman is kept in the knee–chest position and the presenting part is pushed up and held digitally. These measures reduce pressure on the cord.

THE THIRD STAGE OF LABOUR AND THE PUERPERIUM

THE THIRD STAGE OF LABOUR

The third stage of labour begins with the delivery of the baby and ends with the expulsion of the placenta. The uterine muscle contracts after the delivery of the baby constricting the vessels supplying the placental bed and preventing bleeding. In the UK, the management of the third stage is usually active, which involves the administration of an oxytocic agent to enhance uterine contraction (usually Syntocinon® or Syntometrine®, a combination of oxytocin and ergometrine) (**Fig. 8.38**) and the removal of the separated placenta. The active management of the third stage of labour decreases the incidence of postpartum haemorrhage by approximately 60% but is associated with an increase in the risk of a retained placenta. Syntometrine® appears slightly better than oxytocin in preventing postpartum haemorrhage but causes more side effects, such as nausea and vomiting. Furthermore, ergometrine will provoke peripheral vasoconstriction and increase blood pressure and so should be avoided in women with hypertensive problems such as pre-eclampsia.

The placenta is delivered by controlled cord traction (Brandt–Andrews' method) once signs of placental separation are present. This involves placing the left hand suprapubically, and once a contraction has occurred, pushing the uterus upwards, while the right hand applies traction to the cord, pulling the placenta out of the vagina. The potential problems are uterine inversion or avulsion of the cord. Once delivered, the placenta and membranes are examined to check that they are complete. Blood loss is assessed and the genital tract is inspected for damage (**Fig. 8.39**).

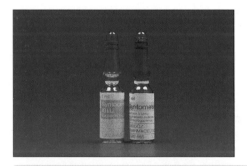

Fig. 8.38 *Vials of Syntocinon® (synthetic oxytocin) and Syntometrine® (a combination of ergometrine and oxytocin) used in the active management of the third stage of labour.*

Management of the third stage of labour

Active
Administer a combination of ergometrine 0.5mg and oxytocin 5 IU, or 10 IU of oxytocin with the delivery of the anterior shoulder
Clamp and divide the umbilical cord
Await signs of placental separation (contraction of uterus, gush of blood, lengthening of cord)
Deliver placenta and membranes by controlled cord traction

Passive
Do not administer oxytocin
Await signs of placental separation
Deliver placenta using maternal effort and gravity
Do not use cord traction

Fig. 8.39 *Management of the third stage of labour.*

THE EXAMINATION OF THE PLACENTA, MEMBRANES AND CORD

The placenta should be suspended by its cord to show the extent and completeness of the membranes (**Fig. 8.40**). The fetal side is examined, paying particular attention to the blood vessels. If any of these run off the edge of the placenta, the possibility of a succenturiate lobe needs to be considered. This may have become detached during delivery and may be retained within the uterus. The maternal side is then examined to ensure that the cotyledons fit together and that none have been left inside the uterus. Finally, the cut end of the cord is assessed and the number of vessels noted. The absence of one umbilical artery can be associated with congenital anomalies in the baby, especially renal abnormalities. The placenta is usually weighed and is usually one sixth to one seventh of the fetal weight (500–600g) in a normal term pregnancy.

PRIMARY POSTPARTUM HAEMORRHAGE

Primary postpartum haemorrhage (PPH) is defined as a blood loss of 500ml or more within 24 hours of delivery. It occurs after 1–2% of all deliveries and remains a significant cause of maternal morbidity (haemorrhage, anaemia, disseminated intravascular coagulation, rarely pituitary necrosis [Sheehan's syndrome]) and mortality. The principles of management are resuscitation, together with the identification and treatment of the cause. Retention of part or all of the placenta, preventing uterine contraction and allowing the placental bed vessels to bleed, and uterine atony, account for 80% of cases. The predisposing factors for uterine atony include overdistension of the uterus (twins, polyhydramnios), multiparity, prolonged labour, deep general anaesthesia, placenta praevia and placental abruption. Any woman with a previous history of postpartum haemorrhage is at an increased risk in subsequent pregnancies (**Fig. 8.41**).

The management of primary postpartum haemorrhage

The management is to stop the bleeding and restore the blood volume. In major haemorrhage, intravenous access should be gained ideally with two wide (14 gauge) bore cannulae and plasma expander administered as required. Blood should be taken to measure the haematocrit and haemoglobin concentration. The patient should be cross matched. The possibility of disseminated intravascular coagulation should be borne in mind. If the placenta has been delivered and is thought to be complete, the first line of action is to ensure that the uterus is well contracted and the bladder empty as a full bladder can be associated with such problems. Uterine contraction can be encouraged by manual stimulation ('rubbing up' a contraction) or by the administration of oxytocic agents including oxytocin, ergometrine, and in refractory cases, the prostaglandin Hemabate®. If

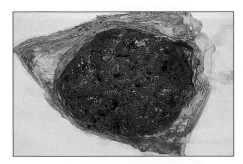

Fig. 8.40 *Normal placenta and membranes. (From Symonds, E. Malcolm and Macpherson, Marion B. A. 'Diagnosis in Color: Obstetrics and Gynecology' (Mosby-Wolfe, 1997), with permission.)*

The causes of primary postpartum haemorrhage	
Retained placenta	Complete or partial retention Morbidly adherent placenta (placenta accreta)
Placenta delivered	Atonic uterus Genital tract trauma
Other causes	Disseminated intravascular coagulation Uterine inversion Uterine rupture

Fig. 8.41 *The causes of primary postpartum haemorrhage.*

bleeding continues despite a well-contracted uterus, a formal examination of the vagina, cervix and uterus may be required under anaesthesia. Ligation of the uterine or internal iliac arteries or even hysterectomy may be necessary in the face of profuse haemorrhage which fails to settle (**Fig. 8.42**).

A RETAINED PLACENTA

If the placenta has separated but has not delivered, delivery can usually be expedited using controlled cord traction. If the placenta cannot be delivered, it should be removed manually. Adequate anaesthesia (general or regional) is required for this procedure. The bladder is emptied. One hand is placed on the abdomen to locate and steady the fundus. The other hand is introduced into the uterus, following the cord to the placenta. The fingers separate

The management of primary postpartum haemorrhage
Alert all relevant medical, midwifery and support staff. 'Rub up' a contraction or give oxytocin intravenously. Empty the bladder (leave Foley catheter in situ). Maintain uterine contraction (oxytocin infusion, ergometrine, Hemabate®). Take blood for cross-match, coagulation screen and full blood count. If placenta is undelivered, remove. Correct hypovolaemia. Check for vaginal, cervical or uterine lacerations. Consider bimanual compression of uterus, packing of uterus, ligation of uterine or internal iliac arteries, or hysterectomy. Deal with coagulation failure.

Fig. 8.42 *The management of primary postpartum haemorrhage.*

the placenta from the uterine wall, with the abdominal hand serving as a guide to prevent tearing of the uterus. Once completely free, the placenta is removed. The uterus is then explored carefully to ensure the cavity is empty. **Figure 8.43** illustrates manual removal of the placenta.

MORBID ADHERENCE OF THE PLACENTA

Placenta accreta is when the chorionic villi invade excessively and are thus morbidly adherent to the myometrium in part or all of the placental site. If the villi penetrate deeper into the muscle, reaching the serosa, the condition is termed placenta increta. These conditions are seen most often after a previous caesarean section, when the placenta implants over the scar. Morbid adherence of the placenta prevents the separation which usually takes place when the uterus contracts after delivery of the baby. Attempts at

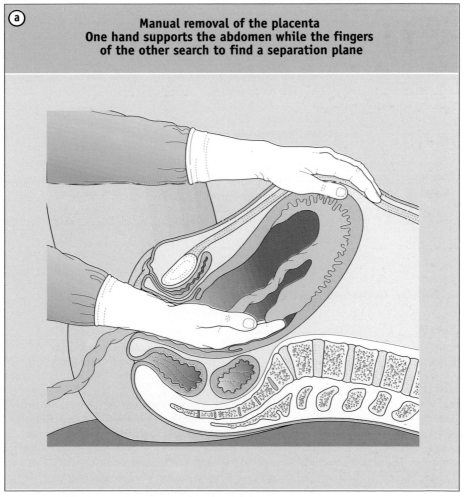

(a)

Manual removal of the placenta
One hand supports the abdomen while the fingers
of the other search to find a separation plane

Fig. 8.43 *Manual removal of the placenta. (a) One hand supports the abdomen while the fingers of the other search to find a separation plane.*

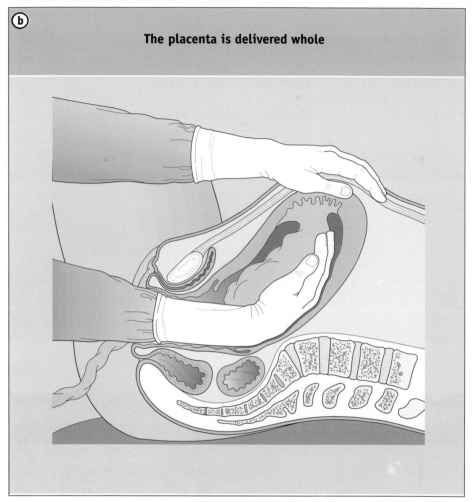

The placenta is delivered whole

Fig. 8.43 *(b)* *The placenta is delivered whole.*

removal can precipitate severe haemorrhage. If the diagnosis is made before there is significant bleeding, the placenta can be left *in utero* and will be absorbed gradually.

GENITAL TRAUMA

Four degrees of perineal tears are recognized. First degree involve the skin at the fourchette. Second degree tears the posterior vaginal wall and the perineal muscle. Third degree involve the anal sphincter, but the rectal mucosa is intact, whereas in fourth degree tears, the anal canal is open. Vaginal haematomas can occur during delivery and there may be no visible blood loss. The patient complains of perineal pain and a continuing desire to bear down. She may require resuscitation and transfusion. Broad ligament haematomas may be palpable abdominally, displacing the uterus laterally. Transfusion is usually required but most resolve spontaneously.

UTERINE INVERSION

Uterine inversion is rare but it can lead to shock, haemorrhage (which can be exacerbated by disseminated intravascular coagulation), sepsis and death. It occurs most commonly when cord traction has been applied in the absence of uterine contractions. The fundus may appear at the introitus or may be felt in the vagina: the uterus will not be palpable in the abdomen. Immediate replacement of the uterus should be attempted. If this is not possible, the patient should be resuscitated and an attempt at manual reduction should be made under general anaesthesia. If this fails reduction may be achieved using hydrostatic pressure. In this procedure, warm saline is run into the vagina, while holding the vulva closed, until the position of the uterus is restored. Reduction by the abdominal route is sometimes required.

SECONDARY POSTPARTUM HAEMORRHAGE

Secondary postpartum haemorrhage is defined as excessive bleeding from the genital tract more than 24 hours after but within 6 weeks of delivery. The most common causes are retained placental fragments and infection. Rare causes include sloughing of a subendometrial fibroid, von Willebrand's disease or choriocarcinoma. The management depends on the severity of bleeding and the cause. After clinical examination, which often reveals a tender, bulky uterus with an open cervix, investigations include a full blood count, C-reactive protein estimation, high vaginal swabs and pelvic ultrasound. If the bleeding is severe, the patient should be resuscitated and given intravenous oxytocics and broad spectrum antibiotics before examination under anaesthesia. Retained products of conception require surgical evacuation of the uterus, under antibiotic cover (**Fig. 8.44**).

THE PUERPERIUM

The puerperium is the time during which the genital tract returns to normal after childbirth. By convention it is said to last 6 weeks. The normal puerperium is characterized by lactation, lochia, involution of the uterus and return of the remainder of the genital tract to normal. Lochia is the term used to describe the uterine discharge after delivery. It is blood for the first few days, serosanguinous for the next 7–10 days and then yellowish-white until it ceases. By the end of the third stage of labour, the uterus has usually contracted down to the level of the umbilicus, and weighs approximately 1kg. Involution occurs by autolysis of the muscle fibres, so that by the end of the first puerperal week, the uterus weighs approximately 500gm and is palpable above the pubis symphysis, and by day 10–12 it is no longer palpable in the abdomen.

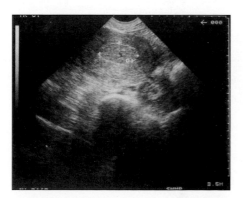

Fig. 8.44 *Ultrasound scan appearance of retained products of conception in a patient who had a secondary PPH following spontaneous vaginal delivery. She was treated with antibiotics and surgical evacuation of the uterus was performed where a piece of placental tissue 5 x 5 x 3cm was obtained.*

The management of the puerperium

The goals of puerperal care are the restoration of optimal maternal health, establishment of infant feeding and bonding, education of the mother and achievement of optimal infant health. Contraception should also be discussed. The length of stay in hospital is governed by a combination of social, manpower and medical factors. There has been a move towards earlier discharge from hospital, which in turn has increased the need for adequate support in the community. In the UK there is a statutory requirement for mothers to be seen daily by a midwife for 10–14 days after delivery (**Fig. 8.45**).

Lactation

Fat is deposited in the breasts during pregnancy. Oestrogen leads to an increase in the size and number of ducts, whereas progesterone increases the number of alveoli. Human placental lactogen also stimulates alveolar development. Lactation is inhibited during pregnancy because of high oestrogen concentrations, which fall rapidly in the 48 hours after childbirth, permitting prolactin to act on the alveolar cells. Lactation itself is encouraged by early and frequent suckling which causes the anterior pituitary gland to secrete prolactin, and which induces the alveolar cells to secrete milk. Suckling also initiates the milk ejection reflex, during which oxytocin is released from the posterior pituitary gland to cause contraction of the myoepithelial cells within the breast.

Breast-feeding

Colostrum is secreted for the first 2 days postnatally. It contains fat globules and antibodies (especially IgA). It has a high mineral content, with moderate protein and low sugar. Milk volumes increase steadily from day 3. By the sixth day, approximately 500ml will be taken by the baby. Feeding is usually on demand. Compared with cow's milk, human milk has a higher energy value. It contains less protein and sodium but more fat and lactose. The anti-infective properties of breast milk are due to specific immunoglobulin IgA, lymphocytes and bacteriocidal enzymes (**Fig. 8.46**).

Management of the puerperium

Observations (temperature, pulse, blood pressure, uterine size, lochia, bladder and
   bowel function, haemoglobin concentration)
Analgesia ('after-pains', perineum, caesarean scar)
Rest, sleep
Infant feeding, mothercraft
Diet
Postnatal exercises
Psychological support

Fig. 8.45 *Management of the puerperium.*

Fig. 8.46 *The advantages of breast feeding.*

The advantages of breast feeding

Simple, safe and free.
More digestible than formula feeds.
Protects against infection (especially gastrointestinal).
Protects against atopic diseases.
Promotes uterine involution.
Decreases the incidence of subsequent breast
    carcinoma in the mother.
Associated with higher infant IQ.
Promotes bonding.

Problems – If cracked nipples occur, fixation of the baby on to the breast should be checked. The affected breast should be rested and the milk expressed manually. Breast engorgement can be very painful. It is seen most often on day 4. Firm support, manual expression and analgesia may be required. The engorgement usually settles within a few days. Acute mastitis usually presents 7–10 days postnatally. The mother develops a fever and a tender, red, firm area in one breast. The organisms involved are usually *Staphylococci* or *Streptococci*. Treatment is with antibiotics and analgesia. Suckling should continue, if possible. If the swelling becomes fluctuant and pus develops, causing a breast abscess, incision and drainage will be required.

Bottle-feeding with artificial formulae

There are a number of formula feeds available, mainly based on cow's milk. Cow's milk contains more protein (predominantly casein) than breast milk, whereas breast milk consists of almost equal parts of casein and lactalbumin. The fat contents are similar, but the quality is different, with breast milk having more polyunsaturated fatty acids. On the first day, feeds start with 60ml/kg and increase by 30ml/kg each day until the baby is receiving 150ml/kg. Fully constituted artificial feeds provide 65–70calories/100ml.

Puerperal pyrexia

Puerperal pyrexia occurs when a woman has a temperature greater or equal to 38°C within 14 days of confinement or miscarriage. A systematic investigation is required to determine the cause and site of the problem. The urinary tract is the most common site, often induced by catheterization and caused by *E. coli*. The genital tract is particularly vulnerable to infection in the days after delivery. The organisms most often responsible for the infection are *E. coli*, *Staphylococcus pyogenes*, *Streptococcus faecalis* and haemolytic streptococci. The patient presents with fever, malaise, lower abdominal pain, offensive lochia and a tender uterus. Swabs (high vaginal and endocervical) need to be taken and any retained products of conception must be excluded. Appropriate broad spectrum antibiotic (e.g. a cephalosporin and metronidazole) therapy is started which can be modified when culture and sensitivity results are available. An evacuation of the uterus will be required if any retained products of conception are suspected. Acute thrombophlebitis is another important cause of puerperal infection which presents 3–4 days after delivery. Localized inflammation, tenderness and thickening in superficial leg veins occurs. Treatment is with anti-inflammatory drugs and support stockings. The possibility of deep venous thrombosis should always be borne in mind. Acute mastitis usually occurs 7–10 days postnatally. Wound infection after caesarean section, although reduced with the use of prophylactic antibiotics, can also be responsible, and chest infection, particularly after general anaesthesia, can occur. Clearly, more than one cause can be present in a patient: for example, urinary and genital tract infection may coexist and deep venous thrombosis is more common in patients with infection particularly after surgery (**Fig. 8.47**).

Fig. 8.47 *Causes of postpartum pyrexia.*

Causes of postpartum pyrexia

Urinary tract infection
Genital tract infection
Thrombophlebitis
Deep venous thrombosis
Acute mastitis or breast abscess
Wound infection
Chest infection

Psychiatric disorders in the puerperium

Minor neurosis	Insidious onset 3–12 months after delivery.
	Composed of 'depression', anxiety, obsessions, phobias and problems with mothering.
	Treatment is to improve social cicumstances, provide support and mobilize self-help groups.
Postpartum	Two peaks of presentation (2–4 weeks and depression 10–14 weeks' postpartum).
	Classic symptoms of depression and anxiety.
	Treatment is with antidepressants and support.
	1:5 recurrence risk.
Postpartum psychosis	Abrupt onset day 3–14.
	Mainly affective (manic depressive) with delusions, hallucinations and impaired perception of reality.
	Requires admission to psychiatric hospital and treatment with psychotropic drugs.
	1:5 recurrence risk.

Fig. 8.48 *Psychiatric disorders in the puerperium.*

Puerperal psychological disorders

Sixteen per cent of women will develop an episode of mental illness during the first 3 months after childbirth. The risk of suffering from a major mental illness in these first 3 months is 16 times greater than it is normally for women. The risk factors include a family or personal history of mental illness, neonatal or maternal disease, caesarean section, unrealistic expectations and social isolation. 'Third-day blues' occur in 50–70% of women, and mainly present with emotional lability and irritability. Symptoms usually last less than a week and respond well to psychological support (**Fig. 8.48**).

Urinary problems

A urinary tract infection occurs in 10–15% of women postpartum. The risk of pyelonephritis also remains high. Voiding difficulties are seen in approximately 10% of women in the 48 hours after delivery. These problems are associated with epidural analgesia, prolonged labour, instrumental delivery and a painful perineum. The traditional methods of encouraging micturition include hot baths, analgesia for perineal pain and local ice packs. If these measures fail, catheterization may be required. Stress incontinence is seen in a significant number of women after childbirth. Pelvic floor exercises should be instituted. If incontinence is present, it must be established whether this is urethral or due to a fistula, particularly after an operative delivery. The instillation of coloured dye into the bladder and a tampon in the vagina can aid diagnosis.

Thromboembolic disease in the puerperium

Thromboembolism remains an important cause of maternal death (**Fig. 8.49**). Not only is there a hypercoagulable state, but there can also be venous stasis (exacerbated by immobility, particularly after operative delivery) and damage to the vessel wall from infection or trauma. The risk of thromboembolism is increased even further by other factors including obesity, a long labour, dehydration, a past history of thrombosis and a family history which may suggest underlying thrombophilia (see below). Prophylactic anticoagulation (usually subcutaneous heparin or low molecular weight heparin postnatally, and sometimes prenatally as well) should be considered for women at risk, in addition to measures including early mobilization and thromboembolic deterrent stockings. Routine prophylaxis at least until discharge from hospital or for 5 days should be considered for women having a caesarean section with any additional risk factors, for example, emergency section during labour or elective caesarean section for a patient with pre-eclampsia. Any patient with either a personal or family history of thromboembolism should be screened for underlying thrombophilia. Blood should be analysed for deficiencies of proteins S and C and antithrombin III, activated protein C resistance (factor V Leiden), prothrombin gene variant, lupus anticoagulant and anticardiolipin antibodies. For patients requiring prolonged prophylaxis, heparin or low molecular weight heparin can be used initially, followed by warfarin. Neither warfarin nor heparin cross the breast and they are safe for breast-feeding.

Diagnosis and management – The importance of an accurate diagnosis of deep venous thrombosis (DVT) in the puerperium cannot be overstressed. The most common clinical features are pain, tenderness, swelling, oedema, a change in leg colour and temperature and a palpable thrombosed vein. Over 80% of DVTs during pregnancy are left-sided and they are usually ileofemoral and therefore at high risk of leading to pulmonary embolus. However, the clinical diagnosis of DVT is unreliable. The investigation of choice is duplex Doppler ultrasound (**Fig. 8.50**). If the diagnosis is still uncertain, venography should be performed. If the diagnosis is confirmed, the patient should be screened for underlying thrombophilia and intravenous or subcutaneous doses of therapeutic heparin should be

Risk factors for thromboembolic disease

Fig. 8.49 *Risk factors for thromboembolic disease.*

Over 35 years
Obesity (>80 kg)
High parity (4 or more)
Gross varicose veins
Emergency caesarean section in labour
Pre-eclampsia
Immobility before delivery
Extended major pelvic or abdominal surgery, e.g.
    caesarean hysterectomy
Previous thromboembolic event
Thrombophilia
Concurrent medical condition, e.g. nephrotic syndrome,
    infection
Paralysis of lower limbs

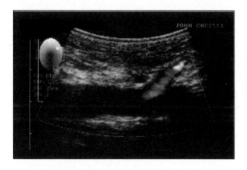

Fig. 8.50 *Duplex colour Doppler ultrasound scan showing a normal saphenous vein with flow present (blue) and an occluded common femoral vein with no flow in patient with left side DVT following caesarean section.*

commenced with monitoring by the activated partial thromboplastin time. Low molecular weight heparins may also be used for treatment of DVT, and for recommended doses no monitoring is required. Warfarin may be introduced after 3–5 days and the clinician should be alert to the possibility of secondary postpartum haemorrhage on warfarin. Patients should remain on anticoagulant therapy for at least 6 weeks after delivery.

FETAL ADAPTATION TO EXTRAUTERINE LIFE

The fetus becomes increasingly hypoxic just before birth. This mild degree of hypoxia stimulates the first gasps for air after the baby is born. During labour and immediately after birth, the lungs are cleared of fluid, one third being squeezed out through the nose and mouth and the remainder being absorbed by the pulmonary lymphatics and circulation. Within 15 minutes the alveoli are distended with air. The lungs expand, open up the pulmonary vascular bed and the pulmonary vascular resistance falls. The systemic arterial pressure rises when the cord is clamped, resulting in a temporary reversal of flow through the ductus arteriosus. The oxygen tension rises and the ductus constricts. The pressure in the right atrium falls. There is an increase in blood flow through the lungs. Together with the increasing systemic resistance, this leads to an increase in the pressure in the left atrium. These changes in turn result in functional closure of the foramen ovale. The ductus arteriosus obliterates eventually by endarteritis. The ductus venosus atrophies, whereas the umbilical vein remains as the ligamentum teres. The umbilical arteries persist as sclerosed remnants.

RESUSCITATION OF THE NEWBORN

The majority of babies are born in good condition and all that may be required is gentle suction to clear mucus and debris from the pharynx, mouth and nostrils. The status of the baby at birth can be quantified using the Apgar score. The score is recorded for five criteria and the total calculated at 1 and 5 minutes (**Fig. 8.51**). If the score is greater than 7 at 1 minute, no resuscitation is required. However, if breathing is impaired or absent, active resuscitation is indicated. With Apgar scores between 4 and 7, the baby usually responds to oxygen via a mask and tactile stimulation. If the Apgar score is less than 3, the newborn requires ventilation, initially with a face mask, followed by endotracheal intubation. When the heart rate is less than 40 beats/minute, external cardiac massage is indicated. Acidosis is corrected by sodium bicarbonate (5mmol/kg) administered via the umbilical vein. If respiratory depression can be attributed to opiates, naloxone should be given.

EXAMINATION OF THE NEWBORN

A check for major abnormalities is made immediately after birth. A more comprehensive examination is usually carried out 24–48 hours later. The Moro reflex is a startle reflex elicited by making a noise, letting the baby's head drop backwards by 1–2 cm or by flexing the head on the trunk. Extension and abduction of the arms should be followed by adduction and flexion. The reflex should be symmetrical and indicates normal

The Apgar score

Score	0	1	2
Colour	Blue/pale	Pink body, blue extremities	Pink
Respiratory effort	Absent	Weak cry, hypoventilation	Good
Muscle tone	Limp	Some flexion of extremities	Active movement
Reflex irritability	None	Grimace	Cry
Heart rate	Absent	Below 100 beats/min	Above 100 beats/min

Fig. 8.51 *The Apgar score.*

Examination of the newborn

Check the identity of baby.
Assess colour and look for skin abnormalities.
Measure occipitofrontal circumference, feel skull and fontanelles.
Palpate the neck for goitre or sternomastoid tumour.
Check for cleft palate by placing a finger in the baby's mouth.
Check for cataracts and that the baby 'follows' movement.
Note respiratory rate.
Listen to the heart and chest.
Palpate the abdomen.
Examine the external genitalia and femoral pulses, and exclude herniae.
Test for Moro and traction reflexes.
Pick up the baby prone: check muscle tone, examine spine and anus.
Exclude dislocation of hips.
Count the fingers and toes.

Fig. 8.52 *Examination of the newborn.*

neuromuscular co-ordination. The traction manoeuvre involves lifting the baby by grasping the hands: the baby should flex the arms and keep his or her head in the plane of the trunk. A mature normal baby has a rectal temperature of 36–36.5°C, a pulse rate of 120–140 beats/minute and a respiratory rate of between 30 and 40 breaths/minute (**Fig. 8.52**).

THE PRETERM INFANT

The use of antenatal steroids and advances in neonatal care have led to dramatic improvements in the survival of infants born before 37 weeks of pregnancy (**Fig. 8.35**). Preterm infants are prone to complications including, hypothermia, respiratory distress syndrome (hyaline membrane disease), jaundice, infection and cerebral haemorrhage. Respiratory distress syndrome is caused by a relative lack of surfactant in the alveoli. It presents within a few hours of birth with expiratory grunting, a respiratory rate of more than 60 breaths/minute, intercostal and sternal indrawing, nasal flaring and cyanosis. The chest radiograph shows a characteristic reticulogranular appearance with an air bronchogram. Treatment involves avoiding heat loss, providing oxygen, the correction of acidosis, the maintenance of blood pressure and the replacement of surfactant.

CRANIAL INJURIES

Caput succedaneum is caused by oedema of the subcutaneous tissues of the scalp due to the impedance of lymphatic and venous drainage in labour. The swelling covers a large area of the scalp and disappears within a few days of delivery. Cephalhaematoma is a subperiostial haematoma which most commonly lies over the parietal bones. It is due to trauma and is

Caput succedaneum (left) and cephalhaematoma (right)

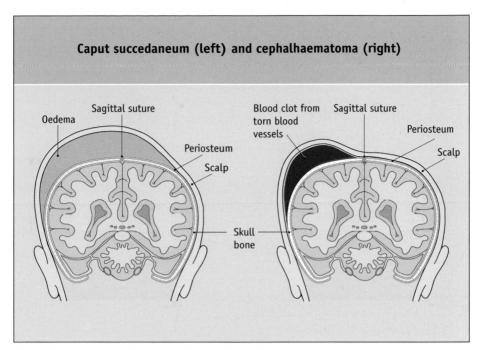

Fig. 8.53 *Caput succedaneum and cephalhaematoma.*

more common after an instrumental delivery with forceps or ventouse. It is confined to the shape of the bone and is fluctuant initially. Ossification takes place later, leaving a hard rim. No treatment is required but the haematoma may take weeks or months to resolve (Fig. 8.53).

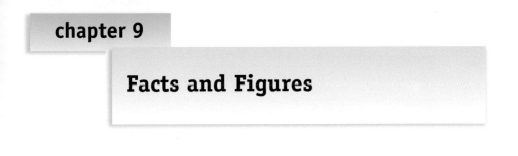

chapter 9

Facts and Figures

Obstetrics and gynaecology has long had as a part of its own clinical analysis a system of audits on maternal and perinatal outcomes. These statistics have documented improvements in maternity care and highlighted areas of concern.

MATERNAL DEATHS

In the UK, there is a system of Confidential Enquiries into each and every maternal death. This has been in place since 1952. Every 3 years, a report of the enquiry is produced detailing numbers of deaths, their causes and areas in which there was substandard care. Maternal deaths, by international agreement, may be subdivided into direct, indirect and fortuitous.

- Direct maternal deaths are "resulting from obstetric complications of the pregnant state (pregnancy, labour and puerperium), from interventions, omissions, incorrect treatment or from a chain of events resulting from any of the above".
- Indirect maternal deaths are defined as "resulting from previous existing disease, or diseases developed during pregnancy and which were not due to obstetric causes or which were aggravated by the physiological effects of pregnancy".
- Fortuitous deaths are "deaths from unrelated causes which happened to occur in pregnancy or the puerperium".

The deaths have to occur during pregnancy or within 42 days of the pregnancy. If death occurs beyond this, it has been termed a "late death". With modern intensive care, it is likely that a proportion of deaths, which would previously have occurred within 6 weeks of delivery, may occur beyond this time and be classified as late deaths.

Deaths are usually reported in terms of the number of maternities, that is, the number of mothers delivered of live or stillborn infants. This is different from the number of babies born which would include multiple pregnancies. In the UK, the maternal mortality rate per 100,000 maternities is approximately six. Elsewhere in the world, however, maternal mortality rates are not so low. Estimates for maternal mortality are shown in **Figure 9.1**.

The main causes of maternal death (**Fig. 9.2**) are pulmonary embolism, hypertensive disease, deaths related to anaesthesia, haemorrhage, sepsis, amniotic fluid embolism, abortion and ectopic pregnancy.

In general terms, the maternal mortality rate has fallen dramatically from the 1950s (**Fig. 9.3**). This improvement has come about through better social conditions and improved population health as much as through relatively specific measures such as improved maternity care, accessibility of blood transfusion and improved management of sepsis. It is noteworthy that deaths from illegal abortion virtually disappeared in the UK after the introduction of the Abortion Act in 1967, despite an increase in legal abortion from

Estimates for worldwide maternal mortality	
Region	**Maternal deaths per 100,000 maternities**
Africa	640
Asia	420
Latin America	270
Europe	<10

Fig. 9.1 *Estimates for worldwide maternal morality.*

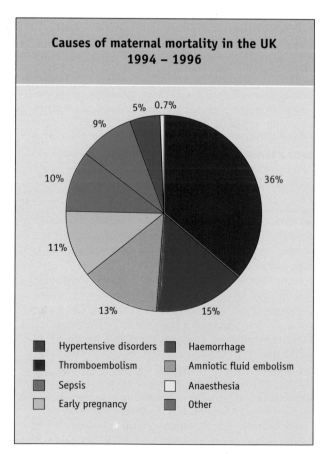

Causes of maternal mortality in the UK 1994 – 1996

0.7%
5%
9%
10%
11%
13%
15%
36%

■ Hypertensive disorders ■ Haemorrhage
■ Thromboembolism ■ Amniotic fluid embolism
■ Sepsis ☐ Anaesthesia
☐ Early pregnancy ■ Other

Fig. 9.2 *Causes of maternal mortality in the UK 1994–1996. The total number of direct deaths was 134. There were another 134 indirect deaths, around 30% due to cardiac causes, in this period. There were also 36 fortuitous deaths and 13 late direct deaths. The maternal mortality rate is approximately 10 per 100,000 for direct and indirect deaths combined.*

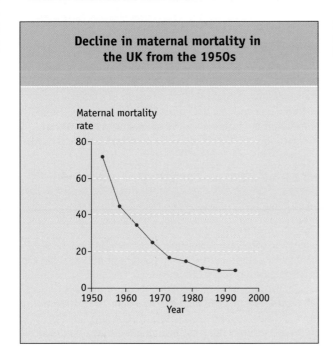

Fig. 9.3 *Decline in maternal mortality in the UK from the 1950s.*

approximately seven out of 1000 women in the early 1970s to approximately 15 out of 1000 women in the 1990s.

PERINATAL AND INFANT DEATHS

BIRTH CERTIFICATION
Each birth must be registered and a period of 6 weeks is allowed for registration to take place in England and Wales and 3 weeks in Scotland. After registration, a birth certificate will be issued. This can either be a certificate of a live birth or a stillbirth.

STILLBIRTH
Stillbirth is defined as the delivery of a baby after the 24th week of pregnancy which has not at any time, after delivery, breathed or shown any sign of life.

PERINATAL DEATH
Perinatal death is defined as a stillbirth or a death occurring in the first week of life.

NEONATAL DEATH
A neonatal death is a death occurring in the first 28 days of life with a further subclassification into early neonatal death which occurs in the first 7 days of life and late neonatal death which occurs during the next 21 days. This subdivision was introduced as a reflection of the fact that causes of early deaths were similar to those of stillbirths, whereas the causes of late deaths often differed.

INFANT DEATH

An infant death is one occurring in the first year of life.

The deaths described are often measured as a rate, which is the number of perinatal, neonatal or infant deaths over the total number of births multiplied by 1000 (Fig. 9.4).

Perinatal death is often used as a measure of establishing the success of obstetric care. However, many of these deaths are now unavoidable due to problems such as congenital abnormality; it may be more important, in the future, to focus on measures of perinatal morbidity. Major factors that have been identified as being associated with perinatal deaths are:

- Low birthweight due to preterm delivery and/or small-for-gestational age/intrauterine growth restriction.
- Intrauterine hypoxia, birth asphyxia and birth injury.
- Congenital abnormality.

Associated factors include socioeconomic deprivation; multiple pregnancy, antepartum haemorrhage, pre-eclampsia, breech presentation, cord accidents and poor maternal health, including medical disorders such as systemic lupus erythematosus.

However, there has been a dramatic improvement in the perinatal death rate in this century with a rate in excess of 60 in 1000 total births in 1930 falling to less than 10 in 1000 births in the 1990s.

Many factors are important in this decline including the introduction of the National Health Service, the introduction of the Abortion Act, improved obstetric care, prenatal diagnosis, the termination of pregnancies with congenital abnormalities, improved care in labour and, perhaps, more strikingly in recent years, improved neonatal care with developments in neonatal intensive care allowing more infants who are born prematurely to survive. Just as with maternal deaths, improvements in socioeconomic conditions have played a major role in the reduction of perinatal mortality (Fig. 9.5). Neonatal deaths occurring out of the perinatal period are attributable to perinatal events, with survival occurring often because of improved neonatal care and the subsequent development of complications related, largely, to prematurity and infant respiratory distress syndrome leading to complications such as intraventricular haemorrhage, necrotizing enterocolitis and infection.

Fig. 9.4 Measurement of perinatal death rate.

Calculating perinatal death rate

Number of perinatal deaths ÷ number of total births × 1000 = Perinatal death rate per 1000 births

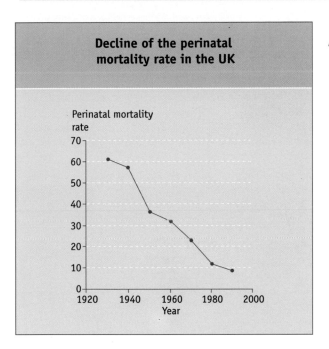

Decline of the perinatal mortality rate in the UK

Fig. 9.5 *Decline of the perinatal mortality rate in the UK.*

In a baby who is born alive, but suffers an early or late neonatal death, both a birth and a death certificate are required to be issued.

Recently, a Confidential Enquiry into stillbirths and deaths in infancy was established in England, Wales and Northern Ireland by the Department of Health to investigate these deaths and provide more detailed information to contribute to a further reduction in death rates.

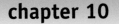

chapter 10

General Gynaecology

VAGINAL DISCHARGE

Most women have problems with vaginal discharge at some time. The common causes can usually be identified clinically and treated without any further investigation.

HISTORY
A description of the woman's symptoms will help you to make a diagnosis. You will need to ask about the onset, duration, colour and texture of the discharge. Does it have an odour? Does it cause itching? Has the woman any other symptoms?

Some women may be very sensitive about their normal vaginal discharge and sometimes this may mask an underlying psychosexual problem.

PHYSIOLOGICAL VAGINAL DISCHARGE
- The vagina produces a normal discharge which is a lubricant, and by maintaining an acidic pH, protects against infection.
- The discharge contains transudated fluid, exfoliated cells from the vaginal walls and cervical mucus. The amount of mucus varies under the hormonal influence of the menstrual cycle. Pregnancy and cervical ectopy may increase the amount of discharge.
- The vagina contains a rich growth of commensal organisms (**Fig. 10.1**). These include potential pathogens but their presence does not indicate infection unless they produce symptoms.

The main commensals are lactobacilli which release lactic acid from the glycogen contained in vaginal squamae. This keeps the vaginal pH at less than 4.5 and prevents an overgrowth of potential pathogens.

Fig. 10.1 *Normal vaginal flora.*

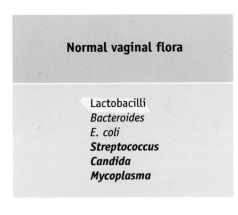

Normal vaginal flora

Lactobacilli
Bacteroides
E. coli
Streptococcus
Candida
Mycoplasma

NONINFECTIVE CAUSES

The age of the woman is an important factor. Vaginal discharge is rarely found in prepubescent girls. The discharge may arise from a foreign body in the vagina; sexual abuse also needs to be considered. Obviously, children need to be treated sensitively and if examination is required, abdominal ultrasound scan can be used to detect a foreign body or examination and swabs may be done under general anaesthetic. During the reproductive era, some discharge is physiological and due to mucus production in the cervical glands.

Cervical ectopy (**Fig. 10.2**) is a common and, again, a physiological finding. It is usually asymptomatic but can produce a heavy, mucous discharge which can be embarrassing. If infection has been exluded, this can be treated by cryocautery or diathermy, although often is best left alone, explaining its essentially physiological nature.

Chronic cervicitis may also produce an excessive endocervical discharge. In addition, the woman may complain of deep dyspareunia. This can be treated by cryocautery or diathermy, with varying degrees of success. Occasionally, a woman with intermenstrual bleeding will complain of a brown or dirty discharge. You should be aware that this is due to altered blood and investigate appropriately. Cervical malignancy is usually advanced before it produces a discharge and this is offensive and blood-stained. A putrid discharge will also be caused by a foreign body, often a forgotten tampon, which will be easily identified on speculum examination and removed.

In the postmenopausal woman, discharge is uncommon. However, due to the loss of natural defence mechanisms secondary to atrophic changes, the woman can develop a nonspecific atrophic vaginitis. This may be pink or blood-stained. If malignancy is excluded, topical oestrogens are often effective in treating this condition. If still sexually active, the women may benefit from a lubricating gel.

INFECTIVE CAUSES

Candida albicans is a common vaginal infection and most women are able to make the diagnosis themselves and self-medicate because antifungal agents such as clotrimazole and econazole can be bought without prescription. These are available both as intravaginal pessaries and creams for topical application; the use of a single dose pessary improves compliance. The discharge is typically thick, white and cloudy and associated with itching (**Fig. 10.3**).

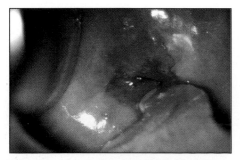

Fig. 10.2 *Colpophotograph showing the columnar epithelium within the squamous epithelium. The squamocolumnar junction is obvious and a smear spatula is being drawn across it.*

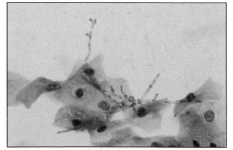

Fig. 10.3 *Cervical smear, Pap. stain: candida hyphae and squamous cells.*

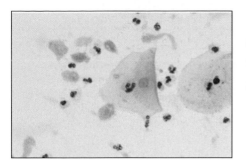

Fig. 10.4 *Cervical smear, Pap. stain: trichomonas vaginalis organisms surrounding squamous cells. A typical pear-shaped organism is seen adjacent to the squamous cell in the centre of the field.*

Some women are prone to recurrent episodes of thrush infections and reinfection can be difficult to prevent. The woman can take general measures such as using cotton underwear, avoiding douching or the use of bubble bath and dietary measures. Specific treatment includes oral fluconazole as a single oral dose or a prolonged topical treatment. Such women are usually screened for underlying diabetic mellitus but this is rarely identified.

Trichomonas vaginalis

Trichomonas is produced by a protozoal organism. Typically, the woman complains of a green, foul-smelling discharge. The discharge is often heavy and can cause irritation. The classic 'strawberry' cervix is not often seen but is due to punctate haemorrhage with cervical infection. The organism can be rapidly identified on a wet slide and is often identified on a cervical smear (**Fig. 10.4**).

Trichomonas infection is treated by a 7-day course of metronidazole. Although not necessarily sexually transmitted, the woman's partner should also be treated as it may cause a symptomless urethritis in men.

Bacterial vaginosis

As the name implies, this is not a vaginal infection but probably an overgrowth of various commensal organisms, usually anaerobes. The discharge is grey or 'dirty' white with a strong fishy odour. The diagnosis is confirmed by 'clue' cells seen on a smear (**Fig. 10.5**). Treatment is with a 7-day course of oral metronidazole. There is no benefit in treating the partner.

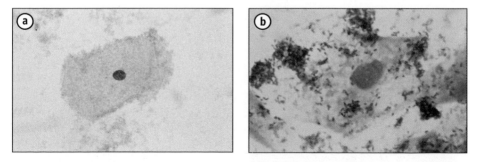

Fig. 10.5 *(a) Cervical smear, Pap. stain: 'clue' cell. This is a squamous cell covered by bacteria, typical of bacterial vaginosis. (b) Gram stain of high vaginal swab showing gram negative coccobacilli covering a squamous cell 'clue' cell.*

EXAMINATION AND INVESTIGATIONS

As always, it is important to examine the external genitalia for evidence of vulvitis, ulceration or genital warts. A speculum examination is necessary to inspect the vaginal walls and cervix and to take a high vaginal swab. Discharge often pools in the posterior fornix and you should use your swab to sample this. With *Candida*, curdy plaques will be seen on the vaginal walls. If you suspect a pelvic infection, endocervical swabs for *Chlamydia* and gonococcus should also be taken. The key points of examination are listed in **Figure 10.6**.

Vaginal discharge: key points

Vaginal discharge is a common problem.
Women may complain of normal physiological discharge.
The diagnosis can often be made on clinical evidence.
Women with recurrent candidiasis will need to take self-help preventive measures.
If a sexually transmitted disease is diagnosed, refer the women to the Genitourinary Medicine Clinic for a full sexually transmitted disease screen and contact tracing.
If a chlamydial or gonococcal infection is suspected, endocervical swabs need to be taken.

Fig. 10.6 *Vaginal discharge: key points.*

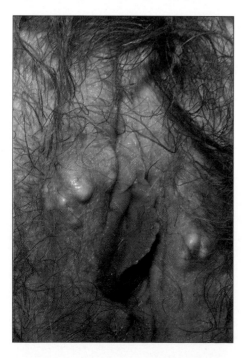

Fig. 10.7 *Multiple sebaceous cysts of the vulva caused by accumulation of sebaceous material behind blocked gland ducts.*

THE BENIGN VULVAL LUMP

An examination of the vulva is an important part of the pelvic examination and if omitted, you may miss an important vulval lesion. Most women presenting with this problem will be able to point out the lesion. Sometimes your findings will be normal, due to a cyst shrinking or abscess discharging, but it may be that the woman has discovered her own normal anatomy such as the hymenal remnants (carunculae myrtiformes) or hypertrophied labia minora.

History

With this problem, inspection rather than history will give you the diagnosis. History will help you gauge the severity of the problem particularly in planning your management. Lumps in this region may be vulval or urethral in origin. Remember that a woman with prolapse may complain of a lump and this should be considered in older women.

Sebaceous cysts are often seen and may be multiple. They are smooth and firm and adherent to the overlying skin (**Fig. 10.7**). Often no treatment is required but they can become infected. The woman often complains of recurrent episodes of pain and discharge. A complete excision of the cyst wall and the overlying punctum is required to prevent recurrence.

Bartholin's cyst

A Bartholin's cyst is easily recognized by its anatomical position lateral to the fourchette (**Fig. 10.8**). The cyst arises from blockage of the duct which opens in the posterio-lateral wall of the vagina between the hymenal ring and the fourchette, and may fluctuate in size. If it becomes infected, an abscess forms which is very tender and painful, although the woman has often endured it for a couple of days before presenting. The abscess may

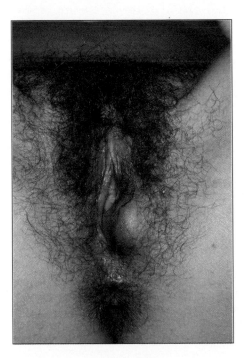

Fig. 10.8 *A Bartholin's cyst sited at the introitus posterolaterally.*

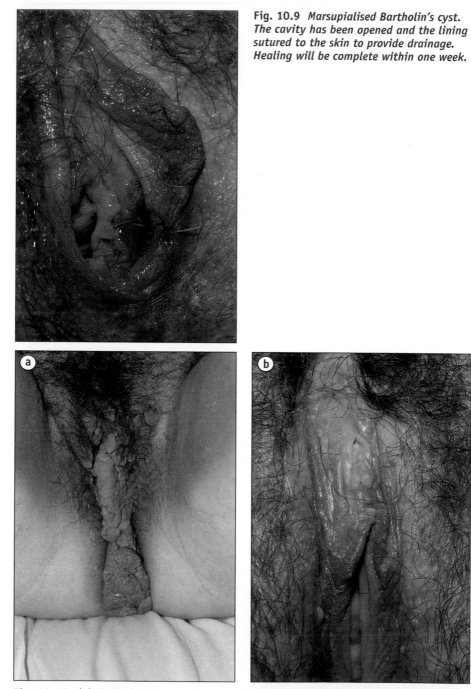

Fig. 10.9 *Marsupialised Bartholin's cyst. The cavity has been opened and the lining sutured to the skin to provide drainage. Healing will be complete within one week.*

Fig. 10.10 *(a) Genital warts may become extremely extensive in pregnancy. This image shows severe vulval and peri-anal warts in a pregnant patient requiring both surgical and medical therapy prior to delivery. (b) Typical genital warts seen on both labia minora and in the clitoral hood.*

Benign vulval lumps: key points

Examination of the vulva should always be part of the pelvic examination.
Pathology is not always present and reassurance may be all that is necessary.
Prolapse presenting at the vulva may look and feel like a lump.
Even when they are an incidental finding, a woman (and her partner) will need
to be treated for genital warts to prevent further transmission.

Fig. 10.11 *Benign vulval lumps: key points.*

discharge spontaneously but surgical management with a general anaesthetic will give rapid relief to the woman and should prevent recurrence. Treatment of both cysts and abscesses is by marsupilization to allow the Bartholin's gland to drain (**Fig. 10.9**). An elipse of skin from the overlying vaginal skin and cyst wall is excised and the two edges sutured together to maintain the patency of the duct.

A vulval abscess will present in the same way but this arises in the hair-bearing skin of the vulva. An early abscess may be managed conservatively with analgesia and a broad spectrum antibiotic but, if fluctuant, it will require incision and drainage.

Genital warts or condyloma acuminata are commonly seen and, may even be an incidental finding. They are generally caused by human papillomavirus (HPV) type 6. They may be extensive involving the vulva, perineum and perianal areas (**Fig. 10.10**). The vagina and cervix should also be inspected for warts. Small warts will often be successfully treated by repeat applications of podophyllin or cryotherapy. Larger or more extensive involvement will require diathermy. Remember to ask if her partner has penile warts, which need treatment to avoid repeated sexual transmission. It is common for women who are immunosuppressed after a renal transplant to suffer from HPV-related changes in the lower genital tract. This can range from florid genital warts to VIN III, or even invasive cancer. The key points of benign vulval lumps are listed in **Figure 10.11**.

UTEROVAGINAL PROLAPSE

Prolapse is a common problem in older women. Both prolapse and stress incontinence arise as a result of pelvic floor weakness but they need not present together. Some causative factors for prolapse are listed in **Figure 10.12**.

THE NORMAL ANATOMY OF PELVIC FLOOR SUPPORT

The main supports for the uterus are the transverse cervical ligaments (cardinal ligaments) and the uterosacral ligaments, both of which insert at the level of the cervix. These keep the uterus above the level of the pelvic floor. The muscles and fascia of the pelvic floor support the bladder and visceral organs (**Fig. 10.13**).

HISTORY

Women with prolapse usually complain of 'something coming down'. They may have a dragging sensation or feeling of a lump in the vagina. They may notice a 'lump' when wiping

Prolapse: casual factors

Childbirth
Menopause (oestrogen deficiency)
Obesity
Constipation
Chronic cough

Fig. 10.12 *Prolapse: causative factors.*

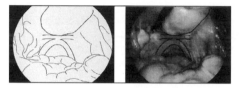

Fig. 10.13 *Laparoscopic view of the pelvis showing the posterior aspect of the uterus and Pouch of Douglas. This demonstrates the ligaments which support the uterus. The uterosacral ligaments and the transverse cervical ligaments both insert at the level of the cervix and the round ligament and broad ligaments which attach to the body of the uterus give no structural support.*

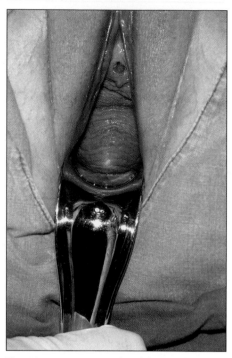

Fig. 10.14 *A cystocoele with the bladder bulging into the vagina.*

or washing themselves. The prolapse may make intercourse difficult or uncomfortable. This discomfort is worse on standing and the prolapse may reduce itself on lying down.

Urinary symptoms

Urinary symptoms are usually associated with a cystocoele. The woman may complain of urinary frequency, stress incontinence or difficulty voiding. Some women will sometimes push the prolapse back themselves to allow them to micturate freely, or to reduce discomfort. Incontinence may present with or without prolapse.

Constipation

A rectocoele may make defecation difficult and the woman may apply pressure through the vaginal wall to empty her bowel. Straining from chronic constipation will aggravate the problem of an already weakened pelvic floor.

When taking a history, these specific details should be sought. In addition, it is important to ask the patient about her general medical condition and whether she is still sexually active, as these factors will influence your management plan.

EXAMINATION

The type and degree of prolapse is determined on examination. Prolapse may be better assessed if the woman is examined in the left lateral position with a Sim's speculum. A cystocoele is due to a weakening of the pubocervical fascia which allows the bladder to bulge into the vagina (**Fig. 10.14**). A rectocoele is due to the rectum bulging into the vagina

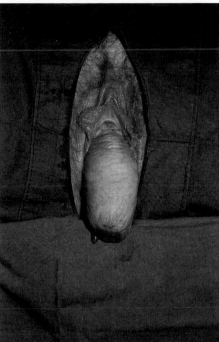

Fig. 10.15 *Complete prolapse (procidentia) of the uterus.*

Classification of prolapse

First degree	Descent within the vagina.
Second degree	Further descent with cervix reaching the introitus.
Third degree	Complete procedentia. The uterine body descends beyond the introitus with inversion of the vaginal walls. The cervix may become swollen with oedema or vascular congestion, and ulceration of the exposed cervix may arise, even causing some bleeding.

Fig. 10.16 *Classification of prolapse.*

posteriorly and is often associated with a deficient perineum where the posterior fourchette is close to the anus. Uterine descent (**Fig. 10.15**) may present on its own or together with vaginal prolapse. The degree of descent is classified in **Figure 10.16**.

The final type of genital prolapse is called an enterocoele which is a peritoneal sac containing the small bowel which bulges into the upper posterior vaginal wall. After hysterectomy, vaginal vault prolapse may arise due to a weakening of the pelvic supports with inversion of the vagina. The relationship of the pelvic organs in the sagittal plane and each type of prolapse are shown in **Figure 10.17**.

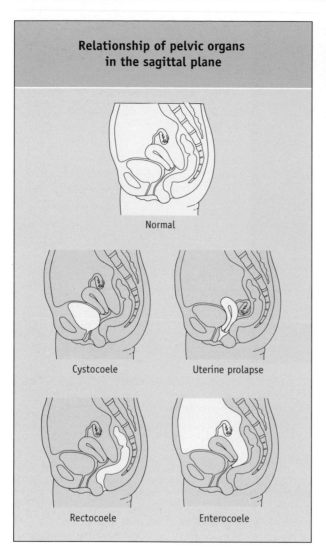

Relationship of pelvic organs in the sagittal plane

Normal

Cystocoele

Uterine prolapse

Rectocoele

Enterocoele

Fig. 10.17 *Relationship of pelvic organs in the sagittal plane. Anticlockwise from top right: sagittal view of pelvic organs; middle left: bladder bulging into vagina to produce a cystocoele; bottom left: rectum bulging into vagina to produce a rectocoele; bottom right: peritoneal sac bulging into vagina to produce an enterocoele; middle right: uterine descent into the vagina.*

MANAGEMENT

When planning the management of a woman with prolapse you will need to consider not only the severity of her symptoms and the degree of prolapse on examination, but her own preferences, her general health and her personal circumstances.

Conservative management

Conservative management is suitable for women with few symptoms, older women unfit for sugery or women unwilling to undergo surgery. Prolapse during pregnancy or immediately postpartum can often be managed expectantly.

With a mild degree of prolapse, the woman may only require reassurance. Physiotherapy may be useful to strengthen the pelvic floor and topical oestrogen therapy may help postmenopausal women.

With a larger degree of prolapse, ring pessaries are often successful in relieving the symptoms of prolapse (**Fig. 10.18**). The ring is inserted and distends the upper vagina, thus keeping the prolapse reduced (**Fig. 10.19**). The ring needs to be replaced every 6–12 months to discourage infection and ulceration of the vaginal wall.

Surgical management

The following procedures may be combined depending on the type of prolapse. For younger women, surgery should be postponed until after their family is complete.

Anterior colporrhaphy for the treatment of cystocoele – The anterior vaginal wall is opened and the prolapsing bladder wall pushed back. The pubocervical fascia is approximated to support the bladder. The excess vaginal skin is excised and the vaginal wall repaired.

Colpoperineorrhaphy for the treatment of rectocoele – The posterior vaginal wall is opened and the prolapsing anterior rectal wall pushed back. The levator ani muscles, which are often very deficient, are sutured together to support the rectum, and the vaginal wall repaired. These women often have a deficient perineum after damage during childbirth and the perineal body can be reconstructed as part of this procedure to lengthen the distance between the vagina and the anus and improve support to the rectum.

'Manchester Repair' for the treatment of uterovaginal prolapse – In this procedure, amputation of the elongated cervix and approximation of the transverse cervical ligaments is performed in addition to an anterior and posterior colporraphy.

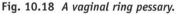

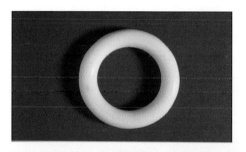

Fig. 10.18 *A vaginal ring pessary.*

Positioning of the ring pessary relative to the pelvic organs

Fig. 10.19 *Positioning of the ring pessary relative to the pelvic organs.*

Alternatively, a vaginal hysterectomy may be performed depending on the woman's reproductive plans or presence of other gynaecological problems such as menorrhagia.

Whatever procedure is performed, there is a significant risk of recurrence both to inadequate healing after the operation or a genuine recurrence due to the same aetiological factors as before. The key points of prolapse are listed in **Figure 10.20**.

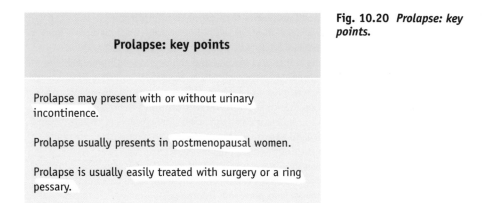

Prolapse: key points

Prolapse may present with or without urinary incontinence.

Prolapse usually presents in postmenopausal women.

Prolapse is usually easily treated with surgery or a ring pessary.

Fig. 10.20 *Prolapse: key points.*

URINARY INCONTINENCE

THE PHYSIOLOGY OF URINARY CONTINENCE

The detrusor muscle of the bladder is a smooth muscle running in longitudinal, circular and spiral bundles. This has a parasympathetic nerve supply from the pelvic nerves. There is also a sympathetic nerve supply, although these do not control micturation (**Fig. 10.21**).

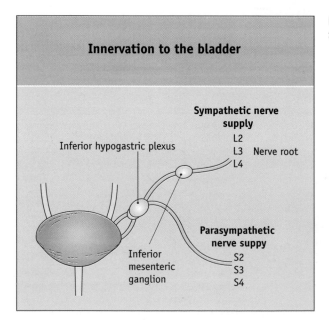

Innervation to the bladder

Inferior hypogastric plexus

Sympathetic nerve supply
L2
L3   Nerve root
L4

Inferior mesenteric ganglion

Parasympathetic nerve suppy
S2
S3
S4

Fig. 10.21 *Innervation to the bladder.*

The parasympathetic nerve supply via the pelvic nerves supplies the main control to the detrusor muscle. The role of the sympathetic innervation is not so well understood. Afferent fibres run chiefly in the pelvic nerves. Stretching of the bladder wall sends a sensory signal to initiate a reflex contraction through the sacral portion of the spinal cord. In infants, this results in voiding but with the development of urinary continence, higher cortical control both inhibiting and facilitating is exerted on the threshold for the voiding reflex.

The adult female bladder has a capacity of 300–400ml. As the bladder fills with urine, there is no pressure increase until the voiding reflex arises. This property of the bladder is called compliance. Above the bladder capacity, the intravesical pressure rises. Continence which is maintained by inhibition of reflex detrusor contractions and by a higher intraurethral pressure until voiding is appropriate, depends on anatomical integrity and neuromuscular co-ordination. Damage to either of these may result in incontinence. The different types and causes of incontinence, and the causal factors in stress incontinence are shown in **Figures 10.22** and **10.23**.

HISTORY

History-taking is important to assess the severity of incontinence and other urinary symptoms, and to aid in reaching a diagnosis. You should ask about the following symptoms.

Stress incontinence

Urine is leaked when intra-abdominal pressure is raised. The severity of this symptom can be assessed by the degree of activity which precipitates incontinence: cough, sneeze, aerobics, running, climbing stairs, walking. When stress incontinence is the only urinary symptom present, the diagnosis is usually genuine stress incontinence. With mixed symptoms it could be caused by detrusor instability or mixed stress and urge incontinence.

Urge incontinence

Urine is leaked because of the inability to delay micturition. Urgency is the sensation of needing to void as soon as bladder fullness is felt. Urgency can be present without urge incontinence if the woman is still able to reach the toilet in time. Although the woman feels her bladder is full, she often only passes small volumes. Typically, shopping trips are planned around the availability of toilets. Urgency or urge incontinence may be precipitated by different triggers, often the sound of running water or arriving home with the key in the door. These symptoms are often found with detrusor instability.

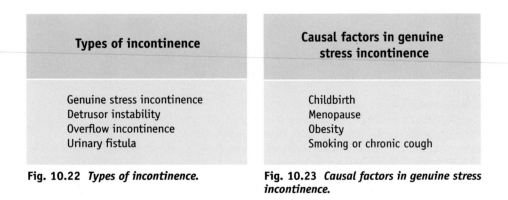

Types of incontinence	Causal factors in genuine stress incontinence
Genuine stress incontinence Detrusor instability Overflow incontinence Urinary fistula	Childbirth Menopause Obesity Smoking or chronic cough

Fig. 10.22 *Types of incontinence.*

Fig. 10.23 *Causal factors in genuine stress incontinence.*

Urinary frequency

With a normal fluid intake, urinary frequency should be more than 2-hourly and no more than twice a night. Women with urgency will pass small, frequent volumes, whereas women with stress incontinence may void frequently to keep the bladder empty to prevent incontinence.

Difficulty voiding

Overflow obstruction is uncommon in women but may be due to uterovaginal prolapse. It is important to take a medical and drug history.

EXAMINATION

An examination of a woman with urinary incontinence includes abdominal and pelvic examination. You will need to exclude any pelvic masses which could be causing urinary symptoms. An unusual cause of incontinence and pelvic mass, in women, is urinary retention with overflow incontinence. You should always examine for any co-existent prolapse, although this is frequently present in the absence of incontinence. When examining for evidence of stress incontinence, severe incontinence will be easily demonstrated. For milder degrees, you will need to ensure that the woman has not just emptied her bladder (most women will have in anticipation of an examination), and you may even need to examine the woman while she is standing.

INVESTIGATION

Except for the woman who complains only of stress incontinence which is demonstrated on examination, most women will require further investigation to diagnose the type of incontinence.

A midstream sample of urine should be taken to exclude a urinary tract infection.

Frequency–volume chart

This simple noninvasive test can provide much information about the severity of symptoms and the possible diagnosis. Over 3 days, the woman records every time she goes to the toilet and measures the volume of urine passed in a measuring jug. Any episodes of incontinence are also recorded. The woman with a stable bladder will have normal bladder capacity and often does not void at night. Some women with stress incontinence will void frequently if they have stress incontinence with a full or nearly full bladder. Women with an unstable bladder or detrusor instability will void frequently, day and night, and pass only small volumes. Women who void frequently because of a large fluid intake will also be obvious from the chart.

Pad test

This test gives some objective evidence of the degree of incontinence and may be helpful in assessing the success of any treatment. After voiding, the woman drinks a standardized volume of fluid and exercises while wearing a pre-weighed pad. The pad is re-weighed to determine the weight of any urinary loss.

Cystometry

Cystometry is the mainstay of assessing bladder function and is used to determine detrusor activity during bladder filling, albeit in an artificial situation. A pressure catheter and a filling catheter are passed into the bladder after emptying. A second pressure catheter is usually introduced into the rectum to measure intra-abdominal pressure. Detrusor pressure is calculated by subtracting the bladder pressure from the intra-abdominal pressure. The detrusor pressure is plotted against the volume of fluid in the bladder.

In a stable bladder, as the bladder volume increases, there is no increase in bladder pressure and no detrusor activity due to normal compliance. In the unstable bladder, unprovoked detrusor activity is seen with pressure rises greater than 15cmH$_2$O. A low compliance bladder will give the same symptoms as detrusor instability but a steady pressure rise is seen with bladder filling.

MANAGEMENT

Stress incontinence

Conservative management will often improve the symptoms of women with mild incontinence. Obese women should be encouraged to lose weight, and for postmenopausal women, oestrogen therapy, in particular, topical oestrogens, may give some benefit. The main stay of conservative management is physiotherapy. Pelvic floor exercises are taught antenatally and postnatally to try to prevent pelvic floor weakness and stress incontinence. In the treatment of incontinence, physiotherapy is only successful when the physiotherapist is enthusiastic and the woman well motivated. Exercises need to be done frequently (a few times each day) and continued long term to maintain improvement. Weighted vaginal cones can be used; these require pelvic floor contraction to hold them in the vagina (**Fig. 10.24**).

Surgical

A surgical procedure may be required when symptoms are severe or conservative measures have failed. Urinary incontinence can interfere severely with a woman's quality of life and any operation that cures the problem is well worthwhile.

The modified colposuspension works by elevating the bladder neck above the pelvic floor. Any increase in intra-abdominal pressure is exerted equally to the bladder and bladder neck to maintain continence. The abdominal wall is opened through a low transverse incision and the retropubic space developed (**Fig. 10.25**). Sutures through the paravaginal tissues are tied to the iliopectineal ligaments on each side to produce elevation of the bladder neck and the vesicourethral angle. Alternatively, sling procedures can be used. An anterior colporrhaphy has a lower success rate but may be used in older women

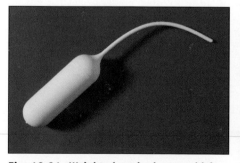

Fig. 10.24 *Weighted vaginal cone which can be used to strengthen the pelvic floor.*

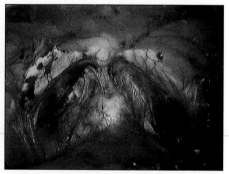

Fig. 10.25 *A view of the retropubic space which is developed during a colposuspension. The bladder is posterior with the urethra and bladder neck in front. Vaginal tissue either side of the urethra is elevated by approximation to the iliopectineal ligaments.*

with prolapse because it is a more minor operation. In skilled hands, surgery for genuine stress incontinence should achieve cure rates of 80%.

Detrusor instability

This condition is more difficult to treat and self-help measure are an important part of the management. Such measures include reducing fluid and caffeine intake, stopping smoking and relaxation techniques; hypnosis may also help. The most effective form of treatment is bladder drill in which the woman is encouraged to suppress unprovoked detrusor activity and regain cortical control of the bladder. This is done by voiding by the clock, starting at half-hourly intervals and increasing the interval until an acceptable frequency such as 3-hourly is achieved. Bladder drill can be conducted over days or even weeks as an outpatient or as an inpatient.

Drug therapy may help some women. Most of the drugs work by an anticholinergic effect on the postganglionic nerve supply to the bladder. This suppresses detrusor activity and raises the threshold for detrusor activity. Probanthine is a very cheap anticholinergic. Oxybutynin is more expensive but more effective and also has a local anaesthetic effect on the bladder wall. Both are limited by their anticholinergic effects: commonly, a dry mouth, blurred vision and constipation. Tricyclic antidepressants may be useful for women for whom nocturia is a significant problem. The key points of urinary incontinence are given in **Figure 10.26.**

Urinary incontinence: key points

Urinary incontinence is a common problem for women.
Genuine stress incontinence and detrusor instability are the most common causes in women.
A careful history may help to differentiate the two conditions.
Further investigation is usually required to make a diagnosis.
Surgery is the treatment of choice for stress incontinence when physiotherapy has not achieved a cure.
Bladder drill is the most effective treatment for detrusor instability.

Fig. 10.26 *Urinary incontinence: key points.*

PELVIC PAIN

HISTORY

The first step is to take a detailed history of the nature, onset and duration of the pain. It is important to establish if the pain is cyclical. Primary dysmenorrhoea (or menstrual pain) will be cyclical, starting with the first period. The cyclical pain of endometriosis often starts days before the period and is worse on the first day of the period, diminishing thereafter. With progressive scarring and adhesions, the duration of the pain may increase to such an extent that the cyclical nature of the pain is lost. The pain of pelvic inflammatory disease may be worse premenstrually but the woman often has a constant lower abdominal ache which may be aggravated by intercourse. Some women with irritable bowel syndrome find it is worse during the second half of their cycle when progesterone levels are high. Middle cycle pain is often due to ovulation.

Mittelschmerz (middle pain)

This pain is related to ovulation and leakage of follicular fluid into the peritoneal cavity. It characteristically occurs in the middle of the cycle, is often unilateral and lasts only a few hours. Some women have it only on alternate months. Often only reassurance and explanation is required. It can be stopped by preventing ovulation by means of the combined oral contraceptive pill.

It is helpful in identifying pelvic pathology to ask about dyspareunia (pain on intercourse). Endometriosis, particularly if the pouch of Douglas, uterosacral ligaments or rectovaginal septum are involved, gives rise to deep dyspareunia which lasts only during intercourse. The deep pelvic pain felt with pelvic inflammatory disease (PID) may be worse the day afterwards than at the time. Primary dysmenorrhoea is not associated with dyspareunia. Some women after a full investigation of pelvic pain will have no cause identified. There may be a psychosexual problem and you should consider this at your initial history. The pain may prevent any sexual activity between the woman and her partner, and superficial dyspareunia and vaginismus may prevent penetration.

The history may be complicated and the woman may have associated menstrual problems. Remember to ask about urinary and bowel symptoms as well as menstrual problems and the method of any contraception. It may help to clarify the details if the woman keeps a symptom diary over two to three cycles.

Women with chronic pelvic pain are commonly seen at the gynaecology outpatient clinic, by which time many will have tried a variety of remedies. Emergency admissions with acute pelvic pain are less common but often are easier to diagnose and to treat (**Fig. 10.27**).

Fig. 10.27 *Differential diagnoses of acute and chronic pelvic pain.*

Differential diagnoses of acute and chronic pelvic pain

Differential diagnosis of acute pelvic pain
Ectopic pregnancy
Acute salpingitis
Appendicitis
Ruptured ovarian cyst
Torsion of ovarian cyst
Urinary tract infection
Unexplained

Differential diagnosis of chronic pelvic pain
Endometriosis
Pelvic inflammatory disease
Primary dysmenorrhoea
Irritable bowel syndrome
'Mittelschmerz'
Psychosomatic
Unexplained

EXAMINATION

Abdominal inspection and palpation is necessary but often unrewarding in a woman with pelvic pain. You should take care to look for previous scars: a subumbilical incision from a previous laparoscopy or low transverse incision from previous pelvic surgery may not be obvious and the information is not always volunteered by the patient. The skin may be reddened or thickened from hot water bottles. The caecum and sigmoid colon may be palpable and tender with irritable bowel syndrome. In PID, tenderness on abdominal palpation tends to be low and deep.

During the pelvic examination, the vulva and vagina should be inspected for signs of sexually transmitted diseases such as ulceration or genital warts. Bimanual and speculum examination may be difficult or not possible in the woman with psychosexual problems. It is better not to persevere at this stage. Endocervical swabs should be taken after inspecting the cervix on speculum examination. You may see endometriotic deposits on the cervix or vaginal wall.

On bimanual palpation you should feel if the cervix feels normal and check for cervical excitation by moving the cervix. You need to check the size, mobility and position of the uterus. A fixed, retroverted uterus suggests pelvic adhesions which may result from endometriosis or PID. The uterus may be bulky and tender with adenomyosis. You should next feel both adnexae for tenderness and swellings. The chocolate cyst will be fixed and more difficult to define than a simple cyst. Tubo-ovarian masses, hydrosalpinges and a full rectum may be felt. The frozen pelvis caused by dense adhesions will feel solid and the pelvic organs fixed, and may be confused with a pelvic malignancy. If the woman is very tender, there is no gain in prolonging the examination.

INVESTIGATIONS

Routine blood tests are not helpful unless there is a specific indication. Cultures of midstream urine or endocervical swabs should also only be taken if clinically indicated. Ultrasound scanning may be useful in identifying pelvic pathology when an adnexal mass is suspected or to exclude pathology when pelvic examination reveals no abnormality (**Figs 10.28** and **10.29**). Unless there are large deposits or chocolate cyst formation, endometriosis will not be seen on ultrasound scanning.

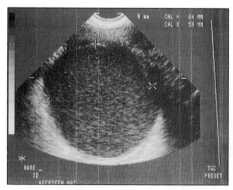

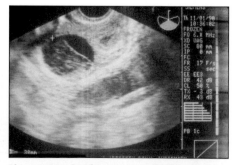

Fig. 10.28 *Ultrasonogram which reveals a cyst 6.5cm across which was found at laparotomy to be an endometrioma, full of altered blood: the so-called 'chocolate cyst'. This may cause cyclical or chronic pelvic pain.*

Fig. 10.29 *Cystic space partly filled with clot caused by bleeding into the cyst.*

Fig. 10.30 *Pelvic pain: key points.*

Pelvic pain: key points

A detailed history is essential.
Physical findings are not always present.
Ultrasound scan and laparoscopy are
   useful methods of investigation.
The cause may be psychosexual in origin.
Frequently no cause is found.

Fig. 10.30 *Pelvic pain: key points.*

Laparoscopy

Laparoscopy will allow direct inspection of the outer surfaces of the pelvic organs and will identify pathology such as adhesions or endometriosis which will not be found on an examination or a scan. This is an invasive procedure and requires a general anaesthetic. Although it will not always be necessary, it may bring to an end a long saga of investigations. There is often no evidence of pathology in cases of pelvic pain, which women may find difficult to accept. In these circumstances, gentle but firm advice is required and pointless treatment is best avoided.

Benign ovarian cysts

Simple ovarian cysts are often asymptomatic and may be an incidental finding. Cyst 'accidents' give rise to acute severe pelvic pain. Such accidents include torsion, rupture and haemorrhage. The woman is often generally unwell with severe constant pain, although it may be intermittent but progressively more severe with a torsion. The site of pain and physical signs may be localized to one side of the pelvis. Irritation from spilled cyst fluid, blood or inflammatory exudate may be localized but may involve both sides of the pelvis. The woman may have a low-grade pyrexia and a raised white cell count. Continued bleeding from a cyst haemorrhage can result in shock and the woman will require resuscitation with fluid replacement and surgery to oversew the bleeding cyst wall. Usually, cyst rupture can be managed conservatively. With cyst torsion the ovary, and often the tube, will become progressively congested, ischaemic and eventually necrotic, in which case releasing the torsion is not sufficient and oophorectomy is required.

Benign ovarian cysts may be physiological or pathological. Most are epithelial in origin, either serous or mucinous (**Fig. 10.31**). One interesting type of benign cyst is the so-called

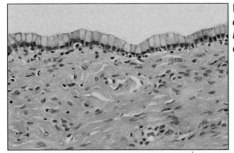

Fig. 10.31 *Benign mucinous cystadenoma of the ovary. The cyst is lined by a single layer of mucin-secreting columnar epithelium. Haematoxylin–eosin.*

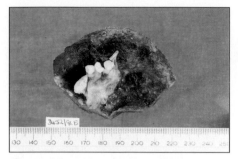

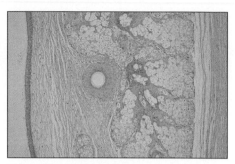

Fig. 10.32 *Mature cystic teratoma or dermoid cyst. The cyst has been opened to reveal tooth-like structures. The diagnosis is sometimes made incidentally on an abdominal X-ray.*

Fig. 10.33 *Mature cystic teratoma. The cyst is lined by stratified squamous epithelium and the wall contains mature sebaceous glands. Haematoxylin–eosin.*

dermoid cyst or mature cystic teratoma. It may contain any tissues derived from ectoderm (**Fig. 10.32**) including teeth and hair seen by naked eye examination. Histopathology reveals a typical appearance (**Fig. 10.33**).

ENDOMETRIOSIS

Endometriosis is the presence of tissue histologically similar to that of the endometrium at sites outside the uterine cavity. In this histopathology section (**Fig. 10.34**) of an endometrioma of the recto vaginal septum glandular cells can clearly be seen within an area of loose stroma which itself is surrounded by the pink staining fibromuscular tissue of the recto vaginal septum. Ectopic endometrium is found both within the myometrium where it is termed adenomyosis, and at other sites where it is correctly termed endometriosis. The current thinking is that the presence of ectopic endometrium is a ubiquitous phenomenon and the term endometriosis should be restricted to patients for whom the ectopic endometrium is associated with either a specific symptom complex or anatomical distortion. The classic symptoms of endometriosis are pelvic pain, dysmenorrhoea and deep dyspareunia.

Many theories have been proposed to explain the aetiology and pathogenesis of endometriosis. The generally accepted view is that endometriosis is the consequence of the dissemination and implantation of endometrium at ectopic sites. This theory was first proposed by Sampson in the 1920s. Endometrium is most commonly disseminated at the time of menstruation either in a retrograde manner along the fallopian tubes or less commonly through the vasculature or lymphatics. The dissemination of the endometrium

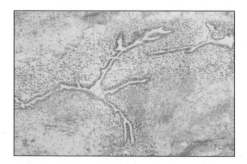

Fig. 10.34 *Histopathology section of an endometrioma.*

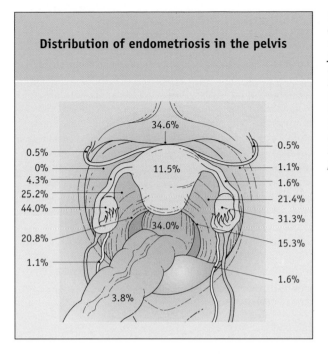

Distribution of endometriosis in the pelvis

34.6%

0.5%

0.5%

0%

11.5%

1.1%

4.3%

1.6%

25.2%

44.0%

21.4%

31.3%

34.0%

20.8%

15.3%

1.1%

1.6%

3.8%

Fig. 10.35 *Distribution of endometriosis in the pelvis illustrating the frequency for various anatomical sites as determined in a laparoscopic study. (From the American College of Obstetricians and Gynecologists (Obstetrics and Gynecology, 1986; 67: 335–338), with permission.)*

along the fallopian tubes explains the distribution of endometriosis in the female pelvis (**Fig. 10.35**). The endometrium may also be disseminated surgically, particularly when the uterine cavity is opened, but also after hysteroscopy and infertility investigation.

A number of factors have been implicated in the aetiology of endometriosis, including genetic and racial predisposition, increased incidence at particular ages and an association with infertility. There is an increased incidence of the disease in first degree relatives of sufferers but apart from an increased incidence among Japanese women there is no specific racial predisposition.

More important than any of these factors, however, is the role of endogenous oestrogens and peritoneal soiling at the time of menstruation. Endometriosis is a hormonally dependent condition (**Fig. 10.36**). It occurs only in women during their reproductive years, has not been described in premenarchal girls and rarely occurs in postmenopausal women. Symptoms are often cyclical, reflecting the cyclical fluctuations during the menstrual cycle, and usually resolve during pregnancy and after the menopause. Endometriosis is found more often in women who have frequent and/or prolonged menstrual loss.

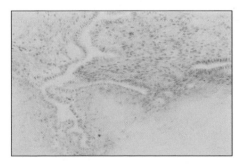

Fig. 10.36 *Histological section (from the same specimen as Fig. 10.34) stained with a monoclonal antibody to the oestrogen receptor. Positive staining for the oestrogen receptor, within the nuclei of the cells is only seen in the glands and stroma of the endometriotic lesion and not in the surrounding connective tissue.*

CASE HISTORY

The patient is a 27-year-old nulliparous woman who presents with secondary dysmenorrhoea of increasing severity and a recent history of deep dyspareunia.

What other history would you request? The history is aimed at identifying the probable differential diagnosis. Enquiry should be made about other symptoms of endometriosis (**Fig. 10.37**) and symptoms that suggest other pelvic pathology. As a result of its myriad presentations many patients allege that doctors are poor at recognizing the condition. The clue is usually the cyclical nature of the symptoms. The history should specifically enquire about vaginal discharge, fever, gastrointestinal symptoms (constipation, diarrhoea and cyclical rectal bleeding) and urinary symptoms (including cyclical haematuria). In addition, some estimation of the severity of the symptoms and the patient's analgesic requirements should be made.

What examination would you perform? A full assessment of the patient is required. In particular, abdominal, pelvic and rectal examination should be undertaken. For this patient, the pelvic findings are of a normal-sized uterus fixed in retroversion with tenderness and nodularity in the posterior fornix and an adnexal mass (**Fig. 10.38**).

What is the differential diagnosis and how would the provisional diagnosis be confirmed? The diagnosis lies between endometriosis with an ovarian endometrioma, an ovarian mass or pelvic mass with a collection. Further information could be obtained by ultrasound but the definitive diagnosis of endometriosis can only be made by direct visualization either at laparoscopy or laparotomy.

Symptoms of endometriosis	
Reproductive tract	Dysmenorrhoea Pelvic pain (lower abdominal) Dsypareunia Acute accident to endometrioma (torsion or rupture) 'Infertility'
Gastrointestinal tract	Lower abdominal pain Cyclical tenesmus Cyclical rectal bleeding Bowel obstruction
Urinary tract	Cyclical pain (ureteric colic) Cyclical haematuria Ureteric obstruction
Other sites	Pain swelling and bleeding in surgical and episiotomy scars Cyclical haemoptysis from respiratory tract

Fig. 10.37 *Symptoms of endometriosis. The precise clinical presentation of endometriosis will depend upon the sites affected.*

Clinical findings of the patient
with endometriosis

Fig. 10.38 *Clinical findings of the patient with endometriosis. Precise clinical findings will depend upon the site and extent of disease.*

Lower abdominal tenderness
Fixed retroverted uterus
Tender nodules on uterosacral ligaments
Generalized pelvic tenderness
Adnexal swelling (ovarian endometrioma)
Tender swelling in surgical scar (more pronounced at
time of menstruation)

THE DIAGNOSIS OF ENDOMETRIOSIS

Endometriosis can only be suspected from history and examination. The cyclical nature of a history together with supporting clinical findings should always raise suspicion but diagnosis requires direct visualization of the disease, usually at laparoscopy (**Fig. 10.39**) and ideally a biopsy. Endometriosis has many different appearances (**Figures 10.40 and 10.41**) which represent different stages in the natural history of the endometriotic lesion. Lesions progress from fresh, biologically active, red lesions to fibrosed, inactive lesions which may contain haemosiderin. These latter lesions which appear blue–black to the eye were

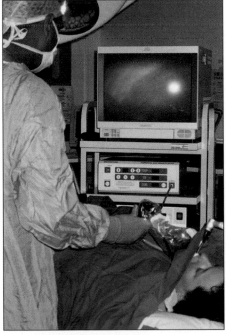

Fig. 10.39 *Laparoscopy of pelvis using video equipment.*

Visual appearances of endometriosis in biopsy specimens

Blue-black nodules
White plaques
Flame-like lesions
Clear papules
Petechial haemorrhages
Yellow-brown plaques
Endometrioma:'chocolate cysts'
Fibrosis
Strawberry-like lesions
Peritoneal defects
Normal peritoneum

Fig. 10.40 *Visual appearances of endometriosis in biopsy specimens.*

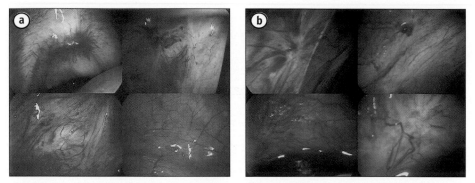

Fig. 10.41 *(a) Endometriosis is associated with many different visual appearances. One of the features of the disease is angiogenesis. Top left: active endometriosis with angiogenesis between the uterosacral ligaments; Top right: classical blue-black lesions; Bottom left demonstrates no pigmentation. The blue-black colour results from the deposition of haemosiderin. Bottom right: normal peritoneum for comparison.*
(b) Further visual appearances of endometriosis. In patients with endometriosis there is often an increased volume of peritoneal fluid (bottom two images). This peritoneal fluid contains an increased number of macrophages of which many are in a state of increased activation.

previously thought to be the only type of endometriotic lesion (**Fig. 10.41**). Other atypical lesions are now widely recognized and this has resulted in an increased incidence of the diagnosis of the disease. The exact incidence of the disease is difficult to determine because not every women of reproductive age is laparoscoped. Best estimates suggest that the overall incidence in the population is approximately 5% but the incidence in patients investigated for pain may be as high as 60% and in those investigated for infertility, 80%.

Endometriosis on the ovarian surface may invaginate to give rise to cysts known as endometriomas (**Fig. 10.42**). The contents of these cysts are typically dark brown in colour and viscous in nature resembling thick chocolate. The contents are also extremely irritant and if these cysts rupture, an inflammatory response and adhesion formation may occur. These cysts are also known as chocolate cysts but this naked eye appearance can also be obtained from other pathologies such as bleeding into a functional cyst.

MANAGEMENT

Endometriosis is diagnosed in three groups of patients. It may be an incidental finding in an asymptomatic patient undergoing another procedure, it may present with symptoms of pain or it may be diagnosed during infertility investigation. Patients who are asymptomatic require no further treatment. The symptomatic patient may be treated either medically or surgically. Medical treatment is usually the first line therapy giving a better response than local ablation of visible lesions. Symptomatic relief may be obtained using nonsteroidal anti-inflammatory drugs such as ibuprofen, mefanamic acid or diclofenac. This approach however does not influence the underlying source of the symptoms.

Medical therapies are based on the principle that endometriosis is hormonally dependent, improves during pregnancy and is rarely found after the menopause. Medical therapy therefore induces a pseudopregnancy or menopausal state.

Pseudopregnancy approaches

Historically, patients were treated with high doses of oestrogen and progestogens, the forerunners of the modern low-dose pill. Current low-dose oral contraceptives have not been evaluated as a specific treatment for endometriosis but are known to relieve dysmenorrhoea and a low incidence of endometriosis is found among pill users. They may be a useful first line therapy when the diagnosis is suspected and contraception is required. The alternative pseudopregnancy approach is high-dose progestogens (medroxyprogesterone acetate 30mg daily) The side effects of progestogens include weight gain, breast tenderness, bloating, fluid retention and depression.

Pseudomenopausal approaches

Pseudomenopausal regimens use either the gonadotrophin-releasing hormone (GnRH) analogues or the drugs danazol and gestrinone, which in addition exert an androgenic effect which is also beneficial.

The GnRH analogues differ from the naturally occurring hormone by amino acid substitutions at positions six and 10 of the natural decapeptide. They are administered as either subcutaneous depot injections or nasal sprays (**Fig. 10.43**). Natural GnRH is released by the pituitary in a pulsatile manner and the pituitary gonadotrophe responds by releasing both follicle-stimulating hormone (FSH) and luteinizing hormone (LH). Constant stimulation of the gonadotrophe results in a downregulation with a consequent reduction in production of FSH and LH. The GnRH analogues have a greater affinity for the receptor and are less susceptible to enzymatic breakdown and thus the gonadotrophe is constantly stimulated (**Fig. 10.44**).

Danazol and gestrinone act in a number of different ways as well as inhibiting secretion of FSH and LH by negative feedback. Both compounds are intrinsically androgenic and in addition, reduce the production of sex hormone binding globulin thus increasing the

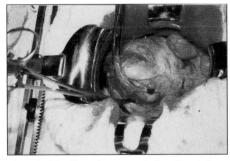

Fig. 10.42 *Chocolate cyst being freed from adhesions and removed at laparotomy.*

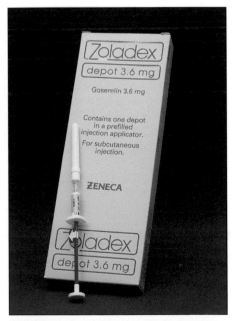

Fig. 10.43 *Goserelin (Zoladex®, Zeneca, UK) depot injection usually administered at monthly intervals into the abdominal wall to suppress menstruation.*

269

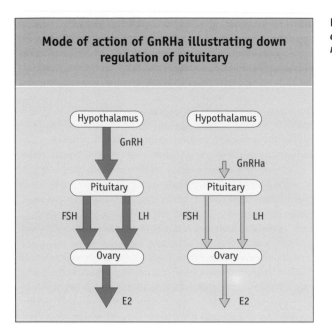

Mode of action of GnRHa illustrating down regulation of pituitary

Fig. 10.44 *Mode of action of GnRHa illustrating down regulation of pituitary.*

amount of free endogenous testosterone within the circulation. The androgenic environment created brings about atrophy of the ectopic endometrium. The side effects are predominately androgenic, in addition to the hypo-oestrogenic effects brought about by the reduced production of the gonadotrophins, with patients complaining of seborrhoea, acne, greasy hair, weight gain, muscle cramps, hirsutism and, rarely, deepening of the voice.

All medical therapies are usually continued for 6 months. Symptomatic relief or improvement should be achieved within 2–3 months.

Surgery may also be used in the treatment of symptomatic endometriosis; a conservative or radical approach may be adopted. The choice of approach will depend to a large extent on whether the patient has completed her child-bearing. Conservative surgery for pain relief is, in general, not as effective as medical therapy. Local ablation, using diathermy or laser, may be employed but will only treat visible deposits. For patients who have been unresponsive to medical therapy, laparoscopic uterine nerve ablation (LUNA), using the CO_2 laser, may give symptomatic relief by disrupting the nerve plexi that run within the uterosacral ligaments (**Fig. 10.45**). For patients with deposits deep within the rectovaginal septum, conservative surgical removal of these deposits may relieve the symptoms of dyspareunia and dyschezia.

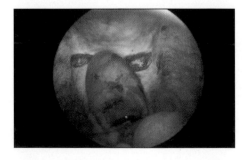

Fig. 10.45 *LUNA (laparoscopic uterine nerve ablation by laser). The utero sacral ligaments have been interrupted by laser. Some of the pain fibres from the uterus run in or in close proximity to these ligaments and are destroyed in the process. This procedure is used to relieve some of the painful symptoms associated with endometriosis.*

When child-bearing is complete more radical surgery can be contemplated. The operation of choice is total abdominal hysterectomy with or without bilateral salpingo-oophorectomy. Removal of both ovaries is advocated by some authorities as further surgery is often required when the ovaries are left behind. However, caution should be exercised before the decision is made to castrate a young woman.

ENDOMETRIOSIS AND INFERTILITY

The association between endometriosis and infertility has long been recognized. Indeed, the increased prevalence of endometriosis in women investigated for infertility has led some to suggest a causal relationship between the two conditions. However, the precise relationship between the two conditions remains unclear and this has led to confusion over the optimum management of the infertile women with coexistent endometriosis.

In women with severe endometriosis, the presence of structural damage, ovarian and tubal adhesions, prevents oocyte release, retrieval and transport, leading to a mechanical disruption in fertility. The severity of disease is established using the American Fertility Society scoring system (**Fig. 10.46**). In women with mild endometriosis and no apparent structural damage, the aetiological basis for the infertility is unclear.

Numerous factors have been investigated to explain how mild endometriosis could affect fertility (**Fig. 10.47**). The endocrine factors that have been implicated include defective follicle development and anovulation, luteinized unruptured follicle syndrome, luteal phase defects and hyperprolactinaemia. However, these factors are also found in women with infertility in the absence of endometriosis. In addition, these abnormalities have not been shown to occur in consecutive menstrual cycles or in patients with endometriosis more commonly than in other infertile patients.

In women with endometriosis inflammatory changes have been observed in the peritoneal fluid. An increase in peritoneal fluid volumes, macrophage numbers, macrophage activity and higher levels of cytokines and prostanoids are observed. The inflammatory changes are thought to interfere with fertility by a direct cytotoxic effect on the oocyte, spermatozoa and embryo. Studies using peritoneal fluid from women with endometriosis have found impaired ovum penetration, decreased sperm motility and velocity, and alterations in sperm movement. When women receive treatment for endometriosis, the peritoneal fluid ceases to be embryotoxic but no improvement in fecundibility is seen in women after treatment for endometriosis.

It has been suggested that there is an increased miscarriage rate with endometriosis. However, controlled prospective studies have not confirmed these suggestions and no causal relationship can be shown between endometriosis and spontaneous abortion. An increased pregnancy loss rate is not observed in patients with endometriosis undergoing assisted conception when an early diagnosis of pregnancy is made.

It has also been suggested that mild endometriosis adversely affects fertility but conception rates are comparable in women with mild endometriosis and without endometriosis. Despite extensive research on infertile women with mild endometriosis, there is no evidence for a causal relationship between these two factors, in contrast with severe endometriosis in which mechanical factors can obviously explain the causality of endometriosis in reduced fertility in the incidence of spontaneous abortion.

Treatment for infertility for patients for whom there is no anatomical distortion should be directed against any other specific fertility factor, or when none exists, the couple should be considered to have unexplained infertility.

The American Fertility Society Revised Classification of endometriosis

Patient's Name ___ D Jones ___   Date ___ 30/11/96 ___

Stage I   (Minimal)   1–5   Laparotomy _____ Laparoscopy ✓ Photography _____
Stage II (Mild)   6–15   Recommended treatment _____
Stage III (Moderate) 16–40   _____
Stage IV (Severe)   >40   _____
Total ___ 7 ___   Prognosis ___ Fertility not compromised ___

PERITOMEUM	ENDOMETRIOSIS		< 1cm	1–3cm	> 3cm
		Superficial	1	2	(4)
		Deep	(2)	4	6
OVARY	R	Superficial	(1)	2	4
		Deep	4	16	20
	L	Superficial	1	2	4
		Deep	4	16	20
	POSTERIOR CUL-DE-SAC OBLITERATION		Partial		Complete
			4		40
	ADHESIONS		< 1/2 Exclusive	1/3–2/3 Exclusive	> 2/3 Exclusive
OVARY	R	Filmy	1	2	4
		Dense	4	8	16
	L	Filmy	1	2	4
		Dense	4	8	16
TUBE	R	Filmy	1	2	4
		Dense	4^+	8^+	16
	L	Filmy	1	2	4
		Dense	4^+	8^+	16

If the fimbriated end of the fallopian tube is completely encased, change the patient assignment to 1A

Additional Endometriosis _____   Associated Pathology _____
_____   _____
_____   _____
_____   _____

To be used with normal tubes and ovaries   To be used with abnormal tubes and/or ovaries

L   R   L   R

Fig. 10.46 *American Fertility Society (AFS) scoring system for endometriosis. The extent of disease may not correlate with painful symptoms but is of more value in assessing fertility. Patients with more extensive disease affecting the normal anatomical relationships might benefit from conservative surgery to normalize the anatomy. Reproduced with permission from the American College of Obstetricians and Gynecologists (Obstetrics and Gynecology, 1986, 67: 335–338.)*

Fig. 10.47 *Putative causes of infertility in endometriosis.*

Putative causes of infertility in endometriosis

Anatomical distortion

Disorders of folliculogenesis or endocrinology
Defective folliculogenesis
Anovulation
Luteinized unruptured follicle syndrome
Luteal phase defects
Elevated prolactin

Inflammatory or immunological
Increased peritoneal fluid volume
Increased macrophage number
Increased prostanoid and cytokine levels
Increased miscarriage rate

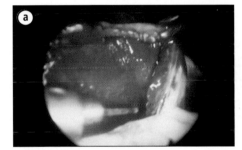 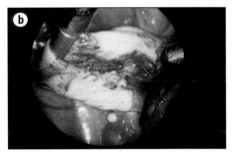

Fig. 10.48 *(a) and (b) Laparoscopy for infertility.*

When anatomical distortion of the pelvis exists, the treatment can either surgically return the pelvis to normal using either laparoscopic or open surgery (**Fig. 10.48**) or patients can be treated by *in vitro* fertilization.

PELVIC INFLAMMATORY DISEASE

PID or pelvic infection of the upper genital tract often begins with a primary infection of the cervix, and with ascending spread, it can involve the endometrium, tubes, ovaries and pelvic peritoneum. At presentation, it is not usually possible to determine which parts are involved and secondary infection with anaerobes often occurs. In the West, the most common primary infective organism is now *Chlamydia trachomatis*, although cases of *Neisseria gonnorhoea* still occur, and in Africa this very commonly causes severe PID.

273

CHLAMYDIA TRACHOMATIS

This obligate intracellular parasite is now the most common organism found in PID in developed countries. Primary infection usually involves the cervix or urethra (in men and women). As many as 70% of women with cervical infection will be asymptomatic. This can spread to involve the tubes, ovaries and pelvis. The infection can be acute, subacute or chronic. Subclinical 'smouldering' infections cause significant long-term morbidity (**Fig. 10.49**). In pregnant women, *Chlamydia* can cause chorioamnionitis or postpartum endometritis. It may be transmitted at birth causing neonatal conjunctivitis or pneumonia. *Chlamydia* is sensitive to doxycycline, tetracycline and erythromycin. *Chlamydia* is detected by an immunofluorescence test or an ELISA test.

NEISSERIA GONORRHOEA

Neisseria gonnorhoea is a Gram-negative diplicoccus and an obligate intracellular parasite of the human urogenital tract. Its presence can be diagnosed on a Gram-stained smear of cervical or urethral discharge (**Fig. 10.50**). These swabs need to be transported in the appropriate medium for laboratory culture. Gonorrhoea has the same route of spread as *Chlamydia*, including transmission during birth. Rarely, haematogenous spread gives rise to septicaemia and arthritis. Penicillin-resistant gonorrhoea will be sensitive to spectinomycin or a third generation cephalosporin.

HISTORY

The threshold for diagnosing pelvic inflammatory disease is low in women of reproductive age with pelvic pain because of the significant sequelae of untreated infection. However, you need to consider other important pathology such as ectopic pregnancy or appendicitis. When taking a gynaecological history, you should always ask for the date of the last menstrual period and method of contraception. The pain is usually bilateral and felt in the lower abdomen. In acute PID, the woman may feel generally unwell with anorexia and vomiting. She may have noticed deep dyspareunia or vaginal discharge in the preceding days. With subacute or chronic PID, the woman may complain of dysmenorrhoea and menorrhagia. Typically, pelvic pain is felt worse after as opposed to during intercourse and may last a few hours or even days afterwards.

Findings in chronic pelvic inflammatory disease

Fallopian tube thickening
Clubbing of fimbrial end
Hydrosalpinx
Tubo-ovarian adhesions
Pouch of Douglas adhesions

Fig. 10.49 *Findings in chronic pelvic inflammatory disease.*

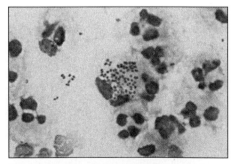

Fig. 10.50 *Gram stain of high vaginal swab showing polymorphs and gram-negative intracellular diplococci typical of neisseria gonorrhoea (oil immersion x 100).*

EXAMINATION

With a severe acute episode of PID, the woman will appear unwell and dehydrated. If an infection has formed a localized abscess, she will have a high, swinging temperature. Signs of peritonitis with guarding and rebound will be found on abdominal palpation. However, the presentation is less dramatic in most women. She may or may not have a low-grade pyrexia. The abdominal findings may be limited to some tenderness, to deep palpation of the lower abdomen.

If peritonitis is present, bimanual pelvic examination will be impossible because of pain and tenderness. A speculum examination will be necessary to obtain endocervical swabs for culture and *Chlamydia* detection. Findings suggestive of pelvic infection are cervical excitation (tenderness elicited by moving the cervix) and adnexal tenderness on bimanual examination. Scarring and adhesions resulting from chronic PID can give rise to fixed retroversion of the uterus or palpable adnexal mass (**Figs 10.49 and 10.51**).

INVESTIGATIONS

PID can be difficult to diagnose on clinical evidence because of absent or nonspecific symptoms and signs.

In acute infections, the woman may have a raised white cell count and C-reactive proteins. Endocervical swabs should be sent for culture and *Chlamydia* detection. Treatment is usually started at this stage on the basis of clinical evidence. However, if there is no clinical improvement after 24–48 hours, you should reconsider the diagnosis and further investigation may be helpful.

Ultrasound scan

Ultrasound scanning may be more useful in subacute and chronic PID. Findings suggestive of PID are free fluid in the pouch of Douglas, thickened fallopian tubes or hydrosalpinges (**Fig. 10.52**). The absence of ultrasonic evidence does not exclude the possibility of PID.

Laparoscopy

Laparoscopy is a valuable means of confirming the diagnosis in the patient with presumed PID not responding to conventional treatment or in the investigation of chronic pelvic pain.

Long-term sequelae of pelvic inflammatory disease	
Tubal damage	Risk of ectopic pregnancy Infertility
Pelvic adhesions	Pain Dyspareunia

Fig. 10.51 *Long-term sequelae of pelvic inflammatory disease.*

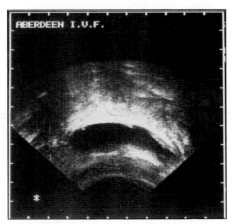

Fig. 10.52 *Ultrasonic image of a hydrosalpinx.*

It offers an opportunity to take intraperitoneal swabs, although if there has been prior antibiotic therapy, there is often no significant growth.

Acute salpingitis

Findings in acute PID can range from reddening and thickening of the tubes to a tubo-ovarian abscess with free pus in the pelvis. However, the pelvis can appear normal with cervicitis, endometritis or interstitial salpingitis. Evidence of chronic PID is best seen at laparoscopy (**Fig. 10.53**).

Tubal clubbing is the result of inflammation of the fimbrial end matting the fimbriae together.

Distension of the tube with fluid causes hydrosalpinx. Tubo-ovarian adhesions are common and may involve the pelvic side wall, pouch of Douglas, omentum or bowel.

Endometritis

Any procedure that breaks down the natural barrier of the cervix to the upper genital tract can result in ascending infection. Often the endometrium is involved but it can spread to other pelvic organs. Endometritis and pelvic infection may arise after childbirth, termination of pregnancy, insertion of an intrauterine contraceptive device or cervical surgery. Typically, the women will have heavy, offensive vaginal bleeding and the uterus will be tender and bulky on bimanual examination.

MANAGEMENT

Many women can be treated as outpatients but some women will require admission for intravenous fluids and antibiotics (**Fig. 10.54**). Antibiotic treatment should start before

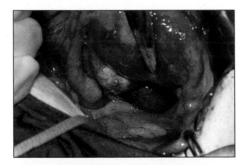

Fig. 10.53 *Laparoscopic view of typical chronic PID. The uterus which is being pushed forward is erythematous. The fallopian tube is thickened, with a clubbed end. A 'pseudocyst' is present deep in the pouch of Douglas.*

Fig. 10.54 *Indications for admission for treatment of PIDs.*

Indications for admission for treatment of pelvic inflammatory disease

Severe illness
Vomiting
Pelvic abscess suspected
Cannot exclude other surgical emergency, e.g. ectopic
    pregnancy
Severe pain

Pelvic inflammatory disease: key points

Fig. 10.55 *Pelvic inflammatory disease: key points.*

Pelvic inflammatory disease is an inflammatory condition of the upper genital tract.

Chlamydia is now the most common infective agent.

Pelvic inflammatory disease may be asymptomatic.

The long-term sequelae include pain, infertility and ectopic pregnancy.

Women with chlamydia or gonorrhoea require a full sexually transmitted disease screen and contact tracing.

Fig. 10.55 *Pelvic inflammatory disease: key points.*

endocervical swab results are available and this should include an anti-*Chlamydia* agent (e.g. doxycycline and metronidazole) to cover secondary infection with anaerobes. If a gonococcal infection is suspected or identified, spectinomycin or cefoxitin should be included.

If the woman has an intrauterine contraceptive device, this should be removed once antibiotic treatment has started.

Surgical treatment is rarely required in the management of acute PID. If laparoscopy is performed for the patient not responding to antibiotics, pelvic swabs can be taken for culture. An acute inflammatory mass should not require resection but pelvic abscess can be drained to aid resolution.

Surgical treatment may be required for the woman with chronic PID that does not respond to analgesia or repeated antibiotic therapy. This can range from laparoscopic division of adhesions to a pelvic clearance. Surgery can be very difficult in the woman with a pelvis 'frozen' by dense adhesions. If *Chlamydia* or gonococcus are identified, the woman and her partner should be referred to genitourinary medicine clinic for a full sexually transmitted diseases screen and contact tracing. The key points of PID are listed in **Figure 10.55**.

POSTMENOPAUSAL BLEEDING

Postmenopausal bleeding (PMB), one of the most important symptoms in gynaecological practice, is generally defined as vaginal bleeding occurring 12 months or more after the menopause. Its importance lies in the fact that 5–10% of women presenting with it will have an underlying gynaecological cancer.

When a women presents with PMB, the history should cover the duration and persistence of the bleeding. Particular attention should be paid to the use of hormone replacement therapy or other hormonal preparations such as oestrogen cream. A history of breast cancer is not uncommon and tamoxifen, which is usually taken as a long-term adjuvant treatment, may result in irregular vaginal bleeding. A careful past medical history is especially important because there is frequently coexisting chronic pathology such as cardiac or respiratory disease.

The examination should begin with a general assessment. Many of these women are elderly, obese, hypertensive or in other ways relatively unfit, which is relevant if anaesthesia is required. An abdominal examination to detect any masses arising from the pelvis is followed by a careful vaginal examination. The external genitalia should be inspected for any vulval lesion. A speculum examination should be carried out and the cervix and vagina carefully inspected. In a significant proportion of women, a speculum examination will not be possible due to vaginal stenosis or patients being simply unable to tolerate a vaginal examination. A bimanual examination is then undertaken to determine uterine size and the presence of an adnexal mass.

The next stage of management is to exclude endometrial cancer, even although, a benign cause such as atrophic vaginitis may be present. Traditionally, examination under anaesthetic with dilatation and curettage has been employed but more recently outpatient endometrial biopsy has largely replaced this. Ultrasound can be used not only to exclude a gross pelvic abnormality, but to examine the endometrial cavity. In the postmenopausal uterus, the endometrium is very thin and atrophic (**Fig. 10.56**). This can be exploited because the endometrial echo is very thin on scanning, and a signal less than 5mm across effectively excludes endometrial cancer (**Fig. 10.57**). When the endometrial cavity is greater

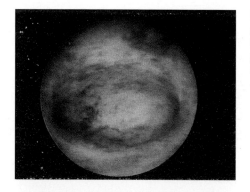

Fig. 10.56 *Hysteroscopic view of a postmenopausal endometrial cavity. Note the pale featureless surface. In the premenopausal woman the surface has a much more velvet appearance (see Fig. 10.60).*

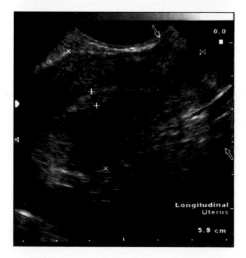

Fig. 10.57 *Ultrasound scan of the endometrial cavity in a postmenopausal uterus showing a very narrow echo. This effectively excludes pathology.*

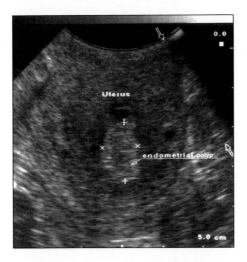

Fig. 10.58 *Ultrasound scan of a postmenopausal uterus showing an abnormal appearance (arrow). This suggests underlying pathology such as a polyp.*

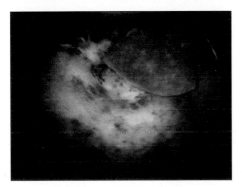

Fig. 10.59 *Hysteroscopic appearance of an endometrial polyp arising from an otherwise unremarkable postmenopausal endometrium.*

than 5mm across, there must be further investigation which may reveal a tumour or possibly a polyp (**Fig. 10.58**). Echoes thicker than 5mm are an indication for further investigation by endometrial sampling. Hysteroscopy may be used and may identify a polyp of the endometrium (**Figs 10.58** and **10.59**). Other causes of PMB include cervical and vulval cancer, both of which are usually clinically obvious. Ovarian cancer is not usually associated with PMB.

If the clinical examination and endometrial assessment are negative, which is the case for 90% of patients, then the woman can be reassured. If atrophic cervicitis or vaginitis is diagnosed, then this can be deemed to be the cause and treated with oestradiol cream. It is common for no pathology to be identified, particularly if the bleeding has occurred relatively soon after the menopause. Should the bleeding recur, then the patient should be re-evaluated under general anaesthetic and dilatation and curettage and hysteroscopy performed.

In a small proportion of patients, there are endometrial changes showing either cystic hyperplasia or atypical hyperplasia. For the former there is little risk of subsequent malignancy but one should question why a postmenopausal woman should have hyperplastic change, and oestrogenic cause should be sought. If atypical hyperplasia is present, then either the architecture of tissue is abnormal or cytological atypia exists. For the latter there is a significant risk of associated endometrial cancer or cancer subsequently and because of this, the best management is hysterectomy. For cystic hyperplasia without atypia, progestogens have to be given over a 3-month period, although treatment is not essential. The key points of PMB are listed in **Figure 10.60**.

Fig. 10.60 *Postmenopausal bleeding: key points.*

Postmenopausal bleeding: key points

Postmenopausal bleeding should always be investigated thoroughly.

Postmenopausal bleeding is associated with cancer in 5–10% of patients.

The endometrium can be investigated in the first instance by ultrasound or endometrial biopsy, rather than dilatation and curettage.

Atrophic changes are the most common cause of postmenopausal bleeding and can be treated with oestrogen therapy in the absence of other pathology.

chapter 11

Oncology

OVARIAN CANCER

EPIDEMIOLOGY

Ovarian cancer is the fourth most common cause of death in women from malignant disease in the Western world after lung, bowel and breast cancer. Although its incidence is not much more than endometrial cancer, the death rate is much higher because it usually presents at an advanced stage, by which time it is generally incurable. In the UK over 5000 new cases occur annually, and with an overall survival of only 30% there are approximately 4000 deaths per annum. The aetiology of epithelial ovarian cancer is not fully understood but recently several strands of epidemiological evidence have emerged. The disease is less common in women who have used oral contraception, who have had several pregnancies and who have an earlier menopause. This suggests that the incidence may be related to the number of ovulatory events that occur. Ovulatory activity leads to increased cell division during repair which may result in mutagenesis. The tumour suppressor gene p53 is frequently mutated in ovarian cancers and an accumulation of such mutations to tumour suppressor genes may be responsible for triggering uncontrolled cell division.

PATHOLOGY

Although malignant tumours can arise from the germinal elements and stroma of the ovary, over 90% of cancers are adenocarcinomas arising from the single layer of epithelial cells on the surface of the ovary. Approximately 50% are serous, 30% endometroid and 20% mucinous. The natural history of ovarian cancer is not well understood and there is no known premalignant lesion. Some tumours grow to large solid cystic structures which remain encapsulated until they present (**Fig. 11.1**), others metastasize widely throughout the perineum with small seedlings over all peritoneal surfaces and an often heavily infiltrated omentum (**Fig. 11.2**). Frequently, a large amount of ascitic fluid secreted by the tumours is found in the peritoneal cavity. There is no convincing evidence to show that benign cysts undergo transition to malignancy, although so-called borderline tumours are described which show malignant epithelial changes without any stromal invasion.

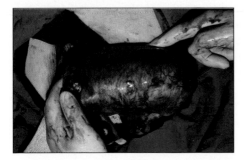

Fig. 11.1 *Large intact cystic ovarian tumour being brought through the abdominal incision. It was a malignant tumour confined to one ovary (Stage 1a).*

Ovarian tumours are a diverse grouping of different pathologies. The epithelial tumours predominate (**Figs 11.3** and **11.4**) and germ cell tumours and tumours arising from the stroma are rarer examples. An example of a germ cell tumour is the endodermal sinus tumour, also known as a yolk sac tumour (**Fig. 11.5**). This tumour secretes α-fetoprotein and is very sensitive to platinum chemotherapy. The granulosa cell tumour (**Fig. 11.6**) is a

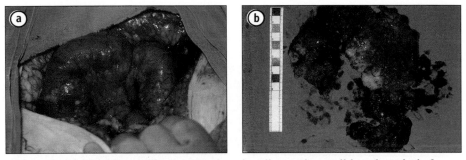

Fig. 11.2 *(a) Multiple seedling tumour deposits all over the small bowel, typical of advanced ovarian cancer with periotoneal spread. (b) Large omental 'cake' heavily infiltrated with ovarian cancer (same case).*

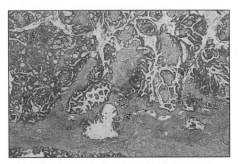

Fig. 11.3 *Serous carcinoma of the ovary. The tumour is papillary and has a complex lace-like pattern. Haematoxylin–eosin.*

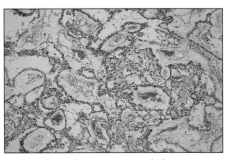

Fig. 11.5 *Yolk sac tumour of the ovary. Haematoxylin–eosin.*

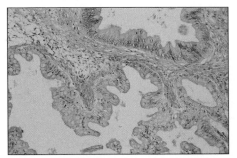

Fig. 11.4 *Mucinous tumour of borderline malignancy. The glandular spaces are lined by a stratified, columnar mucinous epithelium which forms small papillae and infoldings. Haematoxylin–eosin.*

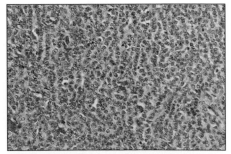

Fig. 11.6 *Granulosa cell tumour with a diffuse pattern. Haematoxylin–eosin.*

stromal tumour, and is interesting in its ability to secrete oestrogen so that it is often accompanied by endometrial hyperplasia or even endometrial neoplasia.

Tumours are staged according to their spread, and vary for different primary sites. For ovarian cancer, the staging system by the degree of spread is shown in **Figure 11.7**, and, of course, prognosis depends very much on stage. When the tumour is confined to a single ovary and remains totally encapsulated, the prognosis is good within 5-year survival of 80% but once the disease has metastasized freely within the abdominal cavity, the prognosis is very poor with approximately only 20% having a long-term survival. Unfortunately, the large majority of cases are advanced at presentation, and the overall 5-year survival for ovarian cancer is only 30%.

Clinical

Ovarian cancer usually occurs in women over the age of 50 years. It presents by virtue of an expanding intra-abdominal mass causing distension or pain. Very often in the earlier stages there are very mild symptoms which are initially ignored by the patient. As a result of the nonspecific nature of these symptoms, the general practitioner may not suspect serious pathology and referral is delayed. These women are often referred to a variety of specialists, such as gastroenterologists, general surgeons or gynaecologists. At presentation, a mass is often palpable arising from the pelvis often with signs of ascites. The mass is usually obvious on pelvic examination, often with a cragginess felt in the pouch of Douglas.

INVESTIGATION AND TREATMENT

A pelvic mass suspicious of ovarian cancer indicates the need for a laparotomy. If there is any doubt, an ultrasound examination of the pelvis should be performed (**Fig. 11.8**). Malignant tumours may be suspected because of solid areas within a cystic lesion, together with the presence of ascites. Preoperatively, blood should be taken to measure the level of CA125, a tumour marker secreted by most serous cystadenocarcinomas.

The FIGO staging for ovarian cancer	
Stage	**Site**
1	Confined to ovaries
2	Involvement of other pelvic sites
3	Involvement above pelvic brim
4	Spread throughout the peritoneal cavity

Fig. 11.7 *FIGO staging (International Federation of Gynaecology and Obstetrics) for ovarian cancer.*

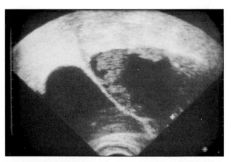

Fig. 11.8 *Ovarian cyst on ultrasonic scan. Within the cyst are solid excrescences suggestive of a malignant lesion.*

Surgery

The aims of laparotomy are threefold: to make a diagnosis, to stage the extent of the ovarian cancer and to debulk it as much as possible. The latter is important because women with minimal residual disease after surgery will have a longer mean duration of survival than those with bulk disease. In addition to debulking, a hysterectomy, bilateral salpingo-oophorectomy and omentectomy should be performed. The omentum is frequently heavily infiltrated with the tumour, and even if not visibly involved, it may be microscopically involved. Disease is often disseminated all around the peritoneal cavity, in 'sago seedling' size deposits (**Fig. 11.2**).

Chemotherapy

Unfortunately, most women will have evidence of spread beyond the primary site, for which chemotherapy is indicated. The most active drugs are platinum, often used in combination with the alkylating agent cyclophosphamide. A new drug, paclitaxel (Taxol®) has shown promise when used in combination with platinum. The drugs used in ovarian cancer and their toxic side effects are shown in **Figure 11.9**. Although the aim is to cure, in advanced disease this is not expected and the best to hope for is a complete remission. Unfortunately, even when the tumour appears to resolve completely and the tumour marker is basal in the serum, disease usually relapses at anything between 6 and 36 months, with a mean of 18 months.

The chemotherapy response rate in ovarian cancer is approximately 70% but unfortunately most women will relapse and the disease is then usually more drug resistant. Response and subsequent relapse are often reflected in the CA125 profile (**Fig. 11.10**).

Toxicity of different chemotherapy drugs used in ovarian cancer	
Drug	**Side effects**
Platinum analogues	
Cisplatin	Vomiting, nephropathy, neuropathy
Carboplatin	Myelosuppression
Taxoids	
Paclitaxel	Alopecia
Alkylating agents	
Cyclophosphamide	Alopecia, myelosuppression
Chlorambucil	Myelosuppression

Fig. 11.9 *Toxicity of different chemotherapy drugs used in ovarian cancer.*

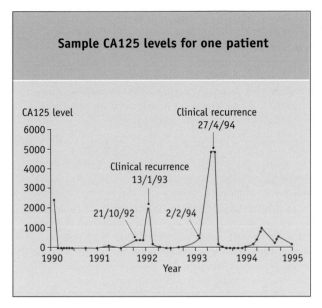

Sample CA125 levels for one patient

Fig. 11.10 *CA125 can act as a tumour marker. Following surgery and primary chemotherapy the level becomes basal and rises and falls with subsequent relapse and chemotherapy responses.*

FAMILIAL OVARIAN CANCER

In approximately 5% of patients, ovarian cancer assumes a familial form sometimes involving breast cancer, and there may also be a history of bowel and uterine cancer. The lifetime risk of a woman developing ovarian cancer is approximately 1%. With one affected first degree female relative who acquired the disease below the age of 55 years, the risk rises to 3%. When there is a family pedigree with a full autosomal dominant pattern, the risk rises to as high as 40%, due to a 50% chance of inheriting the mutation and 80% penetrance.

With such a high risk, many women will wish to be protected, which can only be done effectively by means of prophylactic bilateral oophrectomy. This may seem drastic but provided that reproduction has been completed and hormone replacement therapy is given, then the impact is lessened. This measure, although not providing 100% protection, provides tremendous relief from the anxiety of acquiring the disease. For women at lower risk and for younger women, a more conservative policy involves screening for ovarian abnormalities by means of clinical examination, serum measurement of CA125 and ovarian ultrasound. Another measure is oral contraception which is known in the general population to confer a reduced relative risk of acquiring ovarian cancer, thought to be due to inhibiting ovulation.

Cancer is currently regarded as a loss of control of cell proliferation due to genetic aberrations. In colon cancer this has been shown to involve an accumulation of genetic mutations involving both oncogenes and tumour suppressor genes. In familial cancer, part of the genetic damage is inherited via the germline and part is acquired through somatic mutation. The first example of this is retinoblastoma in which there is damage to Rb1, a tumour suppressor gene. Both tumour suppressor genes have to be affected, and if both are affected at birth, the condition will be congential but for many patients, a somatic mutation in life results in the disease occurring in early childhood. Similarly for familial ovarian cancer, it is now appreciated that inheritance of a mutation of the BRCA-1 gene predisposes women. Mutations to p53, another tumour suppressor gene are common suggesting that in addition to the inherited germline mutation, acquired somatic mutations are necessary to develop ovarian cancer. As fewer somatic mutational events are required, the familial form of the disease will tend to occur much earlier in life.

The benefit of having a genetic marker such as BRCA-1 is that women who are statistically at high risk from a family pedigree will be able to have their individual risk assessed. Thus, individuals who have not inherited the BRCA-1 mutation can be reassured whereas those at high risk will be positively identified and prophylactic measures can be taken.

POPULATION SCREENING FOR OVARIAN CANCER

As most cases of ovarian cancer are advanced at clinical presentation, the question arises: could screening lead to earlier detection, carrying an increased chance of cure and thus a reduction in the death rate? There are several major problems with this strategy which is used in screening for breast cancer in women aged 50–64 years old.

A central axiom of screening is that you should screen for a condition which if detected could be more effectively treated that the clinical condition itself. This applies well to cervical cancer. However, the natural history of ovarian cancer is not well understood, and it is possible that if ovarian cancer metastasizes very early then even cancers discovered by screening before clinical presentation may not be at an earlier stage. As discussed in Chapter 12, other important axioms are acceptability of the screening test, good sensitivity and specificity, avoidance of unnecessary anxiety and reasonable cost effectiveness.

Pelvic examination is not regarded as useful but the other two candidate approaches, serum samples or vaginal scanning have potential. The problems with both of these are the limited sensitivity and specificity. Sensitivity refers to the number of false negative tests and specificity, the number of false positive tests. Too many false negative tests will result in missed cancers and too many false positive tests will result in unnecessary surgery for benign ovarian cysts of no clinical significance. The current feeling is that population screening should not be employed, except for high-risk women but large trials are beginning to evaluate this. It may well be that eventually a genetic test predictive of sporadic ovarian cancer will be developed. The key points of ovarian cancer are listed in **Figure 11.11**.

Fig. 11.11 *Ovarian cancer: key points.*

Ovarian cancer: key points

Ovarian cancer usually presents late.

A poor prognosis is indicated if the cancer is advanced at presentation.

Primary treatment is surgical, usually combined with platinum-based chemotherapy.

The disease is familial in approximately 5% of patients.

CANCER OF THE UTERINE CORPUS

Over 90% of cancers affecting the corpus or body of the uterus are carcinomas of the endometrium. There is a small group who have sarcoma, arising from the myometrium, and other who have carcinosarcoma, or so-called mixed Mullerian tumours, which contain both carcinomatous and sarcomatous elements. The natural history of endometrial cancer is not well understood, which means that unlike cervical cancer, there is no effective screening test for precursor lesions, although certain changes are recognized as carrying a significant risk of subsequent neoplasia.

EPIDEMIOLOGY

Approximately 4000 new cases of endometrial cancer occur annually in the UK or about 15 in 100,000 women per year. Endometrial cancer tends to present early, and as a result carries the best prognosis of the gynaecological cancers with an overall 5-year survival of approximately 70%. It occurs principally in menopausal women, and is rare under the age of 40 years old.

Although the causes of endometrial cancer are ill understood, conditions that result in a relative hyperoestrogenic state are associated with an increased risk. The clearest example of this is unopposed oestrogen for hormone replacement therapy. Introduced in the late 1960s and early 1970s, it was noted that there was an increased incidence of endometrial cancer in women taking this type of therapy. The introduction of a combined oestrogen and progestogen hormone replacement therapy saw this increased risk reduced, probably to the normal incidence. Another classic example is the frequency of endometrial hyperplasia, or even carcinoma, in association with granulosa cell tumours of the ovary, which may produce hyperoestrogenism. Obesity and polycystic ovary syndrome are associated with an increased risk probably through 'physiological' hyperoestrogenism.

Another recent gynaecological factor is tamoxifen, which is used as adjuvant treatment for breast cancer. This is associated with a slightly increased risk of endometrial cancer, and other lesser forms of endometrial pathology. Nevertheless, the beneficial effects of tamoxifen for breast cancer outweigh the small increased risk of endometrial neoplasia.

CLINICAL PRESENTATION

Endometrial cancer generally presents as postmenopausal bleeding. More unusually, before the menopause, the presentation is irregular menstrual bleeding. As the early warning sign of bleeding normally prompts an investigation, the diagnosis is usually made before the disease spreads. As a result, the disease is frequently otherwise asymptomatic.

DIAGNOSIS

As stated, postmenopausal bleeding demands an urgent investigation to exclude among other tumours, endometrial cancer. Frequently, there is no clinical sign of endometrial cancer because the changes lie within the endometrial cavity. It is, therefore, necessary to investigate by obtaining a sample of endometrial tissue. Conventionally, this means examination under anaesthesia and dilatation and curettage. However, increasingly this is being replaced by outpatient procedures involving endometrial biopsy. Although this is reliable, some advocate hysteroscopy to visualize the endometrial cavity directly, which has the potential advantage of seeing any pathology other than cancer, for example, polyps which may be associated with tamoxifen.

A more recent approach has been the use of ultrasound which enables good visualization of the endometrial cavity. Studies have shown that when the endometrial echo is less than 5mm in diameter, then endometrial cancer can be excluded. In expert hands this offers a possible screen for women presenting with postmenopausal bleeding, avoiding the need for biopsy for patients with a normal scan.

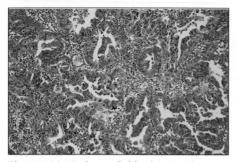

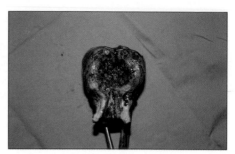

Fig. 11.12 *Endometrioid adenocarcinoma. Haematoxylin–eosin.*

Fig. 11.13 *Hysterectomy specimen showing tumour in endometrial cavity.*

TREATMENT

When endometrial cancer is found on biopsy (**Fig. 11.12**), the standard treatment is surgical, in the form of hysterectomy and bilateral salpingo-oophorectomy (**Fig. 11.13**). If the cancer is more advanced, affecting the cervix or adnexae, then more aggressive surgery may be required. Endometrial cancer spreads initially either as direct spread affecting the cervix, or more indirectly to the pelvic or para-aortic lymph nodes. It is because of the latter that some advocate pelvic lymphadenectomy at the time of the hysterectomy.

When the uterus is examined by the pathologist, particular attention is paid to the depth of myometrial invasion and the degree of differentiation, or grade of tumour, which influences the prognosis. After surgery and pathological evaluation, the tumour can be staged.

The FIGO staging for endometrial cancer is shown in **Figure 11.14** and the relevant prognostic factors in **Figure 11.15**.

The decision of whether more treatment is required rests with the pathological and surgical findings. If positive nodes are identified or if the tumour is high grade, deeply invading or showing other adverse prognostic factors, then adjuvant radiation is usually prescribed as a combination of external beam therapy to control pelvic recurrence, and vault brachytherapy to prevent vault recurrence.

Staging for endometrial cancer

Stage 1	Corpus only
1a	Myometrial
1b	Myometrial invasion less than half
1c	Myometrial invasion greater than half
Stage 2	Involvement of cervix
Stage 3	Involvement of adnexae and pelvic nodes
Stage 4	Involvement of bladder, rectum or distal spread

Fig. 11.14 *Staging for endometrial cancer (FIGO).*

Fig. 11.15 *Adverse prognostic factors in endometrial cancer.*

Adverse prognostic factors in endometrial cancer

Poorly differentiated tumours
Deep myometrial invasion
Positive peritoneal cytology
Pelvic or para-aortic nodes involved
Lymph and vascular spaces involved
Adenosquamous or papillary serous tumours

Adjuvant radiotherapy risks a similar morbidity of that which can occur after radiation for cervical cancer, including bowel and bladder disturbance.

Stage 1 endometrial cancer is associated with an overall 5-year survival of 85%, although within Stage 1 high risk tumours confer a lower survival rate. Survival rates fall the more advanced the stage is.

UTERINE SARCOMA

These tumours are much less common and present as a uterine mass with vaginal bleeding. They may range from low-grade malignancy, sometimes seen as excessive mitosis in 'fibroid' masses, to high-grade, very aggressive tumours often with para-aortic node involvement. The management is again surgical, to remove the uterus if possible, but the effective treatment of any residual disease is difficult and no reliable therapy is available. Combination chemotherapy has been used with varying degrees of success. Radiation is also not very effective in either mixed tumours or pure sarcomas. The key points of uterine sarcoma are shown in **Figure 11.16**.

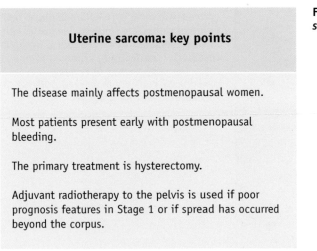

Fig. 11.16 *Uterine sarcoma: key points.*

Uterine sarcoma: key points

The disease mainly affects postmenopausal women.

Most patients present early with postmenopausal bleeding.

The primary treatment is hysterectomy.

Adjuvant radiotherapy to the pelvis is used if poor prognosis features in Stage 1 or if spread has occurred beyond the corpus.

CERVICAL CANCER

EPIDEMIOLOGY

Cervical cancer is a disease affecting more women in total worldwide than any other cancer. It can affect women below the age of 30 years old but usually affects women aged over 35 years. The risk factors for developing cervical cancer are early onset of sexual intercourse, multiple sexual partners and cigarette smoking, although the latter is not commonly practised in countries such as India where cervical cancer is extremely prevalent. These epidemiological facts indicate that a sexually transmitted mutagen is involved in the process of carcinogenesis. This agent is now known to be the human papillomavirus, particularly type 16 (HPV-16). During the 1980s, a large rise in the detection of cervical intraepithelial neoplasia (CIN) occurred in many Western countries. This may have been encouraged by the widespread use of oral or other nonbarrier contraception and more liberal sexual practices.

A PREVENTABLE CANCER

Cervical cancer is unique among the gynaecological cancers because it is largely preventable. This is because the invasive disease is preceded by a detectable preinvasive

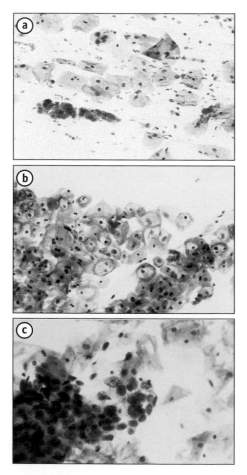

Fig. 11.17 *(a) Normal cervical smear. The slide comprises normal superficial and intermediate squamous epithelial cells together with a row of columnar glandular epithelial cells. Red blood cells and neutrophil polymorphs are present in the background. (b) Borderline nuclear change - HPV infection. The superficial and intermediate squamous epithelial cells show evidence of Human Papillomavirus infection. Koilocytes and binucleate cells are present and the nuclei show enlargement, hyperchromasia and slight irregularity amounting to borderline nuclear change. (c) Severe dyskaryosis. These cells have a high nuclear to cytoplasmic ratio with enlarged nuclei and minimal cytoplasm evident. The nuclei vary in size and shape and have coarse irregular chromatin; nucleoli are visible in some cells. The appearances of severely dyskaryotic cells are in marked contrast to surrounding normal squames.*

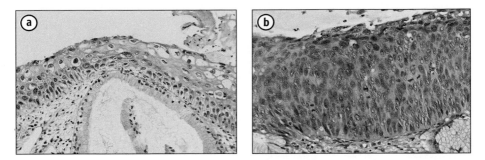

Fig. 11.18 *(a) CIN 1 with koilocytes. The cells in the basal layer of the metaplastic squamous epithelium are enlarged and mildly pleomorphic. Atypical nuclei are present at all layers of the epithelium. Those with perinuclear cytoplasmic clearing are koilocytes. Haematoxylin–eosin. (b) CIN 3. There is no epithelial stratification and minimal cytoplasmic maturation. The epithelial cells have high nucleo-cytoplasmic ratios and abnormally dispersed nuclear chromatin and mitoses are present at all levels in the epithelium. Haematoxylin–eosin.*

disease known as cervical intraepithelial neoplasia (CIN), which in a proportion of patients would develop into cancer over a period of years. This offers a prevention strategy, which is facilitated by the accessibility of the cervix itself, through exfoliative cytology obtained by taking cervical smears. Although regular smears do not provide 100% protection against developing cancer, cytology screening does reduce the death rate from cervical cancer provided there is a wide population coverage. The optimal screening interval balancing prevention and cost is calculated to be 3 years. There is a National Screening Programme in the UK with all women aged 20–65 years being called and recalled every 3–5 years. This is now resulting in a marked reduction in the incidence of cervical cancer.

THE MANAGEMENT OF AN ABNORMAL SMEAR

Each year in the UK, approximately 100,000 women have an abnormal smear. The term used for cellular abnormality in smears is 'dyskaryosis'. The degree of abnormality ranges from mild dyskaryosis to severe dyskaryosis (**Fig. 11.17**). The more marked the cytological abnormality, the more marked the grade of underlying pathology is likely to be. An abnormal smear resulting from a routine screening test requires diagnosis and treatment. This is achieved by using colposcopy to identify any lesion that can be biopsied.

The lesion that is usually responsible for abnormal smears is CIN which is graded as 1, 2 or 3 (**Fig. 11.18**), 3 being the most severe grade. CIN, previously known as dysplasia, develops on the so-called transformation zone of the cervix. At birth the squamous columnar junction (SCJ) is situated at the cervical os. After menarche the SCJ moves on to the ectocervix and the glandular epithelium now visible on the ectocervix (ectopy) undergoes squamous metaplastic to become mature squamous epithelium, and a new SCJ forms. The area between the original and new SCJ is known as the transformation zone and this is where the CIN forms.

The correct way to investigate an abnormal smear is to visualize the cervix using a colposcope (**Fig. 11.19**) – essentially a pair of binoculars on a stand – to achieve a high power view. Abnormal epithelium shows up after the application of acetic acid and a directed biopsy can be taken (**Fig. 11.20**). CIN can be treated by diathermy excision or destruction using a laser or coagulation. For 95% of patients, one treatment is sufficient, and follow-up is essential to ensure that abnormal smears do not recur.

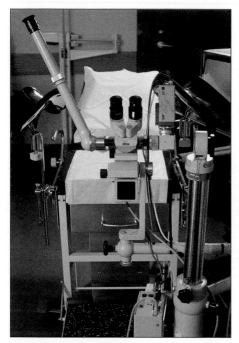

Fig. 11.19 *Colposcope.*

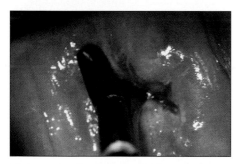

Fig. 11.20 *Directed punch biopsy being taken in an area of acetowhite epithelium.*

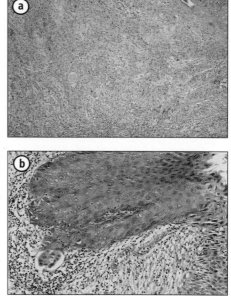

Fig. 11.21 *(a) Moderately differentiated squamous cell carcinoma of the cervix. Haematoxylin–eosin. (b) Microinvasive carcinoma of the cervix. A microscopic tongue of cells with eosinophilic cytoplasm emerges from a crypt lined by CIN and infiltrates directly into a lymphatic in the adjacent stroma. Haematoxylin–eosin.*

PATHOLOGY

The large majority (90%) of cervical cancers are squamous carcinomas (**Fig. 11.21a**), although recently approximately one third of these have been shown to have glandular elements (adenosquamous). Approximately 10% of tumours are histologically pure adenocarcinomas. Very early cancer is sometimes screen detected before the onset of clinical symptoms by routine smears. When a tumour is not more than 5mm deep and 7mm across, it is defined as microinvasion (**Fig. 11.21b**). At this stage radical therapy is unnecessary, and a cone biopsy will usually suffice, provided the excision is complete.

Cervical tumours may be well or poorly differentiated with the latter indicating a worse prognosis. Spread occurs by direct infiltration from the cervix on to the upper vagina and into the parametrial tissues and onward towards the pelvic wall (**Fig. 11.22**).

FIGO staging system for cervical cancer

Stage	Site
1a	Microinvasion (less than 5mm deep and 7mm wide)
1b	Cervix only
Stage 2	Upper two thirds of the vagina and parametrium but not to the side wall
Stage 3	Spread to involve the pelvic side wall
Stage 4	Spread to bladder, rectum or outside pelvis

Fig. 11.22 *FIGO staging system for cervical cancer.*

HPV and cervical cancer

The evidence that HPV-16 and certain other HPV types are involved in the process of cervical carinogenesis is now regarded as compelling. The detection of koilocytosis (the cytopathic effect produced by HPV) is known to increase greatly the risk of subsequent abnormal smears and, as the degree of abnormality increases, so does the prevalence of HPV detection. Virtually all squamous cervical cancers contain HPV DNA. Although there is still an incomplete understanding of how HPV affects cervical cells, it is known that it will inactivate p53 and RB1, two tumour suppressor genes that help to protect against malignant change. It is thought that HPV does not act alone but its early involvement suggests that a preventative strategy involving a HPV vaccine may be possible.

In addition to direct infiltration, the disease progresses by metastasis to the iliac and obturator lymphatic chains and from there up to the para-aortic chain. This pattern of spread often then avoids the direct involvement of the bladder and rectum until very late in the disease process. As the disease advances towards the side wall, it frequently causes ureteric obstruction and renal failure is frequently the terminal event in the disease process. Infiltration of the lumbosacral plexus will cause pain, often affecting the low back and buttock and down the side of the thigh.

Clinical

Cervical tumours are ulcerative, sometimes producing an exophytic cauliflower growth and sometimes a malignant crater (Fig. 11.23). This will eventually cause abnormal bleeding which is frequently the presenting complaint. In premenopausal women this may be postcoital bleeding or intermenstrual bleeding; in older women postmenopausal bleeding will occur. Unfortunately, cervical cancer does not always present early and women may have remarkably extensive disease at presentation.

A speculum examination will unusually reveal an obvious malignant growth at the cervix, although an early tumour may be missed unless a scrupulous technique is used with adequate lighting. Staging should be undertaken by means of examination under anaesthesia with care being taken to assess the degree of adnexal spread. A biopsy should be taken and if the disease is affecting the anterior vagina, a cytoscopy should be done to exclude bladder involvement.

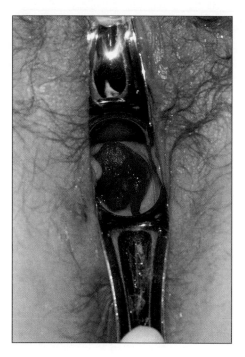

Fig. 11.23 *Typical malignant lesion involving all of the ectocervix.*

TREATMENT

Early stage disease (Stage 1), particularly in young women, is best treated by radical hysterectomy. This has the advantage of conserving the ovaries and leaving the vagina supple, both important for preserving sexual function. However, this surgery requires special expertise, involves pelvic node dissection and deflecting the ureters so that parametrial tissue and a good cuff of vagina can be removed with the uterus (**Fig. 11.24**). Radiotherapy is equivalent to surgery in terms of cure for early stage disease, but it causes ovarian failure and a marked inflammatory reaction which leaves the vagina more rigid and often stenosed. The only treatment for later stage disease is radiotherapy.

Radiotherapy has been exploited to the full in cervical cancer, helped by the fact that even advanced disease often remains confined within the pelvis. Radiotherapy is given in two forms. External radiation using a linear accelerator delivers 5–6000 rads given as 20 fractions (5 each week) over 4 weeks. This is followed by intracavitary caesium treatment which involves placing a caesium source into the uterine and vaginal vault for 2–3 days

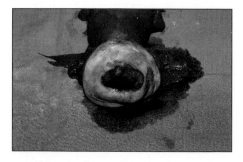

Fig. 11.24 *Uterus with vaginal cuff and parametrial tissue. The tumour can be seen replacing the ectocervix.*

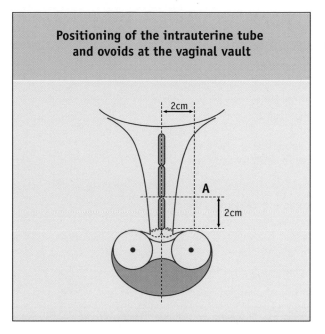

Positioning of the intrauterine tube and ovoids at the vaginal vault

2cm

A

2cm

Fig. 11.25 *Positioning of the intrauterine tube and ovoids at the vaginal vault. Point A is an arbitrary reference point where dose is calculated.*

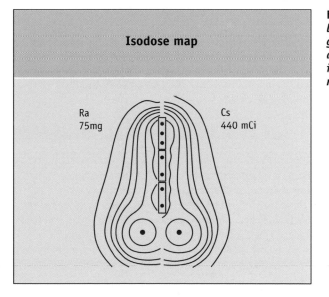

Isodose map

Ra
75mg

Cs
440 mCi

Fig. 11.26 *Isodose map like height contours on a geographical map. As the distance from the source increases, the dose falls off rapidly.*

(**Fig. 11.25**). The external treatment is designed to ablate disease affecting the parametrium and sidewalls, whereas the central sources ablate the primary tumour. In general, treatment is the same whatever the histopathology.

Radiation is subject to the inverse square law, which means that as the distance from the central source increases, the dose falls very rapidly (**Fig. 11.26**). The dose given to the pelvic side wall by the central source is subtherapeutic which is why boosting by external beam treatment is required.

Fig. 11.27 *Cervical cancer: key points.*

Cervical cancer: key points

Cervical cancer is probably initiated by oncogenic human papilloma virus types, e.g. type 16.

Abnormal smears usually indicate underlying cervical intraepithelial neoplasia, diagnosed by colposcopy and biopsy.

Early cervical cancer can be treated surgically or by radiation, with the former offered to younger women.

Advanced disease requires treatment with radiotherapy.

Fig. 11.27 *Cervical cancer: key points.*

PROGNOSIS

Survival is dependent mainly on disease stage. Stage 1 disease (confined to the cervix) carries an 80–90% 5-year survival, whereas stage 3 disease has a 5-year survival of 30–40%. This nevertheless means that this proportion of advanced patients will survive due to the fact that the disease remains confined to the pelvis. The overall 5-year survival in cervical cancer is approximately 60%.

Recurrence is very difficult to treat unless it follows surgery alone, in which case disease confined to the pelvis can be treated with radiotherapy. Chemotherapy is of limited value in cervical cancer. When treatment fails, ureteric obstruction and resultant renal failure lead to death. Pain and occasionally urinary fistula are two very distressing problems. The key points of cervical cancer are listed in **Figure 11.27**.

VULVAL CANCER

GENERAL

Vulval cancer is a relatively uncommon tumour that arises in the keratinized and nonkeratinized skin of the vulva. There are approximately 1000 new cases each year in the UK. It affects mainly older women, being less common in premenopausal women, and tends to occur over the age of 60 years. HPV DNA is present in a significant proportion of tumours but the relationship between vulval cancer and HPV is less clear cut than with cervical cancer.

PATHOLOGY

The lesion can arise anywhere on the vulva but it most often originates on one or other of the lateral aspects. Less commonly it arises in the clitoral area or posteriorly. Vulval cancers are usually very obvious as ulcerated raised lesions, often discoid in the early stages with clearly defined margins (**Fig. 11.28**). Unfortunately, they may be relatively asymptomatic early on and only draw attention when they enlarge and cause bleeding, itch, pain or even foul smell. Older women who may be aware of some of these symptoms may be embarrassed about seeking advice and presentation is delayed until the symptoms worsen.

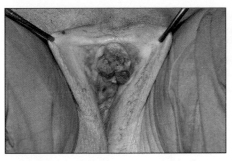

Fig. 11.28 *Fungating tumour replacing the clitoris. The urethral orifice is seen below the tumour.*

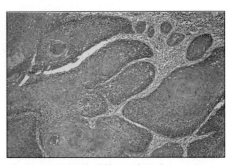

Fig. 11.29 *Well-differentiated squamous carcinoma of the vulva. Note the epithelial 'pearls'. Haematoxylin–eosin.*

As the lesion enlarges, metastases occur to the inguinal and upper femoral nodes which drain the vulva and thereafter spread up the lymphatics above the inguinal ligaments to the iliac nodes. The tumours are usually squamous carcinomas (**Fig. 11.29**), although rare tumours include melanoma and adenocarcinoma of Bartholin's gland.

TREATMENT

The treatment of vulval cancer is surgical and, if necessary, radical comprising excision of the entire vulva, if possible with a clear margin of 1cm around the tumour. The ability to achieve a satisfactory margin may be limited by encroachment of the tumour into the urethral meatus or the anus. Together with the vulvectomy, the inguinal and upper femoral nodes should be excised through separate linear groin incisions. If the tumour is large and anterior, the nodes and tumour may require to be removed *en bloc* but this leaves an unsightly tissue defect over the mons pubis, and still requires removal of the vulval appendages and consequent disfiguration. Fortunately, most cases occur in older women for whom vulval disfigurement is less important, but in young women with small lesions consideration should be given to more limited surgery in an attempt to preserve some of the vulva. This might include wide local excision and unilateral lymphadenectomy.

It is very important not to undertreat vulval cancer because recurrences can be difficult to clear and may cause extreme distress if the tumour cannot be removed. As a result, this surgery should not be compromised even in old women. Vulval cancer should be operated on only by those experienced and practised in its management.

If several lymph nodes are involved, adjuvant radiotherapy may be employed to improve local disease control. Radiotherapy and chemotherapy may be considered as primary treatment for the rare case when the tumour is so advanced that it cannot be tackled surgically.

The prognosis for vulval cancer is very good in the absence of lymph node involvement, with an 80–90% 5-year survival rate, but once the nodes are involved survival falls to approximately 50%.

VULVAL INTRAEPITHELIAL NEOPLASIA

Vulval intraepithelial neoplasia (VIN) is a pathological condition of the vulva characterized by immature cells occupying some of the epithelial layers. It may remain undiscovered but frequently presents as vulval itch. It tends to occur in postmenopausal women but is now

297

increasingly identified in younger women. It can sometimes be seen clinically as white areas on the vulva (**Fig. 11.30**) and is diagnosed by means of colposcopic examination of the vulva and biopsy, which can both be done as an outpatient procedure. The importance of VIN is its potential as a precursor of invasive cancer. As a result of this, VIN is to be distinguished from more benign vulval lesions such as lichen sclerosis (which just means thickened skin) which can also look white (**Figs 11.31** and **11.32**). The natural history of vulval neoplasia is not well understood and although it is generally thought that invasive vulval cancer is preceded by intraepithelial neoplasia, the risk of any given lesion developing

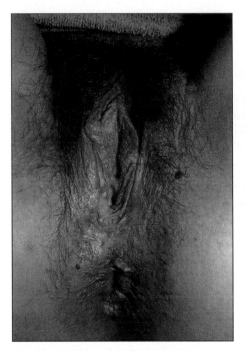

Fig. 11.30 *This vulva demonstrates some patchy white areas posteriorly which colposcopy and biopsy revealed to be vulval intraepithelial neoplasia.*

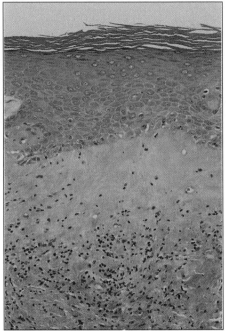

Fig. 11.31 *Lichen sclerosus. The epidermis is shallow and hyperkeratotic. In the underlying dermis there is a superficial hyalinized layer deep to which there is a band-like infiltrate of chronic inflammatory cells. Haematoxylin–eosin.*

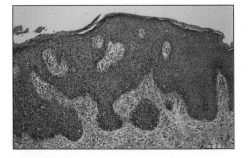

Fig. 11.32 *Vulval intraepithelial neoplasia. The epidermis to the right is normal whilst in that to the left there is no normal stratification or maturation. Haematoxylin–eosin.*

into cancer is impossible to determine. VIN is graded I, II or III according to the extent to which the epithelium is occupied by the immature basiloid cells. In VIN III, the full thickness is affected (**Fig. 11.32**). The overall risk of vulval cancer developing from VIN III is probably approximately 5%.

The management of VIN depends on the grade of disease and the presence of symptoms. VIN I and II can generally be managed conservatively but if pruritis is a problem, this can be managed by topical steroids or excised. VIN III is generally excised because of the risk of cancer developing, although in younger women who are asymptomatic, a careful policy of surveillance may be permissible to avoid the need for surgery which can cause loss of sexual function.

Index